Sexually Transmitted Infections

Editor

JEANNE MARRAZZO

INFECTIOUS DISEASE CLINICS OF NORTH AMERICA

www.id.theclinics.com

Consulting Editor
HELEN W. BOUCHER

June 2023 • Volume 37 • Number 2

ELSEVIER

1600 John F. Kennedy Boulevard • Suite 1800 • Philadelphia, Pennsylvania, 19103-2899.

http://www.theclinics.com

INFECTIOUS DISEASE CLINICS OF NORTH AMERICA Volume 37, Number 2
June 2023 ISSN 0891–5520, ISBN-13: 978-0-443-18302-7

Editor: Kerry Holland
Developmental Editor: Hannah Almira Lopez

Infectious Disease Clinics of North America (ISSN 0891–5520) is published in March, June, September, and December by Elsevier Inc., 360 Park Avenue South, New York, NY 10010-1710. Periodicals postage paid at New York, NY and additional mailing offices. Subscription prices are $368.00 per year for US individuals, $806.00 per year for US institutions, $100.00 per year for US students, $420.00 per year for Canadian individuals, $1,007.00 per year for Canadian institutions, $458.00 per year for international individuals, $1,007.00 per year for international institutions, $100.00 per year for Canadian students, and $200.00 per year for international students. To receive student rate, orders must be accompanied by name of affiliated institution, date of term, and the *signature* of program/residency coordinator on institution letterhead. Orders will be billed at individual rate until proof of status is received. Foreign air speed delivery is included in all *Clinics* subscription prices. All prices are subject to change without notice. **POSTMASTER:** Send address changes to *Infectious Disease Clinics of North America,* Elsevier Health Sciences Division, Subcription Customer Service, 3251 Riverport Lane, Maryland Heights, MO 63043. **Customer Service: 1-800-654-2452 (US). From outside of the US and Canada, call 1-314-447-8871. Fax: 1-314-447-8029. E-mail: JournalsCustomerService-usa@elsevier.com (print support) or JournalsOnlineSupport-usa@elsevier.com (online support).**

Infectious Disease Clinics of North America is also published in Spanish by Editorial Inter-Médica, Junin 917, 1er A 1113, Buenos Aires, Argentina.

Reprints. For copies of 100 or more, of articles in this publication, please contact the Commercial Reprints Department, Elsevier Inc., 360 Park Avenue South, New York, New York 10010-1710. Tel. 212-633-3874, Fax: 212-633-3820, E-mail: reprints@elsevier.com.

Infectious Disease Clinics of North America is covered in *MEDLINE/PubMed (Index Medicus), Current Contents/ Clinical Medicine, Science Citation Alert, SCISEARCH,* and *Research Alert.*

Contributors

CONSULTING EDITOR

HELEN W. BOUCHER, MD, FACP, FIDSA
Dean and Professor of Medicine, Tufts University School of Medicine, Chief Academic Officer, Tufts Medicine, Boston, Massachusetts, USA

EDITOR

JEANNE MARRAZZO, MD, MPH, FACP, FIDSA
Director, Division of Infectious Diseases, C. Glenn Cobbs, MD, Endowed Chair in Infectious Diseases, Executive Vice Chair, Department of Medicine, The University of Alabama at Birmingham Heersink School of Medicine, Birmingham, Alabama, USA

AUTHORS

CATRIONA S. BRADSHAW, MD, PhD
Professor, Melbourne Sexual Health Centre, Alfred Health, Central Clinical School, Faculty of Medicine, Nursing and Health Sciences, Monash University, Melbourne, Victoria, Australia

CHASE A. CANNON, MD, MPH
Department of Medicine, University of Washington, HIV/STD Program, Public Health-Seattle and King County, Seattle, Washington, USA

JOHN M. CURTIN, MD
Department of Medicine, Infectious Disease Service, Walter Reed National Military Medical Center, Bethesda, Maryland, USA

EVAN C. EWERS, MD, MPH
Infectious Disease Service, Fort Belvoir Community Hospital, Fort Belvoir, Virginia, USA; Department of Medicine, Uniformed Services University of the Health Sciences, Bethesda, Maryland, USA

RICARDO A. FRANCO, MD
Associate Professor of Infectious Diseases, Division of Infectious Diseases, Department of Medicine, The University of Alabama at Birmingham Heersink School of Medicine, Birmingham, Alabama, USA

ANURADHA GANESAN, MBBS, MPH
Department of Medicine, Infectious Disease Service, Walter Reed National Military Medical Center, Department of Preventive Medicine and Biostatistics, Infectious Disease Clinical Research Program (IDCRP), Uniformed Services University of the Health Sciences, Henry M Jackson Foundation for the Advancement of Military Medicine, Bethesda, Maryland, USA

WILLIAM M. GEISLER, MD, MPH
Professor, Department of Medicine, The University of Alabama at Birmingham,
Birmingham, Alabama, USA

KEONTE J. GRAVES, MS
Division of Infectious Diseases, The University of Alabama at Birmingham, Birmingham,
Alabama, USA

RONNIE M. GRAVETT, MD
Division of Infectious Diseases, Department of Medicine, The University of Alabama at
Birmingham Heersink School of Medicine, Birmingham, Alabama, USA

EMILY HANSMAN, BA
David Geffen School of Medicine, University of California Los Angeles, Los Angeles,
California, USA

JANE S. HOCKING, PhD
Professor, Head of Sexual Health Unit, Melbourne School of Population and Global
Health, University of Melbourne, Melbourne, Victoria, Australia

CHRISTINE JOHNSTON, MD, MPH
Division of Allergy and Infectious Diseases, Department of Medicine, University of
Washington, Seattle, Washington, USA

MAURICIO KAHN, MD
Infectious Diseases Fellow, Department of Medicine, The University of Alabama at
Birmingham Heersink School of Medicine, Birmingham, Alabama, USA

JEFFREY D. KLAUSNER, MD, MPH
Professor of Clinical Population and Public Health Sciences, University of Southern
California Keck School of Medicine, Los Angeles, California, USA

FABIAN Y.S. KONG, PhD
C.R. Roper Senior Research Fellow, Melbourne School of Population and Global Health,
University of Melbourne, Victoria, Australia

AUDREY R. LLOYD, MD
Infectious Diseases Fellow, Division of Infectious Diseases, Department of Medicine and
Pediatrics, The University of Alabama at Birmingham Heersink School of Medicine,
Birmingham, Alabama, USA

LISA E. MANHART, PhD, MPH
Professor, Department of Epidemiology, University of Washington, Center for AIDS and
STD, Seattle, Washington, USA

CHRISTINA M. MARRA, MD
Department of Neurology, University of Washington, Seattle, Washington, USA

JEANNE MARRAZZO, MD, MPH, FACP, FIDSA
Director, Division of Infectious Diseases, C. Glenn Cobbs, MD, Endowed Chair in
Infectious Diseases, Executive Vice Chair, Department of Medicine, The University of
Alabama at Birmingham Heersink School of Medicine, Birmingham, Alabama, USA

CHRISTINA A. MUZNY, MD, MSPH
Division of Infectious Diseases, The University of Alabama at Birmingham, Birmingham,
Alabama, USA

SKYE A. OPSTEEN
The University of Alabama at Birmingham Heersink School of Medicine, Birmingham, Alabama, USA

ROSALYN E. PLOTZKER, MD, MPH
Clinical Faculty (CAPTC), Assistant Professor (UCSF), California Prevention Training Center, Bixby Center for Global Reproductive Health San Francisco, Department of Epidemiology and Biostatistics, University of California San Francisco, Mission Hall: Global Health and Clinical Sciences, San Francisco, California, USA

UTSAV POKHAREL, MD
Surveillance Officer, California Emerging Infections Program, HPV Impact, Oakland, California, USA

FUAD QUSHAIR, BS
The University of Alabama at Birmignham Heersink School of Medicine, Birmingham, Alabama, USA

MEENA S. RAMCHANDANI, MD, MPH
Department of Medicine, University of Washington, HIV/STD Program, Public Health-Seattle and King County, Seattle, Washington, USA

ELIZABETH A. STIER, MD
Professor, Boston University School of Medicine, Boston Medical Center, Boston, Massachusetts, USA

AKANKSHA VAIDYA, MD, MPH
Clinical Faculty, California Prevention Training Center, University of California San Francisco, Bixby Center for Global Reproductive Health, San Francisco, California, USA

BARBARA VAN DER POL, PhD, MPH
Professor, Department of Medicine, UAB School of Public Health, The University of Alabama at Birmingham Heersink School of Medicine, Birmingham, Alabama, USA

OLIVIA T. VAN GERWEN, MD, MPH
Division of Infectious Diseases, The University of Alabama at Birmingham, Birmingham, Alabama, USA

NICHOLAS VAN WAGONER, MD, PhD
Division of Infectious Diseases, Department of Medicine, The University of Alabama at Birmingham Heersink School of Medicine, Birmingham, Alabama, USA

GWENDOLYN E. WOOD, PhD
Research Assistant Professor, Division of Infectious Diseases, University of Washington, Center for AIDS and STD, Seattle, Washington, USA

Contents

This review presents the epidemiology, pathophysiology, prevention, and management of sexually transmitted human papillomavirus (HPV) and its associated diseases. HPV is the most common sexually transmitted infection worldwide. Prevalence varies regionally. Low-risk strains cause anogenital warts, which can be managed with patient- or provider-applied therapies. High-risk strains cause lower anogenital cancers. Primary and secondary prevention strategies include vaccination and screening for precancerous lesions, respectively. Management of abnormal screening results vary by test result, anatomic site, and individual cancer risk. Approaches include close rescreening, high-resolution visualization with biopsy, and—when biopsy-proven precancer is identified—removal or destruction of the lesion.

Mycoplasma genitalium is a frequent cause of urogenital syndromes in men and women and is associated with adverse sequelae in women. M genitalium also infects the rectum, and may cause proctitis, but rarely infects the pharynx. Diagnosis requires nucleic acid amplification testing. Antibiotic resistance is widespread: more than half of infections are resistant to macrolides and fluoroquinolone resistance is increasing. Resistance-guided therapy is recommended for symptomatic patients, involving initial treatment with doxycycline to reduce organism load followed by azithromycin for macrolide-sensitive infections or moxifloxacin for macrolide-resistant infections. Neither screening nor tests of cure are recommended in asymptomatic persons.

Ongoing sexual transmission presents a significant barrier to viral hepatitis control. Endemic transmission of hepatitis A virus continues through communities of men with male sex partners, despite vaccine availability. Increased incidence of hepatitis B virus from 2014-2018 prompted expanded vaccination guidelines, but uptake and physician awareness remain poor. Hepatitis C virus while strongly associated with injection drug use, is also transmitted by high-risk sexual contact. Despite universal screening recommendations and curative treatment, incidence continues to increase. Even with safe and highly effective vaccinations or treatments, sexual transmission of viral hepatitides must be addressed to achieve disease elimination.

Genital herpes (GH) is a sexually transmitted infection causing recurrent, self-limited genital, buttock, and thigh ulcerations. Symptoms range from unrecognized or mild to severe with frequent recurrences. Herpes simplex viruses (HSV) type-1 or type-2 cause GH. HSV establishes latency in sacral ganglia and causes lifelong infection. Viral reactivation leads to genital ulceration or asymptomatic shedding which may lead to transmission. HSV infection during pregnancy can cause fulminant hepatitis and neonatal transmission. Severe and atypical manifestations are seen in immunocompromised people. Guanosine analogs treat symptoms and prevent recurrences, shedding, and transmission. Novel preventive and therapeutic strategies are in development.

The myriad presentations of ulcerative sexually transmitted infections, other than genital herpes and syphilis, challenge even the most astute clinician given the considerable overlap in clinical presentation and lack of widely available diagnostic resources, such as nucleic acid testing, to confirm the diagnosis. Even so, case prevalence is relatively low, and incidence of chancroid and granuloma inguinale are declining. These diseases still cause substantial morbidity and increased chance for HIV acquisition, and with the recent advent of mpox as a cause, it remains imperative to identify and treat accurately.

Sexually transmitted infections (STIs) are caused by various pathogens, many of which have common symptoms. Diagnostic tests are critical to supporting clinical evaluations in making patient management decisions. Molecular diagnostics are the preferred test type when available, especially in asymptomatic patients for many STIs. However, for some infections, serology offers the best insight into infectious status. Clinicians should be aware of the performance characteristics of the available STI diagnostic tests and understand how to use them. Point-of-care tests are helpful to implement rapid and accurate treatment responses, which are particularly helpful in certain at-risk populations.

Partner management of sexually transmitted infection (STIs) is essential to identify and treat new cases, prevent reinfection in the index case, interrupt chains of transmission, reduce STI-related morbidity, and target STI screening and treatment interventions. The responsibility for partner notification and treatment falls on the health care provider. Approaches to partner management include patient referral, provider referral, contractual referral, and expedited partner therapy (EPT), with EPT and enhanced partner referral outperforming other methods. This article provides an overview of clinical recommendations regarding partner management, with particular emphasis on EPT, and an update on new and emerging evidence in the field.

INFECTIOUS DISEASE CLINICS OF NORTH AMERICA

Preface

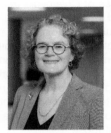

Jeanne Marrazzo, MD, MPH, FACP, FIDSA
Editor

It has been over 20 years since the Institute of Medicine published the landmark report entitled "The Hidden Epidemic: Confronting Sexually Transmitted Diseases." The committee concluded that four major strategies should form the public and private sector response to what was then recognized as the growing (yet still hidden) epidemic of sexually transmitted infections (STIs): (1) overcome barriers to adoption of healthy sexual behaviors; (2) develop strong leadership, strengthen investment, and improve information systems for STI prevention; (3) design and implement essential STI-related services in innovative ways for adolescents and underserved populations; and (4) ensure access to and quality of essential clinical services for STIs.

Since those ambitious goals were published, how has the approach to managing and preventing STIs changed? How has the epidemiology of these important infections changed? And most important for our readers, has the fourth strategy been addressed? Ensuring the quality of essential clinical services directly touches on the skills of providers of clinical care to people concerned about, at risk for, or manifesting STI-related syndromes. In this issue of *Infectious Disease Clinics of North America*, we review salient features of the epidemiology and management of the most important STIs facing our communities today.

The need for effective prevention and management of STIs, including HIV infection, remains urgent, both internationally and domestically. In the United States in 2021, most new HIV infections occurred in men who have sex with men (MSM), a population that also continues to sustain the highest incidence of syphilis—an infection many physicians had experience with primarily in the pre-AIDS era, and one new to many young physicians. As summarized in the article on syphilis, this resurgence has highlighted that clinical recognition of this protean disease—called "the great pretender" by Sir William Osler—continues to present diagnostic and management challenges to those who care for patients at risk, particularly when coinfection with HIV is involved. Persons with HIV are more likely to have atypical manifestations of the genital ulcerations caused by *Treponema pallidum* and atypical results of diagnostic serology tests, and very probably have an increased risk of neuroinvasive disease because of this

Infect Dis Clin N Am 37 (2023) xi–xiii
https://doi.org/10.1016/j.idc.2023.03.001
0891-5520/23/© 2023 Published by Elsevier Inc.

id.theclinics.com

pathogen. We urgently need more precise diagnostic tests for active syphilis, and progress toward a vaccine is welcome.

Rates of other reportable STIs either have not declined or have actually increased in the last decade. In 2020, more than 1.7 million diagnoses of *Chlamydia trachomatis* were reported to the Centers for Disease Control and Prevention (CDC). Despite this, interventions to detect this common infection in populations most at risk are infrequently performed. For example, rates of routine annual screening for genital chlamydial infections in young women, especially adolescents, remain suboptimal, and many women at low risk (primarily those over the age of 30 years without other indications) are tested unnecessarily. Moreover, recommendations to routinely retest infected persons 4 to 6 months after treatment (a practice termed *repeat testing*, which is distinct from test of cure) are not frequently adhered to, despite that this approach detects repeat infection in approximately 15% to 40% of those tested.

As of 2020, the incidence of gonorrhea has increased by 111% in just over 10 years. From 2019 to 2020 alone, gonococcal infections increased 5.7%. Moreover, the relentless evolution of antimicrobial resistance in *Neisseria gonorrhoeae* continues to present a major challenge. Both fluoroquinolones, which offered a new class of effective single-dose oral therapy for this organism in the 1990s, and macrolides (azithromycin) are no longer reliably effective owing to increasing resistance, a trend especially notable in MSM. Providers are now effectively left with only a single class of antibiotics—the cephalosporins—that reliably treat this infection. Concern for nascent development of resistance to this class—a phenomenon that has already been reported—has prompted study of several new alternatives, with at least two hopeful candidates moving into late-phase clinical trials. In 2023, the United States experienced its first cases of gonorrhea with multidrug resistance; while these infections were effectively treated with ceftriaxone, they portend the advent of challenging trends in managing this disease. Sexual transmission of hepatitis C has been increasingly recognized in MSM who report sexual practices involving exposure to blood or even minimal trauma to the rectal mucosa, and most recently, in injection drug users. Finally, the emergence of Mpox (the clinical disease caused by the monkeypox virus) in 2022 raised new challenges for the prevention and management of this infection.

These worrisome trends emphasize the need for physicians to be aware of emerging STI-related challenges and of the availability of guidelines and tools to help manage their patients. The CDC STI treatment guidelines are a great resource (www.cdc.gov/std/treatment). They emphasize emerging evidence of the positive benefits of immunization against several common genital human papillomavirus types for women and men.

The excellent articles that make up this issue cover these developments and more. Against the backdrop of providing key epidemiologic trends for each disease, the authors have emphasized that clinical recognition and diagnosis of these infections are not always straightforward. Moreover, therapeutic management of some STIs can be complicated by limited diagnostic capability, coinfections, and immune compromise resulting from HIV infection or other conditions. In addition to biomedical management of the individual patient who is affected by STIs, clinicians must remember that prevention of these infections requires combinations of biomedical, behavioral, and structural interventions. Among the most promising approaches is expedited partner management, a strategy that allows for treatment of sex partners without in-person evaluation. This approach has been widely adopted and should provide a major tool to control the stubborn epidemics of chlamydia and gonorrhea, in particular. Finally, new technologies have opened up our routes for communicating important information to patients, whether that be point-of-care diagnostic tests results or health promotion messaging through apps, texts, or other electronic platforms.

Although the Institute of Medicine's vision for controlling the hidden epidemic of STIs has not been fully realized, the health care field is in an exciting period of renewed hope for advances in diagnosis, therapy, and prevention of these challenging infections. The state-of-the-art information in the articles that follow will undoubtedly assist clinicians in contributing to the overall goal of improving the community's sexual health through recognition, management, and prevention of STIs.

Jeanne Marrazzo, MD, MPH, FACP, FIDSA
Division of Infectious Diseases
Department of Medicine
University of Alabama at
Birmingham School of Medicine
Tinsley Harrison Tower 215
1900 University Boulevard
Birmingham, AL 35294-0006, USA

E-mail address:
jmarrazzo@uabmc.edu

Syphilis: A Modern Resurgence

Meena S. Ramchandani, MD, MPH[a,b,]*,
Chase A. Cannon, MD, MPH[a,b], Christina M. Marra, MD[c]

KEYWORDS

- Sexually transmitted diseases • Neurosyphilis • Ocular Syphilis • Otosyphilis
- Congenital syphilis • T pallidum • Treponema pallidum • Darkfield microscopy

KEY POINTS

- While syphilis is common among men who have sex with men, rates are increasing among women resulting in an increase in congenital syphilis.
- Syphilis can cause a wide range of sytemic manifestations.
- The hallmark of syphilis diagnosis relies on serologic testing.
- Penicillin G remains the treatment of choice for all stages of syphilis.
- Neurologic, ocular and otologic and congenital syphilis are complications of the disease with great morbidity.

CASE

A 33-year-old man presents to your clinic with a painless penile ulcer that has been present for 2 weeks. It is slightly indurated and shallow with minimal erythema. He has right inguinal lymphadenopathy but otherwise, his examination is unremarkable. He reports 4 sex partners in the last 3 months, 3 are men and one is a woman who is 18 weeks pregnant. He plans to bring in his partners for evaluation.

THINGS TO CONSIDER

What is his stage of syphilis?
What testing would you do?
How would you treat him?
How would you manage each of his male partners?
How would you manage his female partner?
What further evaluation is needed to make sure that none of these individuals has complicated syphilis?

---

[a] Department of Medicine, University of Washington, 1959 NE Pacific Street, Seattle, WA 98195, USA; [b] HIV/STD Program, Public Health-Seattle & King County, 401 5th Avenue, Seattle, WA 98104, USA; [c] Department of Neurology, University of Washington, 1959 NE Pacific Street, Seattle, WA 98195, USA
* Corresponding author. Division of AID, University of Washington, 325 Ninth Ave. Mailstop 359777, Seattle, WA 98104.
E-mail address: meenasr@uw.edu

Infect Dis Clin N Am 37 (2023) 195–222
https://doi.org/10.1016/j.idc.2023.02.006
0891-5520/23/© 2023 Elsevier Inc. All rights reserved.

id.theclinics.com

INTRODUCTION

The rates of syphilis are rising in the United States and many high-income nations despite the availability of screening and effective treatment.[1–4] The diagnosis of syphilis can be challenging due to various clinical manifestations at different stages, some of which can be mistaken for other sexually transmitted infections (STIs). The mainstay of testing relies on serologic tests, of which there are several options. Interpreting serologic tests can be confusing, particularly because of different syphilis screening algorithms.[5] Stigma associated with STIs as well as health care providers' discomfort with taking a sexual history can also make a timely diagnosis and identification of this disease a challenge. In this review geared toward health care practitioners in the U.S., we cover the key clinical findings in syphilis and provide an overview of the diagnosis and management of this disease in adults.

EPIDEMIOLOGY

In the United States, the reported number of cases of syphilis has increased since the early 2000s[6] (**Fig. 1**). Preliminary data for 2021 indicate that there were greater than 171,000 cases of all stages of syphilis, representing a 68% increase from 2017.[3] Just in the 1 year period from 2020 to 2021, there was a 28% increase in cases of syphilis, indicating that, even in the face of the COVID-19 pandemic and probable underreporting, syphilis remains a significant public health concern. The extent of the COVID-19 pandemic's impact on syphilis in the U.S. is unclear, but disruptions to laboratory testing, reassignment of staff, reduced funding, and reduced capacity of sexual health programs may contribute to more drastic increases in the years to come.[7–9]

MSM are disproportionately impacted by syphilis in the U.S, accounting for 53% of all male primary and secondary (P&S) cases in 2020.[6] In 2021, preliminary data show that there were greater than 40,000 men with P&S syphilis, a 19% increase from 2020 and a 49% increase from 2017.[3] The rate of P&S syphilis in men in 2021 was 24 per 100,000 population. However, rates of syphilis among MSM have slowed in the last few years. In contrast, the rates have increased in women in the U.S. In 2021, preliminary data suggest that there were greater than 11,000 women with P&S syphilis, a 49% increase from 2020 and a 216% increase from 2017. Alarmingly, since about 2013, we have witnessed a surge in congenital syphilis. Preliminary estimates suggest

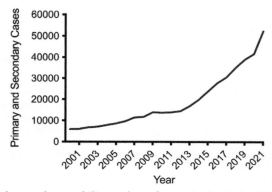

Fig. 1. Primary and secondary syphilis-number of cases in the United States from 2001 to 2021. Numbers for syphilis cases in 2021 are preliminary. (*Adapted from* Centers for Disease Control and Prevention. https://www.cdc.gov/std/statistics/. Accessed December 2022.)

that there were greater than 2600 cases of congenital syphilis in 2021, representing a 24% increase from 2020 and a 184% increase from 2017. In 2020, there were 2148 cases of congenital syphilis, including 149 stillbirths and infant deaths.[6] This is a concerning public health threat that is completely preventable with adequate screening and timely management of syphilis in pregnancy.

Demographic disparities in STI incidence continue to exist and syphilis is no exception. While the number of syphilis cases has increased in almost all race/ethnicity groups since 2019, in 2020, the rates of P&S syphilis were highest among Black or African American persons at a rate of 34 cases per 100,000, followed by American Indian or Alaska Native persons at 27 cases per 100,000.[6] This is much higher than the 7 cases per 100,000 in White persons in the U.S. While the rates of congenital syphilis were highest among American Indian or Alaska Native mothers, followed by Native Hawaiian or other Pacific Islander mothers, the greatest absolute number of reported congenital syphilis cases was among mothers who were Black or African American, followed by Hispanic or Latina mothers.[6,10] Patterns of racial and ethnic disparities vary by geographic location in the U.S. State-level surveillance data from 2016 show rates of syphilis were higher for Black than for White MSM in 42 of 44 states, with Southern states being the most impacted in 2014.[11,12] Reducing these disparities will require increased awareness and both local and national leadership to address a multitude of factors, including stigma, social determinants of health, and barriers to care.

Nondemographic factors also increase the risk of acquiring syphilis. These include multiple sex partners, sex with anonymous partners, while intoxicated/high or with a person who injects drugs, methamphetamine use, injection drug use, exchange of sex for money or drugs, experiencing homelessness, those in correctional facilities, and younger adults.[13] In 2020, 10% of individuals with P&S syphilis reported methamphetamine use (16% among women, 12% among MSW and 8% among MSM).[6] Forty-seven percent of individuals with syphilis reported sex with anonymous partners, and 33% reported sex while intoxicated.

SCREENING RECOMMENDATIONS

The frequency of syphilis screening depends on the patient population, but in general, patients who are sexually active with an increased likelihood of acquiring syphilis as discussed above should be regularly tested.[5,14] Routine syphilis screening is also recommended for MSM, persons with HIV (PWH), and all pregnant persons at least once in pregnancy, ideally at the first prenatal visit. The 2021 CDC STI Treatment Guidelines do not recommend routine screening for syphilis for men who have sex with women and nonpregnant women who have sex with men or women unless there are other risk factors for acquiring an STI.

Syphilis screening is recommended more frequently in some populations based on whether epidemiologic data show a high national or regional STI incidence. The 2021 CDC HIV PrEP Guidelines recommend syphilis screening for all sexually active patients prescribed PrEP both at initial and semi-annual visits, and every 3 months for MSM and transgender women who have sex with men. The 2021 CDC STI Treatment Guidelines recommend syphilis screening every 3 to 6 months for MSM with multiple, anonymous, or concurrent partners.[5,15] In pregnant persons, retesting for syphilis at 28 weeks gestation and at delivery is recommended for those with a history of substance use, an STI during pregnancy, multiple sex partners, a new sex partner or a sex partner with an STI. Testing three times in pregnancy is also recommended if the pregnant person lives in a community with high syphilis rates.[5] Predictive models and risk scores can help identify U.S. counties at elevated risk for the emergence of syphilis in persons who can become pregnant and for congenital syphilis.[16,17] Due to the concerning increase in congenital syphilis cases and syphilis in cisgender women in Seattle & King County, Public Health released recommendations for all sexually active women age 45 and under in Washington state to test for syphilis if not tested in the last year.[18] Clinicians, especially those in infectious diseases, primary care, adolescent medicine, pediatrics, STI specialty care settings, public health clinics, antenatal care, and obstetrics and gynecology should take a detailed sexual history at initial, routine annual visits, and STI-related visits to help guide screening recommendations for syphilis, HIV and other bacterial STIs.[19]

DIAGNOSTIC TESTING

The hallmark of syphilis diagnosis relies on serologic testing, and less on direct detection of *Treponema pallidum* subspecies *pallidum* (hereafter *T pallidum*) in clinical samples. We review the diagnosis of syphilis in adults.

Serology

Serologic tests rely on the detection of treponemal and nontreponemal antigens, which have high sensitivity during the secondary and later stages of syphilis. For PWH, the interpretation of treponemal and nontreponemal tests is the same as those in persons without HIV. Treponemal tests measure IgM and IgG antibodies to treponemal antigens, such as whole organisms or synthetic *T pallidum* proteins; sensitivity is greater than 90% in secondary syphilis.[20] Examples of treponemal tests include the *T pallidum* particle agglutination assay (TP-PA) and fluorescent treponemal antibody absorption (FTA-ABS), enzyme immunoassay (EIA) or chemiluminescent immunoassay (CIA). Once reactive, treponemal tests remain reactive for life in most people, even if they are treated for syphilis. As such, reactive treponemal tests cannot distinguish between previously treated or untreated infection and new infection.[21]

Nontreponemal, or better termed lipoidal, tests measure IgM and IgG antibodies to a cardiolipin-lecithin-cholesterol antigen, which likely cross-react with host lipids incorporated into *T pallidum* membranes.[22] Lipoidal tests can be used qualitatively for screening or quantitatively to provide a titer (in multiples of 2) that can be followed over time. They include the rapid plasma reagin (RPR) and Venereal Disease Research Laboratory (VDRL) tests, and the toluidine red unheated serum test (TRUST). Titers from lipoidal tests increase with re-infection and decrease with successful treatment. A fourfold rise or decrease in titer using the same lipoidal test, equivalent to a change of two dilutions, is considered clinically significant. Different lipoidal tests cannot be compared directly; therefore, follow-up serologic testing after a diagnosis of syphilis should use the same lipoidal test. The different lipoidal tests have approximately the same sensitivity and specificity depending on the stage of infection.[23]

Two algorithms for serologic testing exist in the U.S. to help identify a new diagnosis of syphilis: the traditional algorithm and the reverse screening algorithm.[5] The decision regarding which algorithm to use in a particular community is influenced by laboratory personnel availability, automation, turnaround time, cost, and prevalence of syphilis in the population being tested. In the traditional screening algorithm, laboratory diagnosis of syphilis begins with a lipoidal test. Reactive lipoidal results are confirmed using a treponemal test. If both tests are reactive, this indicates a diagnosis of past or current syphilis. In the reverse screening algorithm, the initial test is a treponemal test. A reactive treponemal test is confirmed by a lipoidal test. If both tests are reactive, a diagnosis of past or current syphilis is made. However, if there are discordant results between the treponemal and lipoidal test, a second, but different treponemal test, ideally using a different assay platform, is performed to confirm past or current infection.[24] The reverse algorithm is increasingly used because some treponemal assays, such as the EIA or CIA are automated and can increase throughput. Discrepant serologic results between the initial treponemal test and the second lipoidal test can be difficult for clinicians to interpret if the full algorithm is not followed and additional treponemal testing is not performed.[24,25] The additional treponemal testing helps to distinguish between past or current syphilis or a false positive initial treponemal screening test. Differentiating between past or current infection requires consideration of syphilis history and treatment and comparison of current with previous serologic test results. Providers should be aware of which algorithm is employed in their local area or practice, and public health staff can often provide syphilis history and past lipoidal titers if not readily available in the medical record.

Syphilis serologic tests may be falsely reactive or falsely nonreactive. Automated treponemal tests can be falsely reactive in the reverse screening algorithm. This is one reason confirmation with a second treponemal test is indicated when there are discordant treponemal and lipoidal test results. Falsely reactive lipoidal tests can occur with viral infections, immunization, autoimmune disease, injection drug use, older age, or pregnancy.[26–31] Falsely nonreactive lipoidal, and sometimes even falsely nonreactive treponemal tests, may occur very early in *T pallidum* infection. Falsely nonreactive lipoidal tests can also result from the prozone phenomenon, whereby high antibody concentration, often in the setting of secondary syphilis, prevents the formation of antigen-antibody complexes and agglutination, which is the basis of the test. Prozone reactions may occur in up to 1% of individuals with primary or secondary syphilis.[32–35] The prozone reaction can be excluded by testing serial dilutions of the serum or plasma sample.[36] The prozone phenomenon does not occur with treponemal serologic tests.

While serologic tests should be performed when any stage of syphilis is suspected, their sensitivity in primary syphilis ranges from 46% to 100%, with treponemal tests yielding reactive results before lipoidal tests.[20,23,37] In a study of 106 individuals, the TP-PA yielded the highest sensitivity (86%) compared with VDRL or RPR confirmed by TP-PA (71%) for patients with darkfield confirmed primary syphilis.[37] These findings highlight the importance of empiric syphilis treatment based on in-depth sexual history and physical examination. Treatment is recommended even before the results of serologic tests are available in primary or secondary stages and for sex partners of a person diagnosed with early syphilis within the past 90 days.[5]

Direct Detection

Darkfield microscopy is often considered the gold standard test to diagnose primary syphilis. It is performed at the point of care and involves examining exudate from a primary or moist secondary lesion under a darkfield microscope to identify *T pallidum* based on characteristic morphology and motility. It is one of the quickest and most definitive ways to diagnose primary syphilis, and the result may be positive before serologic tests becoming reactive. The sensitivity ranges from 75% to 100% in.[23,38,39] However, darkfield microscopy can be challenging as it requires specialized equipment and trained personnel, and therefore, it is rarely performed in clinics today. *T pallidum* can also be directly identified in tissue specimens by histopathologic staining. This technique is invasive or may not always be sensitive depending on sample selection and is not recommended for routine clinical care.

Molecular tests to detect DNA sequences specific to *T pallidum* are promising ways to improve diagnostic sensitivity and can be helpful before serologic tests turning positive in early disease.[40] However, thus far, no molecular tests for syphilis are FDA approved in the U.S., and test performance is limited depending on the stage of syphilis, sample type and target gene used. Sensitivity of molecular tests has ranged anywhere from 20% to 95% based on the type of sample and the molecular target.[41] Primary lesion exudate yields the best sensitivity, ranging from 73% to 100%.[38,42–46] In a meta-analysis of 23 studies from 2009 to 2019, pooled sensitivities for syphilis polymerase chain reaction (PCR) tests were 78% for primary stage and 67% for secondary stage, and the pooled specificities were greater than 97% for both stages.[47] Molecular assays can be helpful to make a diagnosis of syphilis when patients are asymptomatic. Among blood and urine specimens, oropharyngeal and anorectal swabs taken from 293 MSM at a sexual health clinic (SHC) in Amsterdam, T pallidum DNA was detected in 34% with early latent syphilis.[48] DNA was also detected in the anal (14%) or oral (21%) area of men with early syphilis despite no anal or oral primary lesion at that site respectively.[49] This suggests transmission of T pallidum can possibly occur even without visible lesions and during asymptomatic (or latent) disease. A combination screening strategy using a T pallidum transcription-mediated amplification assay on rectal and pharyngeal mucosal swabs with serologic testing might be more sensitive to detect new syphilis in some populations at higher risk.[50] Some guidelines, such as the Australian STI Management Guidelines and 2020 European guideline include a diagnosis of syphilis based on NAAT testing.[4,51]

Complicated Syphilis

The diagnosis of neurosyphilis, otosyphilis, and ocular syphilis, remains a challenge due to nonspecific clinical manifestations and imperfect assays to diagnose the disease. Serologic evidence of T pallidum is required to diagnose complicated syphilis. In neurosyphilis, patients may present with neurologic symptoms such as cognitive impairment, gait imbalance, cranial nerve palsy, meningitis, or stroke. Any patient with a diagnosis of syphilis and neurologic symptoms should have a lumbar puncture to aid in the diagnosis of neurosyphilis.[5] The cerebrospinal fluid (CSF) findings of neurosyphilis may include one or more of the following: CSF pleocytosis and elevated protein, especially in those persons without HIV, or a reactive lipoidal test, typically a CSF-VDRL.[52] In PWH, mild CSF pleocytosis and elevated protein levels can be common in the absence of syphilis. CSF pleocytosis due to HIV is more common in individuals not currently using antiretrovirals, CD4 count greater than 200/μL and detectable plasma HIV RNA.[53,54] Therefore, some experts suggest a higher cutoff of CSF nucleated cell count to make a diagnosis of neurosyphilis in PWH.[55]

Other tests for the diagnosis of neurosyphilis can be used. Although its specificity is high, the sensitivity of the CSF-VDRL test is between 20% to 70% and therefore a negative CSF VDRL does not exclude the diagnosis of neurosyphilis.[56,57] An older treponemal test, the FTA-ABS used for CSF examination is more sensitive than the CSF VDRL but can be less specific.[57–59] A nonreactive CSF FTA-ABS is helpful to rule out neurosyphilis in individuals without neurologic symptoms, but is likely less useful to exclude symptomatic neurosyphilis.[60] Direct detection of T pallidum in CSF using NAAT has been evaluated as an additional tool to aid in the diagnosis of neurosyphilis in research studies. T pallidum was identified by reverse transcriptase PCR in CSF from 21% of patients with untreated early syphilis who were otherwise asymptomatic.[61] However, some studies have indicated T pallidum NAATs on CSF from symptomatic adults and neonates have low sensitivity. In a meta-analysis evaluating 4 studies, sensitivity for PCR-based tests ranged from 42% to 87% and specificity from 92% to 99% for the diagnosis of neurosyphilis.[47] Further research to improve the diagnosis of neurosyphilis is needed.

Ocular syphilis or otosyphilis can occur independently or in association with neurosyphilis. Patients with a new diagnosis of syphilis and ocular symptoms should be evaluated immediately by an ophthalmologist. The 2021 CDC STI Treatment Guidelines recommend that if there are confirmed ocular abnormalities on examination and the patient has no neurologic symptoms, CSF examination is not necessary before treatment.[5] A CSF examination might be helpful in patients with syphilis who have ocular symptoms but no abnormal findings. Patients with syphilis and auditory symptoms concerning for otosyphilis should be managed with an otolaryngologist. If patients have isolated auditory symptoms with a normal neurologic examination, the 2021 CDC STI Treatment Guidelines do not recommend CSF examination before treatment of otosyphilis.[5]

Other Diagnostic Considerations

The diagnosis of syphilis can be challenging when a patient presents from a country whereby other *T pallidum* subspecies are endemic and are not sexually transmitted. The current laboratory methods available in the U.S. cannot distinguish *T pallidum* subspecies *pallidum* from other pathogenic treponemes that cause yaws, pinta, or nonvenereal endemic syphilis (bejel).[62] Patients born in endemic areas might have been infected with endemic treponemes in childhood. Treponemal tests for syphilis are cross-reactive, but lipoidal tests may revert to negative after treatment.[63] In these cases, we recommend treatment of syphilis if no such treatment has been documented, and patients and their partners should be counseled that serologic tests for syphilis cannot discriminate between *T pallidum* subspecies.

Rapid point-of-care tests (POCTs) are now available to aid in the diagnosis of syphilis and to facilitate on-site testing, diagnosis, and prompt treatment. POCTs can use specimens from serum, plasma, and whole blood, are qualitative, and often provide results within 20 minutes. While there are many commercially available POCTs, there are 2 assays for syphilis approved by the US Food and Drug Administration (FDA); the Syphilis Health Check (Diagnostics Direct, Stone Harbor, NJ) and the Dual Path Platform (DPP) HIV Syphilis Assay (Chembio Diagnostics, Hauppauge, NY). The Syphilis Health Check has a sensitivity of 100% compared with samples that are reactive by both RPR and EIA, but 50% to 71% when compared with a reactive EIA test alone.[64,65] A meta-analysis of 10 prospective studies using the Syphilis Health Check across diverse populations showed a pooled sensitivity of 88% and a specificity of 97% when compared with a treponemal test.[66] The DPP assay has a sensitivity of about 94% compared with the TPPA, but there is less experience with this syphilis test in clinical settings as it was approved by the FDA in 2020.[67] Most POCTs, including the Syphilis Health Check and the DPP, rely on treponemal antibodies and therefore can only be used for the initial screening of asymptomatic persons but will not identify new infections for those with previously treated or untreated syphilis. Results of syphilis POCTs should be confirmed with conventional treponemal and lipoidal tests. Given the short turnaround time for results, POCTs are helpful when follow-up cannot be ensured.[68–71] The Australian STI Management Guidelines have implemented a Syphilis Point-of-Care Testing Program to help address the ongoing outbreak in remote areas, predominately in young Aboriginal and Torres Strait Islander people.[51,72] Similarly, the 2020 European Guidelines mention the use of POCTs for on-site testing of outreach populations and in antenatal settings whereby syphilis testing in pregnancy has not been done.[4] A rapid POCT for the diagnosis of neurosyphilis has also been evaluated. The DPP Syphilis Screen & Confirm test (Chembio Diagnostics, Hauppauge, NY) was 80% sensitive and 97% specific for the diagnosis of neurosyphilis in 71 patients with syphilis (35 with confirmed neurosyphilis and 36 without neurosyphilis).[73] Increasing availability and development of accurate POCTs for syphilis is an important area of research to help address the syphilis epidemic in the U.S. and in many parts of the world.[74–77]

CLINICAL MANIFESTATIONS

Syphilis is categorized into stages, depending on the estimated time since infection and the presence or type of symptoms with which a patient presents. A detailed sexual history and thorough physical examination are an important part of the evaluation to identify clinical manifestations. Transmission of *T pallidum* is highest in early syphilis and approximately 30% of persons will develop syphilis after sexual contact with a person with early syphilis.[78–80] The organism can also cross the placenta to cause fetal infection at any stage of the disease and any stage of pregnancy. Complicated syphilis can also occur at any stage of disease.

Primary Syphilis

Primary syphilis usually presents as a single painless, indurated ulcer with a clean base at the site of inoculation by *T pallidum*. The ulcer, also known as a chancre, can be accompanied by regional lymphadenopathy and most often occurs at the ano-genital site (**Fig. 2**). It usually presents 3 to 6 weeks after inoculation, although the incubation period is anywhere from 10 to 90 days.[78,81,82] Atypical chancres can occur and may manifest as multiple ulcers, painful ulcers, fissures, or large denuded areas of the skin, which can result in a secondary bacterial infection[83,84] (**Fig. 3**). Up to 49% of 183 men with anogenital syphilis in Melbourne, Australia, had painful primary lesions and 38% had multiple ulcers.[85] Chancres have been noted on other areas of the body such as the mouth, chin, finger, and chest[86–89] (**Figs. 4** and **5**). Primary syphilis can be mistaken for other ulcerative diseases and the differential might include HSV-1 or 2, mpox or aphthous ulcers.[90–92] The chancre typically lasts 1 to 6 weeks and can heal spontaneously, even without treatment, although the patient will still have an active syphilis that can progress to other stages. If lesions are painless and located in difficult areas to visualize such as the anal region or cervix, the diagnosis can be delayed or missed. Serologic testing, particularly lipoidal tests, can be nonreactive in primary syphilis and therefore, a high clinical suspicion is crucial to initiate empiric therapy and reduce the risk of transmission and progression to later stages.

Secondary Syphilis

The clinical manifestations of secondary syphilis are varied and typically present between 4 to 10 weeks after the appearance of a chancre.[93] Most often, patients present

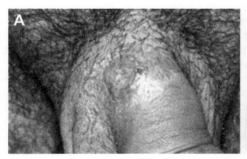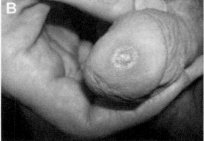

Fig. 2. (*A, B*) penile chancres. (*From* Cohen SE, Klausner JD, Engelman J, Philip S. Syphilis in the modern era: an update for physicians. Infect Dis Clin North Am. 2013;27(4):705 to 722; with permission.)

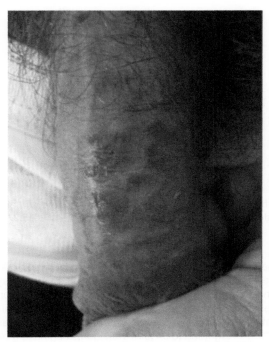

Fig. 3. Multiple penile chancres. (*From* Cohen SE, Klausner JD, Engelman J, Philip S. Syphilis in the modern era: an update for physicians. Infect Dis Clin North Am. 2013;27(4):705 to 722; with permission.)

with a rash, which can be macular, papular, maculopapular, pustular, or with scale, and either disseminated throughout the skin or localized to a particular area (**Figs. 6** and **7**). Of 854 patients with secondary syphilis, 45% had a rash that involved the palms of the hands and 44% included the soles of the feet.[94] Typically, the rash is without associated symptoms, but it may be painful or pruritic, and the median duration is around 14 days in persons without HIV.[95–97] Other secondary syphilis manifestations include condylomata lata, which are moist wartlike lesions, mucous patches in

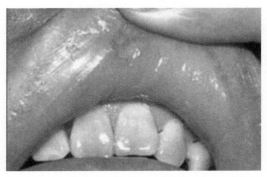

Fig. 4. Chancre on lip. (*From* Cohen SE, Klausner JD, Engelman J, Philip S. Syphilis in the modern era: an update for physicians. Infect Dis Clin North Am. 2013;27(4):705 to 722; with permission)

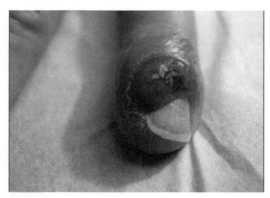

Fig. 5. Chancre on finger. (*From* Cohen SE, Klausner JD, Engelman J, Philip S. Syphilis in the modern era: an update for physicians. Infect Dis Clin North Am. 2013;27(4):705 to 722; with permission.)

the oropharynx, patchy alopecia, and rarely lues maligna, which presents with ulcerating lesions of the skin primarily in PWH (**Figs. 8** and **9**). Systemic symptoms include diffuse lymphadenopathy, fatigue, headache, myalgia, arthralgia or mild fever, or a combination of these symptoms. Renal and liver involvement have also been reported with elevated creatinine or liver enzymes, most commonly an increase in serum alkaline phosphatase.[94,98,99] Eighteen to 34% of individuals can have a persistent chancre with symptoms of secondary syphilis.[78,94] Symptoms from secondary syphilis will resolve after 2 to 6 weeks in an untreated individual but, in the absence of treatment, may recur after resolution in 25% of cases.[100]

Latent Syphilis

Without treatment, patients can progress from secondary syphilis to a latent, or asymptomatic, stage, characterized by infection and lack of symptoms. Often, this stage is diagnosed in the setting of routine serologic screening. In the U.S., early latent

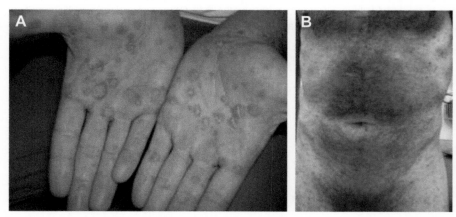

Fig. 6. (*A*) Palmar rash of secondary syphilis. (*B*) Truncal rash of secondary syphilis. (*From* Cohen SE, Klausner JD, Engelman J, Philip S. Syphilis in the modern era: an update for physicians. Infect Dis Clin North Am. 2013;27(4):705 to 722; with permission.)

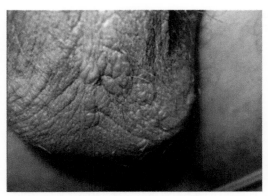

Fig. 7. Papulosquamous scrotal rash of secondary syphilis. (*From* Cohen SE, Klausner JD, Engelman J, Philip S. Syphilis in the modern era: an update for physicians. Infect Dis Clin North Am. 2013;27(4):705 to 722; with permission.)

syphilis is defined as infection within the past 12 months. For example, a diagnosis of early latent syphilis is made if, in the last year, an asymptomatic patient has newly reactive syphilis serology from a nonreactive result or a fourfold or greater increase in lipoidal titers in those with previous syphilis.[5] Early latent disease is also diagnosed if a person with positive serologies had symptoms of primary or secondary syphilis within the last year, a sex partner was documented to have early syphilis within the last year, or if the only possible sexual exposure for a new diagnosis of syphilis occurred in the last year. In the absence of these conditions, a person without symptoms is considered to have the late latent disease. This differs from other international guidelines. For example, the Australian STI Management Guidelines categorize early latent syphilis as those persons with asymptomatic infection acquired within the previous 2 years.[51] However, the 2020 European Guidelines are similar to the U.S. by defining early syphilis as infection acquired in the past 1 year.[4] In the U.S., late latent syphilis is defined as infection lasting greater than 12 months or of unknown duration. Serologic tests are typically reactive in early and late latent syphilis, but with increasing

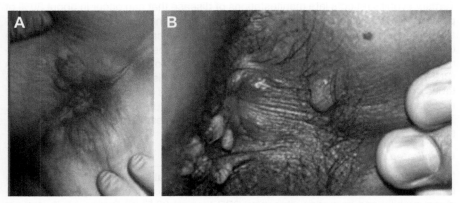

Fig. 8. Perianal condylomata lata shown in (*A* and *B*). (*From* Cohen SE, Klausner JD, Engelman J, Philip S. Syphilis in the modern era: an update for physicians. Infect Dis Clin North Am. 2013;27(4):705 to 722; with permission.)

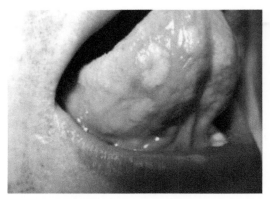

Fig. 9. Mucous patches on the tongue. (*From* Cohen SE, Klausner JD, Engelman J, Philip S. Syphilis in the modern era: an update for physicians. Infect Dis Clin North Am. 2013;27(4):705 to 722; with permission.)

time, lipoidal test titers may decline or revert to nonreactive without treatment despite continued infection.[23] Reactive treponemal tests and a history of lack of treatment can help establish the diagnosis in these cases.

Persons with repeat episodes of syphilis may more likely be asymptomatic in a subsequent syphilis infection.[101] The proportion of individuals diagnosed with early latent syphilis was higher in those with ≥3 syphilis episodes compared with those with 2 or fewer episodes, although the relationship was reduced to a trend when the rate of testing was taken into account.[102] It is unclear whether *T pallidum* is transmitted from asymptomatic people. While historically studies have suggested that *T pallidum* is not transmissible during the latent stages of syphilis, it is possible that some persons with latent infection may be infectious.[78] Shedding of *T pallidum* nucleic acid has been observed in persons with early latent syphilis, and both placental transmission and neurosyphilis can occur during early and latent stages,[48,50,55,103] underscoring the possibility of transmission during asymptomatic syphilis.

Tertiary Syphilis

Tertiary syphilis reflects late manifestations of disease that can occur in about 30% of persons who remain untreated and is rarely seen in the modern era.[93] Symptoms usually occur 10 to 20 years after the onset of infection. Clinical manifestations can include cardiovascular syphilis such as aortic insufficiency or aneurysm, gummas or granulomatous lesions that invade local tissue, and late stages of the central nervous system (CNS) disease.[104,105] In the late stages of neurosyphilis, patients can present with tabes dorsalis: a disease affecting the posterior columns of the spinal cord and dorsal root ganglia, resulting in ataxia and wide-based gait due to loss of proprioception. They can also present with general paresis, which manifests as progressive dementia, seizures, and psychiatric symptoms.

Complicated Syphilis

Neurosyphilis, otosyphilis, and ocular syphilis can occur at any stage of syphilis, even in patients with latent disease. Neurosyphilis is more likely to occur in subjects with early-stage syphilis and in those with serum RPR titer ≥1:32.[55,106] Earlier manifestations of neurosyphilis include meningitis with cranial nerve palsies, and meningovascular disease (stroke).[61] However, symptoms of early and late neurosyphilis may overlap;

for example, patients with early syphilis can have cognitive impairment, gait incoordination, and distal sensory loss.[107,108] Otosyphilis, a serious complication of syphilis, can manifest as tinnitus, hearing decrease, or loss. In a study of 329 participants with syphilis who underwent portable audiometry, 5% had low frequency, 28% high frequency and 17% had combined low and high-frequency hearing loss.[109] Most typically, patients have sensorineural hearing loss, although conductive hearing loss can also occur. Patients with ocular syphilis may have flashes, floaters, unilateral or bilateral vision loss. They can present with uveitis or inflammation of any part of the eye, but anterior uveitis alone is uncommon. In 68 cases of possible neurosyphilis, 8% had vision or hearing changes and 4% had symptoms in addition to abnormal CSF findings or ophthalmologic examination.[110] Untreated, neurosyphilis, otosyphilis, or ocular syphilis can result in permanent neurologic symptoms, vision or hearing loss respectively, therefore timely diagnosis and immediate treatment are critical. Some strains of T pallidum are more common in individuals with neurosyphilis, and certain polymorphisms in toll-like receptor genes are more common in hosts with neurosyphilis.[111–113] Yet, it remains unclear why some patients with syphilis develop neurosyphilis, ocular syphilis, or otosyphilis, and further research is needed in this area.

CSF abnormalities can occur in persons with syphilis in the absence of neurologic findings, also known as asymptomatic neurosyphilis. In the preantibiotic era, asymptomatic individuals with more abnormal CSF were more likely to develop symptomatic neurosyphilis, and this observation justified routine CSF examinations and treatment.[114] The prognosis of asymptomatic neurosyphilis is not known in the current era of antibiotic management for syphilis. While time to cognitive normalization, improvement, or decline did not seem to be affected by treatment based on CSF analysis, individuals with CSF pleocytosis treated for neurosyphilis were less likely to experience cognitive decline than those without CSF pleocytosis who were not treated.[107] The current utility of identifying CSF abnormalities or treating such persons for neurosyphilis is controversial and the 2021 CDC STI Treatment Guidelines advise no variation from recommended diagnosis and treatment according to the syphilis stage, except in the setting of tertiary syphilis, in patients without clinical manifestations of neurologic involvement,.[5]

Persons with HIV

In PWH, the clinical manifestations of syphilis are typically similar to those in persons without HIV. In a study of 541 patients with syphilis, PWH had higher initial serum RPR titers and were more likely to have multiple chancres.[106] PWH with secondary syphilis were also more likely to have concomitant genital ulcers, although there were no differences in other secondary syphilis manifestations in persons with and without HIV.[96] Neurologic complications of syphilis are higher in PWH and one study found 22% of PWH had CSF abnormalities consistent with neurosyphilis.[55] Risk factors for neurosyphilis among PWH include lower CD4 counts ≤350 cells/mL and higher RPR titers.[55] Use of antiretroviral therapy prior to T pallidum infection reduced the odds of neurosyphilis by 65%.[115] Clinicians should evaluate patients thoroughly and ask about neurologic, ocular, or otologic signs or symptoms in any patient with a new diagnosis of syphilis.

Congenital Syphilis

Congenital syphilis can cause adverse birth outcomes and result in early fetal death, stillbirth, neonatal death, preterm birth, low birthweight, and congenital infection in infants.[5] Of those infants born alive, 40% are symptomatic at birth[6] and may present with early or late manifestations. Early symptoms include a morbilliform rash, hepatosplenomegaly, rhinorrhea or snuffles, and signs of neurosyphilis with seizures, bulging fontanelle, and cranial nerve abnormalities. Late symptoms occur after 2 years of life and include tooth abnormalities, saddle nose deformity, and frontal bossing. Late symptoms may also include irreversible ocular and otologic disease.[116] Any infant born to a person with syphilis should have a thorough evaluation, even if no obvious symptoms are present. How to diagnose and conduct congenital syphilis evaluations is beyond the scope of this review; more details can be found in the 2021 CDC STI Treatment Guidelines.[5]

TREATMENT

Syphilis is treated according to the clinical stage of disease. In general, earlier stages of infection are treated for a shorter duration and late stages are treated for a longer course. Based on decades of clinical experience, penicillin (PCN) G is considered the antibiotic of choice for all stages of syphilis. However, not all formulations of PCN G are equivalent, and care must be taken to ensure that the appropriate formulation is used based on the patient's syphilis stage, whether there are complications such as ocular or neurosyphilis, and pregnancy status. Combinations of PCN products (eg, oral amoxicillin with benzathine PCN G) or additional doses of parenteral PCN do not provide additional benefits and are not recommended.[5,106,117] **Table 1** details the recommended and alternative treatment regimens by syphilis stage and population. Several management points merit special consideration and are further detailed in **Table 2**. Particularly in early syphilis, syphilis treatment may result in acute fever, headache, and/or myalgias, known as the Jarisch-Herxheimer reaction. The reaction typically begins within 6 hours after the initiation of treatment and resolves within 24 hours with supportive care (ie, fluids, antipyretics).[5,118] While this potentially can induce fetal distress or early labor in the second half of pregnancy, the benefits of treatment of syphilis in pregnancy and prevention of congenital syphilis must be considered. Women should seek obstetric attention after treatment if any symptoms of fever, contractions, or decrease in fetal movements.[5]

Partners who are exposed to a person diagnosed with syphilis should themselves be evaluated clinically and serologically for incident syphilis.[5] Standard syphilis contact periods are used to inform which partners should be notified. For sexual contact to a person diagnosed with early syphilis (primary, secondary, early latent) within the last 90 days: empiric treatment is indicated before and irrespective of serologic test results. If the last sexual contact was more than 90 days prior, management is based on serologic test results (see **Table 1**). If serologic testing cannot be done and follow-up is not certain, presumptive treatment of early syphilis is appropriate. For sexual contact to a person diagnosed with late syphilis (late latent or unknown duration), management depends on the ability to perform serologic testing and whether the contact can be followed over time.

Alternative treatments for complicated syphilis are not well-studied and most supporting evidence is anecdotal or based on small case series. Current guidelines highlight that some data exist to support the use of ceftriaxone for 10 to 14 days for neurosyphilis. Treatment is more challenging if parenteral therapy is declined or the patient is unable to adhere to a daily injectable medication. Older pharmacokinetic data suggest doxycycline 200 mg by mouth twice daily for 28 days may produce CSF drug levels sufficient to treat neurosyphilis[119]. While there is some observational data using this approach, it's not clear whether all individuals who received doxycycline had confirmed neurosyphilis.[120] Doxycycline use for neurosyphilis is not recommended in 2021 CDC STI Treatment Guidelines. Formal studies to evaluate the

Table 1
Recommended and alternative syphilis treatment regimens

Syphilis stage or population		Primary Recommendation		Alternative Recommendations		Special Considerations
		Medication and Dosage	Duration	Medication and Dosage	Duration	
Early syphilis	Primary	Benzathine PCN 2.4 million units IM	Once	Doxycycline 100 mg PO bid	14 days	Azithromycin not recommended due to high levels of macrolide resistance. Amoxicillin not recommended due to poor bioavailability.
				Tetracycline 500 mg PO qid [b]	14 days	
				Ceftriaxone 1 gm IV/ IM daily [c]	10-14 days	
	Secondary					
	Early latent [a]					
Late syphilis	Late latent	Benzathine PCN 2.4 million units IM	Once weekly for 3 weeks (total of 7.2 million units IM)	Doxycycline 100 mg PO bid	28 days	Ceftriaxone may be effective; optimal dose and duration are unknown
				Tetracycline 500 mg PO qid [b]	28 days	
	Unknown duration					
	Tertiary [d]					
Complicated syphilis	Neurosyphilis, otosyphilis, or ocular syphilis	Aqueous crystalline PCN G 3-4 million units IV every 4 hours or infused continuously (total of 18-24 million units per 24 hours)	10-14 days	Procaine PCN G 2.4 million units IM daily + probenecid 500 mg PO qid	10-14 days	After complicated syphilis treatment, 1-3 additional weekly doses of benzathine PCN G 2.4 million units IM may be considered

(continued on next page)

Table 1
(continued)

Syphilis stage or population	Primary Recommendation		Alternative Recommendations		Special Considerations
	Medication and Dosage	Duration	Medication and Dosage	Duration	
			Ceftriaxone 1–2 gm IM/IV daily [e]		to treat concurrent latent syphilis.[f]
Sex partners	Treat as early syphilis (see above) if sexual contact ≤90 days of partner's diagnosis. No empiric treatment if sexual contact >90 days prior. Treat as above if diagnosis is made through clinical and serological evaluation.				
Late syphilis	Treat empirically if unable to assure follow-up or obtain serologies, or according to the stage if diagnosed by serology.				

[a] Early latent syphilis may also be categorized as early nonprimary, nonsecondary stage in epidemiology reports.

[b] This regimen is uncommonly used due to the frequency of dosing and gastrointestinal side effects.

[c] Previous national guidelines suggested some cases of early syphilis (in the setting of penicillin allergy) have been treated successfully with as few as 8 d of IM ceftriaxone,[134] but overall evidence is scant to support the use of ceftriaxone in early syphilis.

[d] Only if CSF examination is normal. Some experts have opted to treat persons diagnosed with cardiovascular syphilis using a neurosyphilis regimen given concern for possible vascular involvement within the CNS.[135]

[e] Data to support this approach are observational. Some experts reserve this alternative therapy for cases when penicillin cannot be used (eg, unable to desensitize allergic patient).

[f] Since treatment for complicated syphilis is only 10 to 14 d, some experts give additional therapy to provide similar antibacterial coverage for the ≥3-wk duration

Table 2
Treatment of special populations and scenarios

Population	Recommendation
Pregnant persons	• Parenteral PCN is the only recommended treatment option during pregnancy.[5] • Persons with a PCN allergy should be desensitized according to local protocols and receive the recommended regimen for their stage of syphilis. • For early syphilis in pregnancy and in cases whereby the fetal ultrasound detects changes associated with syphilis, some experts and international guidelines recommend administering a second dose of benzathine PCN G 1 week after the first.[5,136] • For treatment of late latent or unknown duration syphilis during pregnancy, weekly benzathine PCN G doses should be administered every 7 days, and up to 9 days in some cases. The 3-dose treatment course must be reinitiated if any doses are missed or the interval between doses is > 9 d.
Persons with HIV	• Syphilis treatment recommendations are the same for persons with and without HIV.[5] • Data on the efficacy of alternative regimens such as doxycycline for late latent syphilis in PWH are limited; thus, close clinical and serologic follow-up is recommended.
Delayed weekly penicillin doses in late latent syphilis or unknown duration	• Weekly benzathine PCN G doses should be administered as close to every 7 d as possible. • For nonpregnant persons, the preferred interval is 7–9 d between doses based on pharmacokinetics, although intervals of 10–14 d may be acceptable based on clinical experience.[5,137,138] • If doses are missed, treatment should be reinitiate
Congenital syphilis and syphilis in children	• Treatment of these populations is beyond the scope of this review. See the 2021 CDC STI Treatment Guidelines for recommendations or consult a local health department or pediatric infectious disease specialist.[5]

optimal dose, duration, and response to oral doxycycline in complicated syphilis are needed.

FOLLOW UP AND POST-TREATMENT MANAGEMENT

The goal of follow-up after syphilis treatment is to confirm that symptoms, if present, have resolved and to ensure serologic response is adequate. In most cases of uncomplicated, early syphilis, lesions improve rapidly within days after treatment and ultimately resolve. Additionally, for all cases of syphilis, including asymptomatic infections, pre and posttreatment lipoidal titers are compared with determine treatment response. Historically, cure has been defined as a two-titer or fourfold reduction in lipoidal titers within the recommended follow-up period. For cases of complicated/neurosyphilis in PWH who are taking antiretroviral therapy or persons who are immunocompetent and are treated with a recommended neurosyphilis regimen, a fourfold lipoidal titer decrease predicts normalization of CSF parameters and obviates the need for repeat CSF examination.[121] Serum treponemal serologic tests are not useful in follow-up as they generally remain reactive for life.

Growing evidence suggests that lipoidal tests can take many weeks to months to decrease after treatment, particularly for persons with prior syphilis.[122,123] Repeat

Table 3
Recommended schedule for syphilis follow-up by stage and HIV status

Syphilis Stage	Recommended Intervals for Clinical and Serologic Follow-Up	
	Persons with HIV	Persons without HIV
Early	3, 6, 9, 12, 24 mo	6, 12 mo
Late latent or unknown duration	6, 12, 18, 24 mo	6, 12, 24 mo
Tertiary	No specific recommendations due to limited data	

testing is indicated to evaluate for reinfection but if lipoidal titers do not decrease immediately, it does not necessarily demonstrate the failure of treatment. The 2021 CDC STI Treatment Guidelines advise that a fourfold decrease in lipoidal tests may take up to 12 months to occur for early syphilis or 24 months for late latent/unknown duration syphilis. Of note, for certain key populations such as people taking HIV PrEP or sexually active MSM living with HIV who may experience the increased risk for syphilis reinfection after treatment, repeat testing (ie, every 3 months) earlier than 12 to 24 months is often recommended. **Table 3** reviews recommended syphilis follow-up testing by stage and HIV status. If reinfection is suspected, treatment should be again administered according to the clinical stage of syphilis.

Follow-up after treatment of syphilis in pregnancy depends weeks of gestational at diagnosis. For cases diagnosed and treated at or before 24 weeks, lipoidal titers should be repeated no sooner than 2 months after treatment, unless reinfection is suspected or signs of primary or secondary syphilis are present. All cases, including those diagnosed and treated after 24 weeks, should have follow-up testing at delivery. As with nonpregnant persons, lipoidal titers may be slow to decline and often will not decrease fourfold by the time of delivery; this does not equate to treatment failure. However, a sustained (for ≥2 weeks) fourfold increase in lipoidal titers is suggestive of possible treatment failure or reinfection.

Up to 44% of lipoidal tests in some populations may not decrease as expected within the recommended evaluation period.[124] Historically, these cases have been collectively referred to as "serofast", but terminology within the field is evolving to be more specific and clearly delineate between 2 clinical entities that are managed distinctly. Such "serofast" cases are better classified as either serologic nonresponse (inadequate serologic response whereby titer fails to decrease fourfold) or non-seroreversion (titer decreases fourfold but remains persistently reactive). Factors associated with serologic cure or an adequate posttreatment lipoidal response include younger age, earlier stages of syphilis, higher initial titers, and HIV-seronegative status.[5,124]

The ideal approach to manage cases of inadequate serologic response to appropriate syphilis therapy is not known. General recommendations are to monitor annually with clinical, neurologic, and serologic examinations. Alternatively, if no follow-up can be reassured or an initial titer was high (>1:32) in late syphilis, retreatment should be offered and a CSF examination can be considered. Though some experts have theorized that failure of titers to decrease fourfold is indicative of treatment failure, repeat treatment in both HIV-negative individuals and PWH who are serofast does not seem to meaningfully change titers or alter the clinical course of previously treated syphilis.[125,126] Occult or asymptomatic neurosyphilis has also been posited as the cause of nonseroreversion.[127] In HIV-negative persons with low titers (<1:32), CSF analysis is unlikely to be helpful in detecting asymptomatic neurosyphilis.[125] However, CSF analysis should be considered for persons with HIV who are not taking ART or with low CD4 counts as asymptomatic neurosyphilis may be more prevalent in this population.[128]

If syphilis signs or symptoms recur or the lipoidal titer increases fourfold or more, interval reinfection or treatment failure is suspected. The clinical history will help to differentiate which is most likely. Persons with neurologic symptoms, or who have persistent signs or symptoms of syphilis without concern for possible interval reinfection, should undergo lumbar puncture for CSF analysis and be treated with additional parenteral therapy if CSF findings are suggestive of neurosyphilis. For persons suspected to have failed an initial treatment course, 3 weekly doses of benzathine PCN G 2.4 million units IM are recommended.[5] In the absence of neurologic findings, additional therapy beyond one retreatment course is not recommended as it is unclear whether further treatment significantly changes serologies or provides any further clinical benefit.

PREVENTION MEASURES AND FUTURE DIRECTIONS

Several strategies have been proposed to reduce the increasing rates of syphilis in the U.S. Some focus on identifying opportunities for early diagnosis to avert syphilis transmissions and others target prevention before exposure using existing and nascent biomedical interventions.

A. Opportunities to curb the congenital syphilis epidemic: CDC evaluated congenital syphilis cases in 2018 and determined that inadequate treatment during pregnancy despite timely diagnosis, lack of antenatal care or testing, and delayed diagnosis late in pregnancy were the most commonly identified missed prevention opportunities[129]. These findings underscore the importance of timely diagnosis and treatment in pregnancy.
B. Antibiotic prophylaxis: Syphilis postexposure prophylaxis (PEP) consists of taking an oral doxycycline dose 24 to 72 hours after sex to prevent infection. Randomized trials including MSM and transgender women in France and the U.S. found that PEP with doxycycline reduced incident syphilis rates by 63% to 87%[130,131]. Questions regarding how to identify populations who could benefit most from the intervention and potential long-term effects such as the development of doxycycline resistance in T pallidum and disturbance of the gut microbiome remain unanswered and will be important considerations for broader real-world implementation.
C. Syphilis vaccine: A human syphilis vaccine could significantly deflect syphilis rates and dramatically reduce morbidity. While no single vaccine candidate has yet proven to be ready for mass distribution, efforts at many sites across the U.S. to identify the optimal T pallidum antigenic targets and adjuvant for an effective syphilis vaccine are underway.[132,133]
D. Diagnostic testing: The development of more sensitive POCTs and molecular assays for the diagnosis of syphilis in each stage is greatly needed. Additional areas of focus should include improved diagnostics for neurosyphilis, otosyphilis, and ocular syphilis. Performance characteristics and interpretation of these assays in different populations are a priority. Increasing the availability and decreasing the cost of sensitive, rapid syphilis tests can help address the current syphilis epidemic.

SUMMARY

The high rates of syphilis and associated complications seen in the U.S. and many parts of the world are concerning. The diagnosis of syphilis is challenging, but timely recognition of clinical manifestations, identifying appropriate diagnostic tests, and adherence to screening recommendations are key to syphilis control and appropriate patient management. Further research is needed to improve diagnostic tests, to better evaluate treatment response, and to expand prevention measures, such as vaccines, for syphilis.

CLINICS CARE POINTS

- Rates of syphilis are rising in the United States and familiarity with clinical findings, diagnosis and management is important for health care practitioners.
- Patients who are sexually active with an increased likelihood of acquiring syphilis should be regularly tested and the hallmark of syphilis diagnosis relies on serologic testing.
- Screening neurosyphilis, otosyphilis, and ocular syphilis should be assessed with each new syphilis diagnosis.
- All persons who are pregnant should be tested for syphilis at least once in pregnancy and more frequently based on risk factors or in communities with high syphilis rates.
- Penicillin G is the antibiotic of choice for all stages of syphilis and care must be taken to ensure that the appropriate formulation is used based on the patient's syphilis stage.

CONFLICTS OF INTEREST

No conflicts of interest are reported by the authors.

ACKNOWLEDGEMENT

MSR: Grants through the Centers for Disease Control and Prevention paid to the institution. CAC and CMM: none.

SOURCES OF FUNDING

None were declared.

REFERENCES

1. Jansen K, Schmidt AJ, Drewes J, et al. Increased incidence of syphilis in men who have sex with men and risk management strategies, Germany, 2015. Euro Surveill 2016;21.
2. Callander DWSL, M oriera C, Asselin J, et al. The Australian Collaboration for Coordinated Enhanced Sentinel surveillance of sexually transmissible infections and blood Borne Viruses: NSW HIV report 2007-2014. Sydney, NSW: UNSW Australia; 2015.
3. Centers for Disease and Prevention. Sexually transmitted disease surveillance: preliminary 2021 data. Atlanta: US Department of Health and Human Services; 2022.
4. Janier M, Unemo M, Dupin N, et al. 2020 European guideline on the management of syphilis. J Eur Acad Dermatol Venereol 2021;35:574–88.
5. Workowski KA, Bachmann LH, Chan PA, et al. Sexually Transmitted Infections Treatment Guidelines, 2021. MMWR Recomm Rep (Morb Mortal Wkly Rep) 2021;70:1–187.

6. Centers for Disease Control and Prevention. Sexually transmitted disease surveillance 2020. Atlanta: U.S. Department of Health and Human Services; 2021. Available at: https://www.cdc.gov/std/statistics/2020/default.htm. Accessed November 2022.
7. Wright SS, Kreisel KM, Hitt JC, et al. Impact of the COVID-19 Pandemic on Centers for Disease Control and Prevention-Funded Sexually Transmitted Disease Programs. Sex Transm Dis 2022;49:e61–3.
8. Ramchandani MS, Bourne C, Barbee LA, et al. The need for sexual health clinics, their future role, and contribution to public health. Sex Health 2022;19: 346–56.
9. Centers for Disease Control and Prevention. Impact of COVID-19 on STDs. Available at: https://www.cdc.gov/std/statistics/2020/impact.htm. Accessed November 2022.
10. Trivedi S, Williams C, Torrone E, et al. National Trends and Reported Risk Factors Among Pregnant Women With Syphilis in the United States, 2012-2016. Obstet Gynecol 2019;133:27–32.
11. Sullivan PS, Purcell DW, Grey JA, et al. Patterns of Racial/Ethnic Disparities and Prevalence in HIV and Syphilis Diagnoses Among Men Who Have Sex With Men, 2016: A Novel Data Visualization. Am J Public Health 2018;108:S266–73.
12. Grey JA, Bernstein KT, Sullivan PS, et al. Rates of Primary and Secondary Syphilis Among White and Black Non-Hispanic Men Who Have Sex With Men, United States, 2014. J Acquir Immune Defic Syndr 2017;76:e65–73.
13. Center for Disease Control and Prevention. Syphilis Surveillance Supplemental Slides, 2016-2020. Available at: https://www.cdc.gov/std/statistics/syphilis-supplement/default.htm. Accessed November 2022.
14. Force USPST, Mangione CM, Barry MJ, et al. Screening for Syphilis Infection in Nonpregnant Adolescents and Adults: US Preventive Services Task Force Reaffirmation Recommendation Statement. JAMA 2022;328:1243–9.
15. Centers for Disease Control and Prevention. US Public Health Service: Preexposure prophylaxis for the prevention of HIV infection in the United States—2021 Update: a clinical practice guideline. 2021. Available at: https://www.cdc.gov/hiv/pdf/risk/prep/cdc-hiv-prep-guidelines-2021.pdf.
16. Kimball AA, Torrone EA, Bernstein KT, et al. Predicting Emergence of Primary and Secondary Syphilis Among Women of Reproductive Age in US Counties. Sex Transm Dis 2022;49:177–83.
17. Cuffe KM, Torrone EA, Hong J, et al. Identification of United States Counties at Elevated Risk for Congenital Syphilis Using Predictive Modeling and a Risk Scoring System, 2018. Sex Transm Dis 2022;49:184–9.
18. Karasz HN. New public health recommendations make a syphilis test routine for women 45 and younger. Available at: https://publichealthinsider.com/2022/11/28/new-public-health-recommendations-make-a-syphilis-test-routine-for-women-45-and-under/#:~:text=All%20sexually%20active%20women%2045,Health%20%E2%80%93%20Seattle%20%26%20King%20County. Accessed December 2022.
19. Barrow RY, Ahmed F, Bolan GA, et al. Recommendations for Providing Quality Sexually Transmitted Diseases Clinical Services, 2020. MMWR Recomm Rep (Morb Mortal Wkly Rep) 2020;68:1–20.
20. Park IU, Tran A, Pereira L, et al. Sensitivity and specificity of treponemal-specific tests for the diagnosis of syphilis. Clin Infect Dis 2020;71:S13–20.
21. Schroeter AL, Lucas JB, Price EV, et al. Treatment for early syphilis and reactivity of serologic tests. JAMA 1972;221:471–6.

22. Matthews HM, Yang TK, Jenkin HM. Unique lipid composition of Treponema pallidum (Nichols virulent strain). Infect Immun 1979;24:713–9.
23. Larsen SA, Steiner BM, Rudolph AH. Laboratory diagnosis and interpretation of tests for syphilis. Clin Microbiol Rev 1995;8:1–21.
24. Centers for Disease Control Prevention. Discordant results from reverse sequence syphilis screening–five laboratories, United States, 2006-2010. MMWR Morb Mortal Wkly Rep 2011;60:133–7.
25. Centers for Disease Control Prevention. Syphilis testing algorithms using treponemal tests for initial screening–four laboratories, New York City, 2005-2006. MMWR Morb Mortal Wkly Rep 2008;57:872–5.
26. Tuffanelli DL. Ageing and false positive reactions for syphilis. Br J Vener Dis 1966;42:40–1.
27. Mmeje O, Chow JM, Davidson L, et al. Discordant Syphilis Immunoassays in Pregnancy: Perinatal Outcomes and Implications for Clinical Management. Clin Infect Dis 2015;61:1049–53.
28. Gu WM, Yang Y, Wang QZ, et al. Comparing the performance of traditional nontreponemal tests on syphilis and non-syphilis serum samples. Int J STD AIDS 2013;24:919–25.
29. Dionne-Odom J, Van Der Pol B, Boutwell A, et al. Limited Utility of Reverse Algorithm Syphilis Testing in HIV Clinic Among Men Who Have Sex With Men. Sex Transm Dis 2021;48:675–9.
30. Ishihara Y, Okamoto K, Shimosaka H, et al. Prevalence and clinical characteristics of patients with biologically false-positive reactions with serological syphilis testing in contemporary practice: 10-year experience at a tertiary academic hospital. Sex Transm Infect 2021;97:397–401.
31. Oboho IK, Gebo KA, Moore RD, et al. The impact of combined antiretroviral therapy on biologic false-positive rapid plasma reagin serologies in a longitudinal cohort of HIV-infected persons. Clin Infect Dis 2013;57:1197–202.
32. Tuddenham S, Katz SS, Ghanem KG. Syphilis Laboratory Guidelines: Performance Characteristics of Nontreponemal Antibody Tests. Clin Infect Dis 2020; 71:S21–42.
33. Jurado RL, Campbell J, Martin PD. Prozone phenomenon in secondary syphilis. Has its time arrived? Arch Intern Med 1993;153:2496–8.
34. el-Zaatari MM, Martens MG, Anderson GD. Incidence of the prozone phenomenon in syphilis serology. Obstet Gynecol 1994;84:609–12.
35. Liu LL, Lin LR, Tong ML, et al. Incidence and risk factors for the prozone phenomenon in serologic testing for syphilis in a large cohort. Clin Infect Dis 2014;59:384–9.
36. Larsen SAPV, Johnson RE, Kennedy EJ Jr. A manual of tests for syphilis. 9th edition. Washington, DC: American Public Health Association; 1998.
37. Creegan L, Bauer HM, Samuel MC, et al. An evaluation of the relative sensitivities of the venereal disease research laboratory test and the Treponema pallidum particle agglutination test among patients diagnosed with primary syphilis. Sex Transm Dis 2007;34:1016–8.
38. Theel ES, Katz SS, Pillay A. Molecular and Direct Detection Tests for Treponema pallidum Subspecies pallidum: A Review of the Literature, 1964-2017. Clin Infect Dis 2020;71:S4–12.
39. Hook EW 3rd, Roddy RE, Lukehart SA, et al. Detection of Treponema pallidum in lesion exudate with a pathogen-specific monoclonal antibody. J Clin Microbiol 1985;22:241–4.

40. Towns JM, Leslie DE, Denham I, et al. Timing of primary syphilis treatment and impact on the development of treponemal antibodies: a cross-sectional clinic-based study. Sex Transm Infect 2022;98:161–5.
41. Salle R, Mayslich C, Grange PA, et al. Specific detection of Treponema pallidum in clinical samples: validation of a qPCR assay combining two genomic targets. Sex Transm Infect 2022;99(2):91–6.
42. Gayet-Ageron A, Laurent F, Schrenzel J, et al. Performance of the 47-kilodalton membrane protein versus DNA polymerase I genes for detection of Treponema pallidum by PCR in ulcers. J Clin Microbiol 2015;53:976–80.
43. Grange PA, Gressier L, Dion PL, et al. Evaluation of a PCR test for detection of treponema pallidum in swabs and blood. J Clin Microbiol 2012;50:546–52.
44. Heymans R, van der Helm JJ, de Vries HJ, et al. Clinical value of Treponema pallidum real-time PCR for diagnosis of syphilis. J Clin Microbiol 2010;48:497–502.
45. Tipple C, Hanna MO, Hill S, et al. Getting the measure of syphilis: qPCR to better understand early infection. Sex Transm Infect 2011;87:479–85.
46. Tantalo LC, Mendoza H, Katz DA, et al. Detection of Treponema pallidum DNA in Oropharyngeal Swabs and Whole Blood for Syphilis Diagnosis. Sex Transm Dis 2021;48:915–8.
47. Simpore A, Bazie BV, Zoure AA, et al. Performance of Molecular Tests in the Diagnosis of Syphilis From 2009 to 2019: A Systematic Review and Meta-Analysis. Sex Transm Dis 2022;49:469–76.
48. Nieuwenburg SA, Zondag HCA, Bruisten SM, et al. Detection of Treponema pallidum DNA During Early Syphilis Stages in Peripheral Blood, Oropharynx, Ano-Rectum and Urine as a Proxy for Transmissibility. Clin Infect Dis 2022;75:1054–62.
49. Towns JM, Chow EPF, Wigan R, et al. Anal and oral detection of Treponema pallidum in men who have sex with men with early syphilis infection. Sex Transm Infect 2022;98:570–4.
50. Golden M, O'Donnell M, Lukehart S, et al. Treponema pallidum Nucleic Acid Amplification Testing To Augment Syphilis Screening among Men Who Have Sex with Men. J Clin Microbiol 2019;57.
51. Australasian Sexual Health Alliance. Australian STI Management Guidelines For Use in Primary Care. Available at: http://www.sti.guidelines.org.au/. Accessed November 2022.
52. Hooshmand H, Escobar MR, Kopf SW. Neurosyphilis. A study of 241 patients. JAMA 1972;219:726–9.
53. Marshall DW, Brey RL, Cahill WT, et al. Spectrum of cerebrospinal fluid findings in various stages of human immunodeficiency virus infection. Arch Neurol 1988;45:954–8.
54. Marra CM, Maxwell CL, Collier AC, et al. Interpreting cerebrospinal fluid pleocytosis in HIV in the era of potent antiretroviral therapy. BMC Infect Dis 2007;7:37.
55. Marra CM, Maxwell CL, Smith SL, et al. Cerebrospinal fluid abnormalities in patients with syphilis: association with clinical and laboratory features. J Infect Dis 2004;189:369–76.
56. Ho EL, Marra CM. Treponemal tests for neurosyphilis–less accurate than what we thought? Sex Transm Dis 2012;39:298–9.
57. Davis LE, Schmitt JW. Clinical significance of cerebrospinal fluid tests for neurosyphilis. Ann Neurol 1989;25:50–5.
58. Marra CM, Critchlow CW, Hook EW 3rd, et al. Cerebrospinal fluid treponemal antibodies in untreated early syphilis. Arch Neurol 1995;52:68–72.

59. Harding AS, Ghanem KG. The performance of cerebrospinal fluid treponemal-specific antibody tests in neurosyphilis: a systematic review. Sex Transm Dis 2012;39:291–7.
60. Tuddenham S, Ghanem KG. Neurosyphilis: knowledge gaps and controversies. Sex Transm Dis 2018;45:147–51.
61. Marra CM. Neurosyphilis. Continuum 2015;21:1714–28.
62. Giacani L, Lukehart SA. The endemic treponematoses. Clin Microbiol Rev 2014; 27:89–115.
63. Mitja O, Asiedu K, Mabey D. Yaws. Lancet 2013;381:763–73.
64. Fakile YF, Brinson M, Mobley V, et al. Performance of the syphilis health check in clinic and laboratory-based settings. Sex Transm Dis 2019;46:250–3.
65. Matthias J, Dwiggins P, Totten Y, et al. Notes from the field: evaluation of the sensitivity and specificity of a commercially available rapid syphilis test - escambia county, Florida. MMWR Morb Mortal Wkly Rep 2016;65:1174–5.
66. Bristow CC, Klausner JD, Tran A. Clinical test performance of a rapid point-of-care syphilis treponemal antibody test: a systematic review and meta-analysis. Clin Infect Dis 2020;71:S52–7.
67. Leon SR, Ramos LB, Vargas SK, et al. Laboratory evaluation of a dual-path platform assay for rapid point-of-care hiv and syphilis testing. J Clin Microbiol 2016; 54:492–4.
68. Unemo M, Bradshaw CS, Hocking JS, et al. Sexually transmitted infections: challenges ahead. Lancet Infect Dis 2017;17:e235–79.
69. Bronzan RN, Mwesigwa-Kayongo DC, Narkunas D, et al. On-site rapid antenatal syphilis screening with an immunochromatographic strip improves case detection and treatment in rural South African clinics. Sex Transm Dis 2007;34: S55–60.
70. Mabey DC, Sollis KA, Kelly HA, et al. Point-of-care tests to strengthen health systems and save newborn lives: the case of syphilis. PLoS Med 2012;9: e1001233.
71. Terris-Prestholt F, Vickerman P, Torres-Rueda S, et al. The cost-effectiveness of 10 antenatal syphilis screening and treatment approaches in Peru, Tanzania, and Zambia. Int J Gynaecol Obstet 2015;130(Suppl 1):S73–80.
72. Australian Government Department of Health. Syphilis Point-of-Care (POC) Testing Program. Available at: https://www.syphilispoct.com.au/. Accessed November 2022.
73. Gonzalez H, Koralnik IJ, Huhn GD, et al. A dual-platform point-of-care test for neurosyphilis diagnosis. Sex Transm Dis 2021;48:353–6.
74. Gaydos CA, Manabe YC, Melendez JH. A narrative review of where we are with point-of-care sexually transmitted infection testing in the United States. Sex Transm Dis 2021;48:S71–7.
75. Satyaputra F, Hendry S, Braddick M, et al. The laboratory diagnosis of syphilis. J Clin Microbiol 2021;59:e0010021.
76. Brandenburger D, Ambrosino E. The impact of antenatal syphilis point of care testing on pregnancy outcomes: A systematic review. PLoS One 2021;16: e0247649.
77. Angel-Muller E, Grillo-Ardila CF, Amaya-Guio J, et al. Diagnostic accuracy of rapid point-of-care tests for detecting active syphilis: a systematic review and meta-analysis. Sex Transm Dis 2021;48:e202–8.
78. Garnett GP, Aral SO, Hoyle DV, et al. The natural history of syphilis. Implications for the transmission dynamics and control of infection. Sex Transm Dis 1997;24: 185–200.

79. Schober PC, Gabriel G, White P, et al. How infectious is syphilis? Br J Vener Dis 1983;59:217–9.
80. Schroeter AL, Turner RH, Lucas JB, et al. Therapy for incubating syphilis. Effectiveness of gonorrhea treatment. JAMA 1971;218:711–3.
81. Magnuson HJ, Thomas EW, Olansky S, et al. Inoculation syphilis in human volunteers. Medicine (Baltim) 1956;35:33–82.
82. Moore MB Jr, Price EV, Knox JM, et al. Epidemiologic Treatment of Contacts to Infectious Syphilis. Public Health Rep (1896) 1963;78:966–70.
83. Ramoni S, Genovese G, Pastena A, et al. Clinical and laboratory features of 244 men with primary syphilis: a 5-year single-centre retrospective study. Sex Transm Infect 2021;97:479–84.
84. Babu CS, Vitharana S, Higgins SP. Primary syphilis presenting as balanitis. Int J STD AIDS 2007;18:497–8.
85. Towns JM, Leslie DE, Denham I, et al. Painful and multiple anogenital lesions are common in men with Treponema pallidum PCR-positive primary syphilis without herpes simplex virus coinfection: a cross-sectional clinic-based study. Sex Transm Infect 2016;92:110–5.
86. Ma DL, Vano-Galvan S. Images in clinical medicine. Syphilitic chancres of the lips. N Engl J Med 2013;368:e8.
87. Zhang Q, Chen S, Chai B, et al. Extragenital Chancre in Men Who Have Sex with Men: Six Cases from China. Arch Sex Behav 2022;51:3211–7.
88. Zhou X, Wu MZ, Jiang TT, et al. Oral Manifestations of Early Syphilis in Adults: A Systematic Review of Case Reports and Series. Sex Transm Dis 2021;48: e209–14.
89. Chapel TA, Prasad P, Chapel J, et al. Extragenital syphilitic chancres. J Am Acad Dermatol 1985;13:582–4.
90. Veraldi S, Lunardon L, Persico MC, et al. Multiple aphthoid syphilitic chancres of the oral cavity. Int J STD AIDS 2008;19:486–7.
91. Turco M, Mancuso FR, Pisano L. A monkeypox virus infection mimicking primary syphilis. Br J Dermatol 2022;187(6):e194–5.
92. Grange PA, Jary A, Isnard C, et al. Use of a Multiplex PCR Assay To Assess the Presence of Treponema pallidum in Mucocutaneous Ulcerations in Patients with Suspected Syphilis. J Clin Microbiol 2021;59.
93. Gjestland T. The Oslo study of untreated syphilis; an epidemiologic investigation of the natural course of the syphilitic infection based upon a re-study of the Boeck-Bruusgaard material. Acta Derm Venereol Suppl 1955;35:3–368. Annex I-LVI.
94. Mindel A, Tovey SJ, Timmins DJ, et al. Primary and secondary syphilis, 20 years' experience. 2. Clinical features. Genitourin Med 1989;65:1–3.
95. Hourihan M, Wheeler H, Houghton R, et al. Lessons from the syphilis outbreak in homosexual men in east London. Sex Transm Infect 2004;80:509–11.
96. Rompalo AM, Joesoef MR, O'Donnell JA, et al. Clinical manifestations of early syphilis by HIV status and gender: results of the syphilis and HIV study. Sex Transm Dis 2001;28:158–65.
97. Balagula Y, Mattei PL, Wisco OJ, et al. The great imitator revisited: the spectrum of atypical cutaneous manifestations of secondary syphilis. Int J Dermatol 2014; 53:1434–41.
98. Mullick CJ, Liappis AP, Benator DA, et al. Syphilitic hepatitis in HIV-infected patients: a report of 7 cases and review of the literature. Clin Infect Dis 2004;39: e100–5.

99. Tsai YC, Chen LI, Chen HC. Simultaneous acute nephrosis and hepatitis in secondary syphilis. Clin Nephrol 2008;70:532–6.

100. Clark EG, Danbolt N. The Oslo study of the natural history of untreated syphilis; an epidemiologic investigation based on a restudy of the Boeck-Bruusgaard material; a review and appraisal. J Chronic Dis 1955;2:311–44.

101. Kenyon C, Osbak KK, Apers L. Repeat Syphilis Is More Likely to Be Asymptomatic in HIV-Infected Individuals: A Retrospective Cohort Analysis With Important Implications for Screening. Open Forum Infect Dis 2018;5:ofy096.

102. Marra CM, Maxwell CL, Sahi SK, et al. Previous Syphilis Alters the Course of Subsequent Episodes of Syphilis. Clin Infect Dis 2022;74:e1–5.

103. Lafond RE, Lukehart SA. Biological basis for syphilis. Clin Microbiol Rev 2006; 19:29–49.

104. Devanand NA, Sundararajan K. Gummatous neurosyphilis in an elderly patient in the Australian outback: a case report. J Med Case Rep 2021;15:552.

105. Miller SA, Ladich ER. Syphilitic Aortitis. N Engl J Med 2022;386:e55.

106. Rolfs RT, Joesoef MR, Hendershot EF, et al. A randomized trial of enhanced therapy for early syphilis in patients with and without human immunodeficiency virus infection. The Syphilis and HIV Study Group. N Engl J Med 1997;337:307–14.

107. Davis AP, Maxwell CL, Mendoza H, et al. Cognitive impairment in syphilis: Does treatment based on cerebrospinal fluid analysis improve outcome? PLoS One 2021;16:e0254518.

108. Davis AP, Stern J, Tantalo L, et al. How Well Do Neurologic Symptoms Identify Individuals With Neurosyphilis? Clin Infect Dis 2018;66:363–7.

109. Marra CM, Maxwell CL, Ramchandani M, et al. Hearing loss in individuals at risk for neurosyphilis. Int J STD AIDS 2020;31:1178–85.

110. Dombrowski JC, Pedersen R, Marra CM, et al. Prevalence Estimates of Complicated Syphilis. Sex Transm Dis 2015;42:702–4.

111. Marra C, Sahi S, Tantalo L, et al. Enhanced molecular typing of treponema pallidum: geographical distribution of strain types and association with neurosyphilis. J Infect Dis 2010;202:1380–8.

112. Marra CM, Sahi SK, Tantalo LC, et al. Toll-like receptor polymorphisms are associated with increased neurosyphilis risk. Sex Transm Dis 2014;41:440–6.

113. Johns DR, Tierney M, Felsenstein D. Alteration in the natural history of neurosyphilis by concurrent infection with the human immunodeficiency virus. N Engl J Med 1987;316:1569–72.

114. Moore JEHH. Asymptomatic Neurosyphilis VI. The Prognosis of Early and Late Asymptomatic Neurosyphilis. JAMA 1930;95:1637–41.

115. Ghanem KG, Moore RD, Rompalo AM, et al. Neurosyphilis in a clinical cohort of HIV-1-infected patients. Aids 2008;22:1145–51.

116. Keuning MW, Kamp GA, Schonenberg-Meinema D, et al. Congenital syphilis, the great imitator-case report and review. Lancet Infect Dis 2020;20:e173–9.

117. Ganesan A, Mesner O, Okulicz JF, et al. A single dose of benzathine penicillin G is as effective as multiple doses of benzathine penicillin G for the treatment of HIV-infected persons with early syphilis. Clin Infect Dis 2015;60:653–60.

118. Miller WM, Gorini F, Botelho G, et al. Jarisch-Herxheimer reaction among syphilis patients in Rio de Janeiro, Brazil. Int J STD AIDS 2010;21:806–9.

119. Yim CW, Flynn NM, Fitzgerald FT. Penetration of oral doxycycline into the cerebrospinal fluid of patients with latent or neurosyphilis. Antimicrob Agents Chemother 1985;28:347–8.

120. Girometti N, Junejo MH, Nugent D, et al. Clinical and serological outcomes in patients treated with oral doxycycline for early neurosyphilis. J Antimicrob Chemother 2021;76:1916–9.
121. Marra CM, Maxwell CL, Tantalo LC, et al. Normalization of serum rapid plasma reagin titer predicts normalization of cerebrospinal fluid and clinical abnormalities after treatment of neurosyphilis. Clin Infect Dis 2008;47:893–9.
122. Ghanem KG, Erbelding EJ, Wiener ZS, et al. Serological response to syphilis treatment in HIV-positive and HIV-negative patients attending sexually transmitted diseases clinics. Sex Transm Infect 2007;83:97–101.
123. Sena AC, Wolff M, Martin DH, et al. Predictors of serological cure and Serofast State after treatment in HIV-negative persons with early syphilis. Clin Infect Dis 2011;53:1092–9.
124. Sena AC, Zhang XH, Li T, et al. A systematic review of syphilis serological treatment outcomes in HIV-infected and HIV-uninfected persons: rethinking the significance of serological non-responsiveness and the serofast state after therapy. BMC Infect Dis 2015;15:479.
125. Zhang X, Shahum A, Yang LG, et al. Outcomes From Re-Treatment and Cerebrospinal Fluid Analyses in Patients With Syphilis Who Had Serological Nonresponse or Lack of Seroreversion After Initial Therapy. Sex Transm Dis 2021;48:443–50.
126. Sena AC, Wolff M, Behets F, et al. Response to therapy following retreatment of serofast early syphilis patients with benzathine penicillin. Clin Infect Dis 2013;56:420–2.
127. Zhou P, Gu X, Lu H, et al. Re-evaluation of serological criteria for early syphilis treatment efficacy: progression to neurosyphilis despite therapy. Sex Transm Infect 2012;88:342–5.
128. Pastuszczak M, Sitko M, Bociaga-Jasik M, et al. Lack of antiretroviral therapy is associated with higher risk of neurosyphilis among HIV-infected patients who remain serofast after therapy for early syphilis. Medicine (Baltim) 2018;97:e13171.
129. Kimball A, Torrone E, Miele K, et al. Missed Opportunities for Prevention of Congenital Syphilis - United States, 2018. MMWR Morb Mortal Wkly Rep 2020;69:661–5.
130. Molina JM, Charreau I, Chidiac C, et al. Post-exposure prophylaxis with doxycycline to prevent sexually transmitted infections in men who have sex with men: an open-label randomised substudy of the ANRS IPERGAY trial. Lancet Infect Dis 2018;18:308–17.
131. Luetkemeyer A, Dombrowski J, Cohen S, et al. Doxycycline post-exposure prophylaxis for STI prevention among MSM and transgender women on HIV PrEP or living with HIV: high efficacy to reduce incident STI's in a randomized trial. The 24th International AIDS Conference. July 29-August 2. Montreal, Canada. Available at: https://programme.aids2022.org/Abstract/Abstract/?abstractid=13231. Accessed November 2022.
132. Cameron CE. Syphilis Vaccine Development: Requirements, Challenges, and Opportunities. Sex Transm Dis 2018;45:S17–9.
133. Kojima N, Konda KA, Klausner JD. Notes on syphilis vaccine development. Front Immunol 2022;13:952284.
134. Stoner BP. Current controversies in the management of adult syphilis. Clin Infect Dis 2007;44(Suppl 3):S130–46.
135. St John RK. Treatment of late benign syphilis: review of the literature. J Am Vener Dis Assoc 1976;3:146–7.

136. Zhu L, Qin M, Du L, et al. Maternal and congenital syphilis in Shanghai, China, 2002 to 2006. Int J Infect Dis 2010;14(Suppl 3):e45–8.
137. Hagdrup HK, Lange Wantzin G, Secher L, et al. Penicillin concentrations in serum following weekly injections of benzathine penicillin G. Chemotherapy 1986;32:99–101.
138. Collart P, Poitevin M, Milovanovic A, et al. Kinetic study of serum penicillin concentrations after single doses of benzathine and benethamine penicillins in young and old people. Br J Vener Dis 1980;56:355–62.

Challenges in Managing Gonorrhea and New Advances in Prevention

Evan C. Ewers, MD, MPH[a,b], John M. Curtin, MD[c],
Anuradha Ganesan, MBBS, MPH[c,d,e],*

KEYWORDS

- Gonorrhea • Antimicrobial resistance • Point-of-care testing
- Expedited partner therapy

KEY POINTS

- Incident gonorrhea cases continue to increase and previously observed ethnic disparities remain; in the United States (US) young African American men are at the highest risk for acquisition of GC.
- In the US, 35% of the gonococcal isolates exhibit resistance to quinolones, 28% to tetracycline, just over 5% to azithromycin, however, ceftriaxone non-susceptibility remains rare.
- Based on the changing antimicrobial susceptibility, the 2021 US treatment guidelines recommend ceftriaxone monotherapy at a dose of 500 mg for the treatment of uncomplicated genitourinary, pharyngeal and rectal GC.
- Expedited partner therapy, use of point of care testing, pre- and post-exposure chemoprophylaxis, and the use of the group B meningococcal vaccine are all being evaluated as prevention strategies.

INTRODUCTION

Gonorrhea, caused by the human pathogen *Neisseria gonorrhoeae* (NG), is the second most common bacterial sexually transmitted infection (STI) in the United States. In 2020, there were an estimated 82 million new infections globally, with about 677,000

The authors have no conflicts of interest to disclose.
[a] Infectious Disease Service, Fort Belvoir Community Hospital, 9300 DeWitt Loop, Fort Belvoir, VA 22060, USA; [b] Department of Medicine, Uniformed Services University of the Health Sciences, 4301 Jones Bridge Road, Bethesda, MD 20814, USA; [c] Department of Medicine, Infectious Disease Service, Walter Reed National Military Medical Center, Building 7, 1st Floor (Liberty Zone), 8960 Brown Drive, Bethesda, MD 20889, USA; [d] Department of Preventive Medicine and Biostatistics, Infectious Disease Clinical Research Program (IDCRP), Uniformed Services University of the Health Sciences, Bethesda, MD 20814, USA; [e] Henry M Jackson Foundation for the Advancement of Military Medicine, Bethesda, MD 20817, USA
* Corresponding author.
E-mail address: anuradha.ganesan.ctr@health.mil

Infect Dis Clin N Am 37 (2023) 223–243
https://doi.org/10.1016/j.idc.2023.02.004
0891-5520/23/© 2023 Elsevier Inc. All rights reserved.

infections reported to the US Centers for Disease Control (CDC) alone.[1] The last 10 years have witnessed the continued emergence of antimicrobial-resistant (AMR) NG, with increasing prevalence of multidrug-resistant (MDR) strains and case reports of extensively drug resistant (XDR) isolates, even as the development of new effective antimicrobials lags behind. This has prompted changes to national treatment guidelines, and a call to pursue more sophisticated means of prevention, diagnosis, and treatment.[2] Such advances include the development of novel point-of-care diagnostic tests (POCTs) that allow for rapid diagnosis and early treatment initiation, new strategies for screening and expedited partner therapy, evaluation of group B meningococcal vaccine for prevention, doxycycline for postexposure prophylaxis (PrEP), and several promising antibiotics that have reached advanced stages of clinical study.

Microbiology

NG is a pathogen of mucosal surfaces appearing as a gram-negative diplococcus on standard microscopy. Although most men with gonococcal urethritis are symptomatic, cervicitis in women is typically asymptomatic or present with subtle/nonspecific signs and symptoms.[3,4] In women, ascending genital infection is responsible for morbid sequelae, such as infertility and ectopic pregnancy. The oropharynx, anorectum, and conjunctiva are sites of extragenital infection. Gonorrhea increases risk for both transmission and acquisition of human immunodeficiency virus (HIV) infection, both by shared exposure risks as well as mechanisms that directly enhance transmissibility.[5,6]

Two features of NG are of particular importance: the propensity to establish asymptomatic infection and its ability to acquire new genetic material. NG is capable of both conjugation and transformation of free environmental deoxyribonucleic acid (DNA), allowing it to readily acquire resistance genes directly from other bacteria as well as its environment.[4] Owing to the prevalence of asymptomatic infection, such transfer of resistance can occur unimpeded, presenting a major obstacle to halting the propagation and spread of AMR strains.

Epidemiology

As with other STIs, gonorrhea rates in the United States have been increasing over the last decade, continuing the epidemiologic trends noted in the early 2010s.[7] As of 2020, the incidence rate has increased to 206.5/100,000, a 111% increase in just over 10 years.[8] From 2019 to 2020 alone, gonococcal infections increased 5.7%. Increases have affected both sexes, with men experiencing a 132% increase and women a 60% increase over the last decade. Young adults 20 to 24 years old make up the highest burden of new infections (844/100,000 women and 819/100,000 men). Geographically, prevalence has increased in virtually every state, but the southeastern United States continues to have the highest rates in the nation.

The burden of infection is not shared equally, and data from the CDCs STD Surveillance Network (SSuN; established 2005) demonstrate marked disparities in prevalence by age, gender, sexual preferences, geography, and race (**Table 1**). SSuN data for 2019 demonstrated that 42% of all gonorrhea infections occurred among men who have sex with men (MSM), and in certain areas such as San Francisco, MSM accounted for 85% of cases. African American males are the most affected group, with an incidence of approximately 724/100,000 persons, 8.8-fold greater than their White male counterparts.[8]

The causes of increasing incidence for NG and other bacterial STIs remain elusive. Potential contributors include evolving perception of lesser concern for HIV acquisition in the setting of increasingly available and highly effective HIV PrEP, accompanied by greater willingness to engage in riskier sexual activities.[9,10] A recent study demonstrated

Table 1
Epidemiologic trends of gonococcal infection in the United States[a]

Characteristics	Incidence, 2019	Incidence, 2010
Overall	188.4	100.2
Women	157.7	98.7
MSW	122.7	72.4
MSM	5,165.6	1,421.5
Ethnicity		
African American/Black	581.0	512.2
American Indian/Alaskan	355.8	125.7
Hispanic	117.8	63.2
White	73.8	26.0
Asian	39.0	18.1
Region		
South	205.4	132.7
Midwest	197.2	108.3
West	185.2	61.4
Northeast	144.4	77.4

[a] Values reported as cases per 100,000 population.
(*Data from* CDC. Sexually Transmitted Disease Surveillance: National Overview. US Department of Health and Human Services. https://www.cdc.gov/std/statistics/2020/overview.htm)

that the rates of condomless sex among MSM are increasing, reaching greater than 70% among both HIV-positive and HIV-negative populations.[11] It is also likely greater numbers of asymptomatic NG infections are being captured due to guideline-directed routine screening of high-risk populations, such those taking PrEP. Together, increased rates of screening combined with changing societal perception of sexual risk may be contributing to the rising rates of gonorrhea seen over the last decade, particularly given the increasing incidence in MSM.

ANTIMICROBIAL RESISTANCE

AMR remains a major problem with gonorrhea, and surveillance is necessary to combat this threat. International surveillance is conducted by the World Health Organization's (WHO) Gonococcal Antimicrobial Surveillance Program (GASP) and Enhanced GASP.[12,13] The Euro-GASP network is involved in surveillance across the European Union/European Economic Area (EEA). Within the United States, the CDCs Gonococcal Isolate Surveillance Project (GISP; established 1986) and SSuN monitor resistance rates to inform national guidelines. Mirroring the WHO, CDC has also introduced the Enhanced Gonococcal Isolate Surveillance Program, focusing on surveillance of non-urethral sites to determine if these niches may be fostering resistance.[14]

Evolution of Antimicrobial-Resistance and Contemporary Cephalosporin Resistance

NG has proven itself capable of rapid acquisition of AMR. Widespread resistance to sulfonamides occurred within a decade of their introduction in the 1930s, and this pattern has repeated itself with each subsequent class of antibiotics introduced. Penicillins, aminoglycosides, tetracyclines, macrolides, and fluoroquinolones all experienced rising resistance until each became unreliable for empirical treatment.[15] By

2007, neither ciprofloxacin nor azithromycin was reliable as monotherapy. The 2017 to 2018 WHO GASP surveillance report noted widespread azithromycin and ciprofloxacin resistance among sampled specimens, with 72% and 77% (respectively) of contributing countries reporting a resistance rate of greater than 5%.[12]

Since 2006, cephalosporins have been considered the only reliable first-line empirical therapy, but even within this class treatment, failures have been reported, threatening the future of these agents. Cefixime, an oral third-generation cephalosporin, has seen increasing minimum inhibitory concentration (MIC) values and documented clinical failures. Early incidences of non-susceptibility occurred in Japan between 1999 and 2002 and have now been seen in Europe, Canada, Americas, and South Africa.[16–21] The 2017–2018 GASP report notes that 47% of countries reporting cefixime testing had at least one isolate with decreased susceptibility.[22] Although most countries reported an overall non-susceptibility rate of less than 5%, nine detected rates greater than 5%.[22]

High level ceftriaxone non-suscebtility was seen in Japan in 2011, followed by case reports from other locations around the world.[19,23–27] GASP data from 2017 to 2018 reported that 31% countries had detected isolates with reduced ceftriaxone susceptibility, an increase from 24% in 2015 to 2016. Among these countries, six reported a greater than 5% prevalence of ceftriaxone non-susceptibility.[22] Isolates with decreased susceptibility to both ceftriaxone and azithromycin have been detected in the United Kingdom, Australia, and Hawaii.[27–30]

In the United States, CDC GISP data from 2019 are published, as are preliminary data from 2021. **Table 2** reports the established data from 2019, but it is important to remember that these data continue to be periodically updated. As of 2019, 35.4% of US NG isolates were resistant to ciprofloxacin, 27.8% were resistant to tetracycline, and 5.1% had decreased susceptibility to azithromycin. After an increase to 1.4% in 2011, rates of decreased susceptibility to cefixime declined to 0.3% in 2019, corresponding with updated guidelines deemphasizing a role for routine cefixime use.[31] Ceftriaxone non-susceptibility has fortunately remained rare in the United States, which present in only 0.1% of isolates in 2019.[14] Overall, 44.5% of isolates were susceptible to all tested antimicrobials, whereas 4.6% demonstrated reduced susceptibility or resistance to ≥3 different agents. In 2019, no isolates from the mainland US reported to the CDC had decreased susceptibility to both ceftriaxone and azithromycin; however, cases with this profile have been recognized in Hawaii.[28] For nearly all antimicrobials, the rates of resistance are higher in the MSM population compared with heterosexual men who have sex with women (MSW) peers, particularly for non-cephalosporin agents. In 2019, the azithromycin non-susceptibility rate among MSM was 8.8%, as compared with 3.3% among MSW. For ciprofloxacin, 44.8% of MSM isolates were resistant (30.6% MSW), and for ceftriaxone non-susceptibility, rates were 0.2% (0.1% MSW).[14] Confronting MDR and XDR NG may increasingly become part of the therapeutic landscape.

Resistance Mechanisms, Pharmacodynamics, and Antimicrobial Stewardship

Table 3 summarizes the mechanisms of resistance, pharmacodynamics, and tissue penetrance of important anti-gonococcal medications. Resistance acquisition may be by transformation and/or *de novo* mutation, and NG has a remarkable variety of potential mechanisms at its disposal, including enzymatic destruction or modification of drugs, modification of drug targets, and changes to drug influx and efflux.[32] The appropriate antibiotic use has been shown to not only slow the development of resistance, but in some cases to reverse such trends altogether, something that is of particular importance for gonorrhea.[33] Responsible antibiotic stewardship is a key component of health care delivery. Over half of antibiotic prescriptions in the United States may not be consistent with recommended guidelines, and oral antibiotics with potential anti-NG activity are some

Table 2
Selected antibiotics with comparative definitions of minimum inhibitory concentration breakpoints and prevalence of resistance in the United States

	Cefixime (μg/mL)	Ceftriaxone (μg/mL)	Azithromycin (μg/mL)	Ciprofloxacin (μg/mL)	Tetracycline (μg/mL)
CLSI	≤0.25[a]	≤0.25[a]	≤1.0[a]	≥1.0	≥2.0
EUCAST	>0.125	>0.125	>1.0[a]	>0.06	>1.0
CDC	≥0.25[b]	≥0.125[b]	≥2.0[b]	≥1.0	≥2.0
WHO[c]	Variable	Variable	Variable	Variable	Variable
US prevalence of decreased susceptibility or resistance[d]	0.3%	0.1%	5.1%	35.4%	27.8%
No (%) of countries reporting rates of decreased susceptibility or resistance ≥5%[e]	6 (9.0%)	9 (18.0%)	44 (72.0%)	54 (77.0%)	NR

Abbreviations: CDC, US Centers for Disease Control and Prevention; CLSI, US Clinical Laboratory Standards Institute; EUCAST, the European Committee on Antimicrobial Susceptibility Testing; NR, not reported; WHO, World Health Organization.

[a] No defined MIC cutoff for resistance. Values represent susceptibility breakpoints only.

[b] CDC alert value and breakpoint for "elevated MIC"; resistance cut-off not defined.

[c] WHO recommends that quantitative methods be used to determine the MIC, and values should be interpreted using internationally validated interpretative criteria such as those recommended by EUCAST or CLSI.

[d] Based on 2019 data reported from the CDC GISP, using CDC alert values.

[e] Based on 2017 to 2018 data reported from the WHO GASP network, using the interpretative criteria of the reporting country.

(*Data from* Refs[1,22,31,32])

Table 3
Summary of antimicrobial mechanisms of resistance, genetic determinants, and pharmacodynamics in the treatment of gonococcal infection

Antibiotic	Mechanism of Resistance[a]	Major Genetic Determinants[a]	Pharmacodynamics/Tissue Penetrance	Empirical Utility for Pharyngeal Infection
Ciprofloxacin	Reduced target binding affinity	gyrA	Good intracellular activity; $t_{1/2}$ 4–6 hours; 70% bioavailable; 20–40% protein bound; moderate penetration into saliva	Not recommended
Tetracycline	Release of tetracycline from ribosome; change in influx/efflux	tetM; mtrR	Good intracellular activity; $t_{1/2}$ 6–11 hours; 77–88% bioavailable; 55% protein bound; moderate penetration into saliva	Not recommended
Azithromycin	Modification of ribosomal target; change in influx/efflux	erm genes; mtrR	Good intracellular activity; protein binding varies by dose; $t_{1/2}$ 68–72 hours; high penetration into saliva and tonsils	Not recommended
Cefixime	Modification of transpeptidase target; change in influx/efflux	penA; mtrR; and penB	Poor intracellular activity; 40–50% bioavailable; 65% protein bound; $t_{1/2}$ 3–4 hours; low penetration into saliva	Not recommended
Ceftriaxone	Modification of transpeptidase target; change in influx/efflux	penA; mtrR; and penB	Poor intracellular activity; $t_{1/2}$ 6–8 hours; 85–95% protein bound; low penetration into saliva and tonsils	Recommended

[a] Major mechanisms of resistance and genetic determinants are listed; however, this table is not exhaustive and other additional mechanisms exist. For a more comprehensive review, please refer to references cited above.
(Data from Refs[15,30,32])

of the most prescribed in the outpatient setting. For example, in 2020, the top two most-prescribed outpatient antibiotics in the United States were amoxicillin and azithromycin with doxycycline ranking fourth.[34] The combination of frequent, and often inappropriate, use of these medications, with the inherent propensity of NG to acquire resistance, is a dangerous combination. Asymptomatic gonorrhea coupled with suboptimal dosing or duration suggests that NG is being exposed to subtherapeutic quantities of drug, creating an ideal environment for fomenting resistance. There has been an increased push from multiple government agencies and professional societies for hospitals to establish antibiotic stewardship programs with the purpose of educating providers, ensuring appropriate antibiotic selection and duration and preventing AMR development.[33,35]

Fortunately, there have been some successes. After cefixime non-susceptibility rates increased to 1.4% in 2011, these rates have since declined to 0.3% as of 2019, in large part due to better adherence to guideline-based therapy. This success emphasizes the need for ongoing vigilance in antibiotic prescribing both to preserve current therapies and potentially reverse resistance trends.

Treatment and Pharmacodynamic Considerations

In response to changing antimicrobial susceptibility data, the CDC updated the US STI Treatment Guidelines in 2021 (**Table 4**).[2] These recommendations contain several important changes from the previous iteration published in 2015.[2,31] Dual therapy with ceftriaxone and azithromycin is no longer recommended for first-line treatment; rather, ceftriaxone monotherapy with 500 mg (increased from 250 mg) is recommended. This change was made after US NG isolates crossed the 5% non-susceptibility threshold for azithromycin set by the WHO for determining when a medication should no longer be considered first line for STI treatment.

Although first-line antimicrobial therapy for uncomplicated urethral, cervical, and rectal gonorrhea likely has cure rates of greater than 99%, pharyngeal infection bears special mention. Pharyngeal infections are often asymptomatic and are thought to play an important role in community transmission and transfer of antimicrobial resistance.[36] In addition, eradication of gonorrhea from this site is notoriously difficult with cure rates for most non-ceftriaxone-based regimens estimated at around 90% or lower.[2,37] The reasons for this are not fully understood, but are hypothesized to be related to ease of resistance gene transfer from commensal nonpathogenic *Neisseria* species, colonization of tonsils and tonsillar crypts that may allow for high bacterial burden, and lack of concomitant inflammation that curtails antibiotic penetration into oropharyngeal tissue.[38,39] Although ceftriaxone is efficacious and the only recommended treatment for pharyngeal infection, the pharmacodynamic reasons for this are also unclear. Ceftriaxone is highly protein bound and has relatively low penetrance into saliva and tonsillar tissue, two areas that would seem to be of importance for oropharyngeal eradication. It is not known if salivary or plasma concentrations of antibiotics reliably reflect antimicrobial exposure in the oropharynx, and it seems likely that the interplay between bug, drug, and tissue is more complex than our current understanding.[39,40] For these reasons, current guidelines recommend treatment with ceftriaxone followed by a test of cure at 7 to 14 days posttreatment for all cases of pharyngeal gonorrhea.[31] Culture and nucleic acid amplication tests (NAATs) are acceptable, though clinicians should be mindful of the potential for false-positive NAAT assays if they are obtained too soon after therapy (within the first 5 days of treatment). Repeat testing ensures microbiologic cure and early identification of potential non-susceptible isolates, limiting asymptomatic community spread. Strategies for treatment of oropharyngeal infection following ceftriaxone failure or unavailability are uncertain; potential options

Table 4
Summary of treatment recommendations

Syndrome	Treatment Recommendations
Uncomplicated Infections[a]	
Urethritis, Cervicitis, Rectal	Ceftriaxone 500 mg IM, single dose (preferred)[b] Gentamicin 240 mg IM, single dose PLUS Azithromycin 2000 mg PO, single dose (alternative) Cefixime 800 mg PO, single dose (alternative)
Pharyngeal[c]	Ceftriaxone 500 mg IM, single dose[b]
Conjunctivitis	Ceftriaxone 1000 mg IM, single dose
Epididymitis	Ceftriaxone 500 mg IM once, PLUS: Doxycycline 100 mg BID for 10 d, OR Levofloxacin 500 mg daily for 10 d, as dictated by risk for concomitant chlamydia and/or enteric infection
Complicated/Invasive Infections	

Septic Arthritis or Arthritis/
   Dermatitis Syn.[e]
Disseminated
   Gonococcal infections
	Ceftriaxone 1000 mg IM or IV every 24 h for ≥7 d (preferred)
	Cefotaxime 1000 mg IV every 8 h (alternative)
	Ceftizoxime 1000 mg IV every 8 h (alternative)

Complicated/Invasive Infections	
Pelvic Inflammatory Disease	
Outpatient	Ceftriaxone 500 mg IM once, as part of appropriate combination regimen[b]
Inpatient	Ceftriaxone 1000 mg IV every 24 h, as part of appropriate combination regimen
Complicated/Invasive Infections	
Meningitis, osteomyelitis, endocarditis[d]	Ceftriaxone 1000–2000 mg IV every 24 h

[a] If chlamydial infection has not been ruled out, then empiric co-treatment with either doxycycline (preferred) or azithromycin (alternative) is recommended.
[b] In persons weighing ≥150 kg, the dose should be increased to 1000 mg IM in a single dose.
[c] Test of cure should be performed with culture or NAAT 1–2 weeks following treatment.
[d] Duration of therapy should be prolonged and determined on individual basis.
[e] Once substantial clinical improvement is noted, switch to oral therapy can be considered for treatment completion

Data from Workowski KA, Bachmann LH, Chan PA, et al. Sexually Transmitted Infections Treatment Guidelines, 2021. MMWR Recomm Rep. Jul 23 2021;70(4):1–187. https://doi.org/10.15585/mmwr.rr7004a1.

include rechallenge with a higher dose of ceftriaxone or attempted use of an alternative regimen, such as a quinolone if susceptible. For clinical nonresponse, therapy should be guided by the results of antimicrobial susceptibility testing.

Cephalosporin treatment failure warrants prompt attention, and suspicion should be prompted when symptoms do not resolve within 3 to 5 days of treatment and/or there is a positive test-of-cure via appropriately timed culture or NAAT. Reinfection must be ruled out but performing culture and antimicrobial sensitivities is imperative if treatment failure is suspected.[2] Infectious disease consultation is encouraged, and prompt notification to public health authorities for case reporting and contact tracing is necessary.

Novel or Repurposed Antibiotics for Gonorrhea

New antimicrobial development targeting NG is a national strategic priority given the increasing rates of AMR. Within the past 10 years, several therapies including solithromycin, zoliflodacin, and gepotidacin have entered advanced clinical trials, and investigations into other Food and Drug Administration (FDA)-approved antibiotics are ongoing. The results from these recent clinical trials are shown in **Table 5**.

Despite initial promising studies, solithromycin, a fourth-generation macrolide, was found to be not non-inferior in a Phase III trial assessing eradication in comparison with ceftriaxone and azithromycin.[41]

Zoliflodacin and gepotidacin are two additional promising agents. These are novel DNA topoisomerase II inhibitors formulated for oral therapy.[42,43] Although their mechanism of action is similar to quinolones, these agents have distinct binding sites affected by *gyrB* or *parE* (zoliflodacin) or *gyrA/parC* (gepotidacin). A Phase II clinical trial of zoliflodacin (ETX0914) assessing 179 participants with uncomplicated urogenital NG infection showed promising results for genitourinary and rectal infection with both 2 and 3 g doses.[44] However, pharyngeal infection only had an 82% cure rate to the 3 g dose, compared with 100% for ceftriaxone. Subsequently, a multicenter Phase III non-inferiority trial comparing 3 g zoliflodacin with 500 mg ceftriaxone + 1 g azithromycin is ongoing, with primary completion estimated in mid-2023 (NCT03959527). Similarly, gepotidacin (GSK2140944) also demonstrated high efficacy in small Phase II trial of urogenital gonorrhea.[45] Of the 69 patients given gepotidacin, the three treatment failures were associated with gepotidacin MIC greater than 1 µg/mL. A phase III clinical trial comparing two doses of oral gepotidacin (3gram) with 500 mg ceftriaxone and 1 gram azithromycin for the treatment of uncomplicated urogenital gonorrhea in 600 participants is ongoing and also set to end mid-2023 (NCT04010539).

Repurposing currently approved therapies for the treatment of gonorrhea is also being studied the recently published NABOGO trial, which compared 1000 mg of IM ertapenem, IM gentamicin 5 mg/kg (up to 400 mg), and oral fosfomycin (6 g) to IM ceftriaxone (500 mg) found that ertapenem was non-inferior to ceftriaxone, but

Table 5 Novel antimicrobial agents			
Antimicrobial	**Mechanism of Action**	**Efficacy**	**Stage of Development**
Solithromycin	Macrolide/ketolide	Phase III: 80% eradication vs 84% ceftriaxone and azithromycin; did not meet non-inferiority	Further studies for gonococcal infections (GC) have been halted
Zolidoflacin	DNA topoisomerase II inhibitors (gyrB, parE)	Phase II: 96% eradication of urogenital with 2 g and 3 g doses. 100% rectal eradication, only 50% and 60% eradication of pharyngeal infection ($n = 179$)	Phase III Trial comparing 3 g zoliflodacin vs 500 mg ceftriaxone and 1 g azithromycin. Completion estimated mid-2023 (NCT03959527).
Gepotidacin	DNA Topoisomerase II inhibitor (gyrB, gyrC)	Phase II: 96% for urogenital infection ($n = 69$)	Phase III: 3 grams gepotidacin vs 500 mg ceftriaxone and 1 g azithromycin. Completion estimated mid-2023 (NCT04010539).

(Data from Refs[41–47])

fosfomycin and gentamicin were inferior.[46] Ceftriaxone non-susceptible strains were not included in this trial, although the results suggest that in that ertapenem might be an option in that setting. There is interest in the novel pleuromutilin agent lefamulin for the treatment of MDR NG. Lefamulin had potent activity against NG isolates in vitro, including MDR strains with efflux pumps.[47] To date, however, no clinical trials have evaluated its efficacy in humans.

Testing as a strategy for both prevention and reducing antimicrobial-resistance

Routine diagnosis in the United States is typically established using NAAT.[48] When compared with cultures, NAAT-based testing offers several advantages including faster time to results (potentially about 2–3 hours), greater sensitivity for diagnosing extragenital and asymptomatic infections, higher throughput, and potential identification of more than one pathogen.[48–54] Samples for NAAT can be self-collected, potentially overcoming some of the reluctance associated with testing.[55] As discussed previously, culture is necessary for comprehensive antibiotic susceptibility data, making it a key part of the evaluation of suspected treatment failures and epidemiologic surveillance.

Samples for NAAT testing are usually batched and runs occur either daily or every other day. This method is highly efficient, but requires follow-up appointments for treatment, underscoring the need for POCTs. POCTs that provide results within 30 minutes (ie, during an office visit) could allow for near simultaneous testing, treatment, and initiation of the partner notification process, thereby reducing transmission. An ideal POCT would follow the WHO-defined ASSURED guidelines (ie, the test should be Affordable, Sensitive, Specific, User Friendly, Equipment Free and Deliverable), be CLIA waived, couple diagnosis with AMR information, and allow for collection at home.[56] A recent study from South Africa suggests that POCT significantly reduced the time to treatment in comparison with central laboratory based testing (adjusted hazard ratio of 39.62; 95% CI 15.13–103.74) highlighting the significant potential for POCT in STI prevention.[57]

In the last decade, there have been significant advances in POCT, as detailed in Chapter ("Advances in Diagnostics of Sexually Transmitted Infections" by Mauricio Kahn and Barbara Van Der Pol). These vary in the platform used, size, portability, voltage-needs, turn-around time, specimens approved for testing and organisms identified.[58] The FDA has currently cleared three POCT for the diagnosis of NG but these tests do not meet all the ASSURED criteria, highlighting significant room for growth in this area.[59] In general, POCT have been approved for urethral, vaginal, urine, or endocervical specimens, with only one POCT approved for use with extragenital specimens: the GeneXpert *Chlamydia trachomatis*/NG Platform (Xpert CT/NG).[60] However, the lack of CLIA waiver approval, cost, and the turn-around time of ~90 minutes limits the use of the Xpert CT/NG in a STI clinic/office setting, and the GeneXpert is more a near-patient test rather than a true POCT. Two POCTs, Visby Medical Sexual Health Click Test (Visby diagnostics, San Jose, CA) and the binx health io CT/NG assay (binx health inc, MA), have received 510 (k) clearance and are allowed for use in any health care setting with a CLIA certificate of waiver, so non-laboratory personnel can run the test. Although the binx health io CT/NG assay requires a small instrument, the Visby click test is portable and disposable and is meant for single use. The Visby Medical Sexual Health Click test was approved based on a study of 1555 women, with 97.4% sensitivity and 99.4% specificity for NG when compared with standard NAAT testing.[61] The Visby click test is approved for use in women with both self and physician collected vaginal swabs. The binx io platform was approved based on a study of 1523 women (~50% symptomatic) and 922 men (~33% symptomatic). Sensitivity estimates were 100.0% (95% CI, 92.1%–100.0%) for women and 97.3% (95% CI, 90.7%–99.3%) for men; specificity was 99.9% (95% CI, 99.5%–

100%) for women and 100% (95% CI, 95.5%–100%) for men.[62] The binx io test was approved for use with urine in men and self or provider collected vaginal swabs in women. Neither test is yet approved for extragenital samples.

An ideal POCT would combine identification and resistance detection; however, the complexity of NG resistance determination presents a major barrier to development.[32,63] For example, resistance to extended spectrum cephalosporins is predicted by four principal genes (penA, penB, mtrR, and ponA), with the main determinant being the mosaic penA alleles.[63] Strains with different penA mosaic alleles circulate in different parts of the world; hence, developing a universal assay is challenging and would require constant adaptation, reducing its commercial potential.[64–67] The prediction of resistance based on genetic characterization in NG is most accurate for fluoroquinolones, as the absence of mutations in serine codon 91 of the gyrA gene predicts susceptibility. Resistance-guided therapy for treatment with quinolones has demonstrated success.[68,69] In one prospective study, treatment with a quinolone was successful in 100% of the infections examined (30 genitourinary, 14 pharyngeal, and 73 rectal samples).[69] Results of this and other studies suggest that in the right patient population, quinolones could be useful for treatment.[68,69] The use of oral quinolones would simplify treatment, allow for expedited partner therapy (EPT), and slow down AMR generation by reducing exposure to cephalosporins. In fact, a permissive strategy for quinolone use has been adopted by the British guidelines.[70] A commercial test that combines pathogen identification with quinolone resistance determination is now available in Australia and Europe and is under breakthrough designation by the FDA (Speed-Dx ResistancePlus NG).[71]

PREVENTION
Screening as a Tool to Prevent New Infections

Screening for gonorrhea is an effective and important public health tool. NAAT is the preferred method of screening, either using first catch urine or swabs depending on anatomical site. As previously noted, genitourinary infections in women are often asymptomatic, whereas 90% of men with urethritis are symptomatic.[3,4,72] Extragenital infections are often asymptomatic and can be frequent additional sites of infection in patients diagnosed with urogenital gonorrhea (particularly MSM) with rates ranging from 12% to 30%.[72–75] The high rate of asymptomatic infections in women and MSM provides opportunities for ongoing transmission.

Both the US Preventive Services Task Force (USPSTF) and the CDC updated screening recommendations in 2021 (**Table 6**).[2,76] For women, urogenital NG screening is recommended for sexually active women under the age of 25 and those over 25 at increased risk. Female extragenital screening should be based on patient risk factors and discussions between the patient and their provider. The CDC and USPSTF found insufficient evidence for asymptomatic urogenital screening in males at standard risk. However, in certain groups such as MSM and those taking HIV PrEP, screening extragenital sites is recommended at 3 to 6-month intervals, especially if there are new sexual partners. Transgender and gender diverse persons should be screened based on anatomy and sexual risk factors, at intervals varying from 3 to 12 months.

An area of emphasis involves extragenital screening in the MSM population, particularly those on HIV PrEP. Extragenital NG infection is disproportionately high in this community, and routine screening of extragenital sites varies.[72,77] In an assessment of extragenital screening for STI in MSM, Patton and colleagues[77] reported higher rates for urogenital screening (83.9%) than for rectal (50.4%) or pharyngeal (65.9%) sites. In addition, they demonstrated that 70% of extragenital NG infections had negative urethral testing. More recently, Assaf and colleagues[78] found that solely following

Table 6
Summary of current screening recommendations

Population	Timing	Anatomic Site[c]
Women		
Sexually active, age <25 y	Annual	Urine or vaginal swab; other sites based on risk following shared decision-making
Increased risk, age ≥25 y[a]	Annual	Urine or vaginal swab; other sites based on risk following shared decision making
Pregnancy Age <25 y	All during first trimester; rescreen in third trimester	Urine or vaginal swab; other sites based on risk
Age ≥25 y	During first trimester if at increased risk; third trimester screen if at risk	Urine or vaginal swab; other sites based on risk
MSM		
No specific risk factors	Annual	All sites of contact (urethral, rectum, pharynx) regardless of condom use
Increased risk[b]	Every 3–6 mo	All sites of contact (urethral, rectum, pharynx) regardless of condom use
Persons with prior known infection	Screen at 3 mo post-treatment	Site of prior infection and/or new exposure
All others at low risk	No recommendation	N/A

[a] Women considered to be at increased risk include those who have a new sex partner, more than one sex partner, a sex partner with concurrent partners, or a sex partner who has an STI.
[b] MSM considered to be at increased risk include those with multiple anonymous partners, history of substance abuse, or those otherwise at risk for HIV acquisition.
[c] In general, both physician-collected and patient self-collected specimens are permissible within the clinic setting.
(*Data from* Refs[2,76])

the minimum screening recommendations in MSM would result in missed or delayed diagnoses of extragenital gonorrhea in up to 65% of those who underwent urogenital testing, and 35% of combined extragenital CT/NG infections would be missed if testing is solely based on patient-reported sexual behaviors.

Despite the current CDC and USPSTF recommendations for NG screening, significant challenges remain. Screening relies heavily on provider-collected, in-person office visits, which require time, and both patient and provider familiarity and comfort with screening procedures.[79] Self-collection of screening swabs has been proposed to help alleviate some of these barriers and has a high accuracy when compared with provider-collection in both men and women (including MSM and people with HIV).[80–83] Clinicians can encourage patients to self-collect swabs at home, although some patients might be apprehensive about self-collection, particularly related to perceived efficacy and delays in diagnosis.[84]

Pooled specimen processing has been proposed as a cost-control measure that retains diagnostic accuracy. A meta-analysis including 17 studies, with a majority including MSM, found that the pooled sensitivity for NG infection was retained at 94.1%, with significant cost savings between 33% and 66%.[85] One of the limitations of this method is an inability to differentiate between sites of infection, potentially having adverse implications on treatment or follow-up/test of cure strategies.

Expedited Partner Therapy is a Prevention Tool

Identification and treatment of sexual partners is one of the most important public health tools available for limiting the spread of STIs. EPT allows treating clinicians to provide antibiotic prescriptions to the patient to give to their partner(s) to ensure that all partners are treated, thereby reducing the risk of repeat infections and transmission. The implementation of EPT has been shown to decrease rates of persistent or recurrent Chlamydia Trachomatis (CT) or NG infection and has contributed to greater partner notification.[86,87] It has also been shown through modeling to reduce both health care and societal cost by 32% to 37% for female partners of male patients and greater than 29% for male partners of female patients.[88] Since 2005, the CDC has continued to recommend consideration of EPT in women and heterosexual men for CT, including the 2021 guidelines. Owing to concerns about increasing antimicrobial resistance in NG, EPT is only recommended if it is unlikely the partner would be screened and treated through standard referral in a timely manner.[2] However, there has been relatively slow adoption of EPT by treating providers. Data analysis from the SSuN from 2010 to 2012 found that only 5.4% of patients diagnosed with NG were given EPT and that heterosexual males were twice as likely to receive EPT compared with MSM (6.6% vs 2.6%).[89]

Additional challenges in implementation of EPT include legal complications limited by local state laws. Currently, 45 states allow EPT, and in Alabama, Kansas, Oklahoma, and South Dakota it is "potentially allowable." Only South Carolina bans EPT.[90] There are also regional differences in implementation. For example, in Washington state 35.5% of heterosexual patients with NG were offered EPT, compared with only 2% in New York City.[89] Regional differences are potentially due to population demographics in major metropolitan areas that disfavor EPT in accordance with the CDC guidelines at the time. Currently, EPT is not routinely recommended for MSM due to concerns about missed opportunities for screening for other sexually transmitted diseases given the high coinfection incidence.[2] Thus, using EPT is recommended under shared clinical "decision making." Although limited data exist regarding outcomes of EPT in MSM, it has been shown to increase partner notification and in a modeling study potentially reduced STI incidence by between 27% and 32% if given to 20% of the cases.[91,92] Despite concerns regarding coinfection screening, EPT is a potential, perhaps underused, option for decreasing rates of NG. Concerns about AMR and missed opportunities for HIV and STI screening and prevention represent barriers for expansion of EPT. Information specific to individual state regulations is updated regularly at www.cdc.gov/std/ept.

Primary Prevention with Vaccines

Primary prevention against gonococcal disease could be a vital tool in curbing the spread of resistant strains without impacting AMR rates. Implementation of a vaccination program, even with moderate efficacy, has been predicted have a substantial impact on overall disease burden. In a modeling study of NG vaccination in heterosexual populations, a durable vaccine with 20% efficacy could decrease prevalence by 40%, and a vaccine with 50% efficacy could decrease prevalence by 90% over 20 years if given to all 13 year olds.[93] In MSM, modeling predicted that a vaccine with 50% efficacy could reduce incidence by 62% if given to only 30% of patients who present for STI testing.[94] Despite decades of research, developing an effective vaccine has remained elusive despite multiple different vaccination strategies. Recently, vaccination against NG Group B outer membrane vesicle has been shown in retrospective analyses to confer some level of protection against infection with NG. A case-control study in New Zealand in those who had receive the MeNZB vaccine against NG group B found protection against NG infection with 31% efficacy.[95] Two subsequent studies demonstrated similar efficacy for those who had received the MenB-4C vaccine in both Australia (32.7%) and the United States (40%), providing the platform for the development of randomized clinical trials assessing the efficacy of commercially available MenB-4C vaccines in the United States and abroad.[96,97]

Preexposure and Postexposure Chemoprophylaxis

The success of HIV PrEP coupled with rising STI rates has renewed a discussion about chemoprophylaxis against other STIs. Given the biologic differences in bacterial STIs, finding a single effective prophylactic agent is difficult. Doxycycline is considered a frontrunner, with broad coverage of multiple different STIs. Bolan and colleagues[98] found that daily 100 mg doxycycline reduced rates of select bacterial STI when compared with monetary incentives for remaining STI free in a small pilot study in HIV-infected men with recurrent syphilis (OR 0.27; CI 0.09–0.83, $P = 0.02$). However, the reductions in NG or CT were not statistically significant (OR 0.36; CI 0.08–1.56, $P = 0.18$). Similarly, a substudy of the ANRS IPERGAY trial assessed the efficacy of 200 mg doxycycline as postexposure prophylaxis no later than 72 hours after sex and found no difference in gonorrhea infections after 10 months.[99] In contrast, Leutkemeyer and colleagues[100] reported that 200 mg doxycycline taken within 72 hours following condomless sex reduced rates of all bacterial STIs, including NG. Although the latter trial is promising, the results of future planned or ongoing studies will likely be needed to determine the efficacy of doxycycline for gonorrhea prophylaxis.

SUMMARY

The increasing rates of gonorrhea over the past decade highlight many of the challenges with its management. Threats from AMR are at the forefront, including rising rates of azithromycin non-susceptibility and increasing ceftriaxone MICs, posing challenges to clinical management. There is immediate need for increased screening, further development of rapid POCT to allow prompt diagnosis and treatment, and new antimicrobials to combat AMR strains. Future success in the management of gonorrhea will rely on preventive efforts drawing from a wide range of tools including primary prevention with vaccines, chemoprophylaxis, and broader utilization of EPT.

CLINICS CARE POINTS

- In the US, a single dose of ceftriaxone (500 mg) administered intramuscularly is recommended for the treatment of uncomplicated genitourinary, pharyngeal, and rectal gonococcal infections.

- For pharyngeal infections, most non-ceftriaxone-based regimens have less than 90% cure rates. Following treatment of pharyngeal infections, a test of cure is recommended. Both culture and nucleic acid-based testing (NAAT) can be used, NAAT based testing maybe falsely positive if performed within 5 days of treatment.

- For the diagnosis of gonococcal infection, currently, three POCTs are licensed by the US Food and Drug Administration (FDA), GeneXpert (Xpert CT/NG), Visby Medical Sexual Health Click test and the binx io CT/NG assay. The three POCTs differ in turn-around times and samples that they can be used with.

- Routine annual screening for genitourinary infections is recommended for all sexually active women under 25 years of age. Routine screening for men in the same age group is not recommended. For those at increased risk, screening every 3 to 6 months, based on sites of contact, is recommended for those at increased risk.
- Several new prevention strategies are being evaluated including the use of the Group B meningococcal vaccine to prevent gonococcal infections and the use of a single dose of doxycycline within 72 hours of exposure as post-exposure prophylaxis.

DISCLAIMER

DISCLOSURE

This project was conducted by the Infectious Disease Clinical Research Program (IDCRP), a Department of Defense (DoD) program executed by the Uniformed Services University of the Health Sciences (USU) through a cooperative agreement with The Henry M Jackson Foundation for the Advancement of Military Medicine, Inc (HJF).

FUNDING

This project has been supported with federal fund from the National Institute of Allergy and Infectious Diseases, National Institutes of Health under Inter-Agency Agreement Y1-AI-5072, the Defense Health Program, US DoD under award HU0001190002.

REFERENCES

1. WHO. Sexually transmitted infections (STIs) Factsheet. Available at: https://www.who.int/news-room/fact-sheets/detail/sexually-transmitted-infections-(stis. Accessed 10 1, 2022.
2. Workowski KA, Bachmann LH, Chan PA, et al. Sexually transmitted infections treatment guidelines, 2021. MMWR Recomm Rep (Morb Mortal Wkly Rep) 2021;70(4):1–187.
3. McCormack WM, Stumacher RJ, Johnson K, et al. Clinical spectrum of gonococcal infection in women. Lancet 1977;1(8023):1182–5.
4. John E., Bennett R.D. and Martin J., Blaser. mandell, douglas, and bennett's principles and practice of infectious diseases, 9 ed., 2020, Elsevier/Saunders, Philadelphia, PA.
5. Laga M, Manoka A, Kivuvu M, et al. Non-ulcerative sexually transmitted diseases as risk factors for HIV-1 transmission in women: results from a cohort study. AIDS 1993;7(1):95–102.
6. McClelland RS, Lavreys L, Katingima C, et al. Contribution of HIV-1 infection to acquisition of sexually transmitted disease: a 10-year prospective study. J Infect Dis 2005;191(3):333–8.
7. Barbee LA, Dombrowski JC. Control of Neisseria gonorrhoeae in the era of evolving antimicrobial resistance. Infect Dis Clin North Am 2013;27(4):723–37.

8. CDC. Sexually Transmitted disease surveillance: national overview. US Department of Health and Human Services. 2022. Available at: https://www.cdc.gov/std/statistics/2020/overview.htm. Accessed 10/1/2022.

9. Vanable PA, Ostrow DG, McKirnan DJ, et al. Impact of combination therapies on HIV risk perceptions and sexual risk among HIV-positive and HIV-negative gay and bisexual men. Health Psychol 2000;19(2):134–45.

10. Brooks RA, Landovitz RJ, Kaplan RL, et al. Sexual risk behaviors and acceptability of HIV pre-exposure prophylaxis among HIV-negative gay and bisexual men in serodiscordant relationships: a mixed methods study. AIDS Patient Care STDS 2012;26(2):87–94.

11. Zhang Kudon H, Mulatu MS, Song W, et al. Trends in condomless sex among MSM who participated in CDC-funded HIV risk-reduction interventions in the United States, 2012-2017. J Public Health Manag Pract 2022;28(2):170–3.

12. WHO. Gonococcal AMR surveillance programme (WHO-GASP). World Health Organization. 2022. Available at: https://www.who.int/data/gho/data/themes/topics/who-gonococcal-amr-surveillance-programme-who-gasp. Accessed 10/1/2022.

13. WHO. Enhanced gonococcal antimicrobial surveillance programme (EGASP): general protocol. . World Health Organization. 2022. Available at: https://www.who.int/publications/i/item/9789240021341. Accessed 10/1/2022.

14. CDC. Gonococcal isolate surveillance project (GISP), 2020. US Department of Health and Human Services. 2022. Available at: https://www.cdc.gov/std/gisp/default.htm. Accessed 10/1/2022.

15. Unemo M, Shafer WM. Antibiotic resistance in Neisseria gonorrhoeae: origin, evolution, and lessons learned for the future. Ann N Y Acad Sci 2011;1230: E19–28.

16. Allen VG, Mitterni L, Seah C, et al. Neisseria gonorrhoeae treatment failure and susceptibility to cefixime in Toronto, Canada. JAMA 2013;309(2):163–70.

17. Ison CA, Hussey J, Sankar KN, et al. Gonorrhoea treatment failures to cefixime and azithromycin in England, 2010. Euro Surveill 2011;16(14):19833.

18. Ito M, Yasuda M, Yokoi S, et al. Remarkable increase in central Japan in 2001-2002 of Neisseria gonorrhoeae isolates with decreased susceptibility to penicillin, tetracycline, oral cephalosporins, and fluoroquinolones. Antimicrobial Agents Chemother 2004;48(8):3185–7.

19. Unemo M, Golparian D, Potocnik M, et al. Treatment failure of pharyngeal gonorrhoea with internationally recommended first-line ceftriaxone verified in Slovenia, September 2011. Euro Surveill 2012;17(25).

20. Lewis DA, Sriruttan C, Muller EE, et al. Phenotypic and genetic characterization of the first two cases of extended-spectrum-cephalosporin-resistant Neisseria gonorrhoeae infection in South Africa and association with cefixime treatment failure. J Antimicrob Chemother 2013;68(6):1267–70.

21. Starnino S, Galarza P, Carvallo ME, et al. Retrospective analysis of antimicrobial susceptibility trends (2000-2009) in Neisseria gonorrhoeae isolates from countries in Latin America and the Caribbean shows evolving resistance to ciprofloxacin, azithromycin and decreased susceptibility to ceftriaxone. Sex Transm Dis 2012;39(10):813–21.

22. Unemo M, Lahra MM, Escher M, et al. WHO global antimicrobial resistance surveillance for Neisseria gonorrhoeae 2017-18: a retrospective observational study. Lancet Microbe 2021;2(11):e627–36.

23. Ohnishi M, Saika T, Hoshina S, et al. Ceftriaxone-resistant Neisseria gonorrhoeae, Japan. Emerg Infect Dis 2011;17(1):148–9.

24. Tapsall J, Read P, Carmody C, et al. Two cases of failed ceftriaxone treatment in pharyngeal gonorrhoea verified by molecular microbiological methods. J Med Microbiol 2009;58(Pt 5):683–7.
25. YC M, Stevens K, Tideman R, et al. Failure of 500 mg of ceftriaxone to eradicate pharyngeal gonorrhoea, Australia. J Antimicrob Chemother 2013;68(6):1445–7.
26. Golparian D, Ohlsson A, Janson H, et al. Four treatment failures of pharyngeal gonorrhoea with ceftriaxone (500 mg) or cefotaxime (500 mg), Sweden, 2013 and 2014. Euro Surveill 2014;19(30). https://doi.org/10.2807/1560-7917. es2014.19.30.20862.
27. Fifer H, Natarajan U, Jones L, et al. Failure of dual antimicrobial therapy in treatment of gonorrhea. N Engl J Med 2016;374(25):2504–6.
28. Papp JR, Abrams AJ, Nash E, et al. Azithromycin resistance and decreased ceftriaxone susceptibility in Neisseria gonorrhoeae, Hawaii, USA. Emerg Infect Dis 2017;23(5):830–2.
29. Eyre DW, Town K, Street T, et al. Detection in the United Kingdom of the Neisseria gonorrhoeae FC428 clone, with ceftriaxone resistance and intermediate resistance to azithromycin, October to December 2018. Euro Surveill 2019; 24(10). https://doi.org/10.2807/1560-7917.ES.2019.24.10.1900147.
30. Unemo M, Golparian D, Eyre DW. Antimicrobial resistance in Neisseria gonorrhoeae and treatment of gonorrhea. Methods Mol Biol 2019;1997:37–58.
31. Workowski KA, Bolan GA, Centers for Disease C, Prevention. Sexually transmitted diseases treatment guidelines, 2015. MMWR Recomm Rep 2015; 64(RR-03):1–137.
32. Unemo M, Shafer WM. Antimicrobial resistance in Neisseria gonorrhoeae in the 21st century: past, evolution, and future. Clin Microbiol Rev 2014;27(3):587–613.
33. Barlam TF, Cosgrove SE, Abbo LM, et al. Implementing an antibiotic stewardship program: guidelines by the infectious diseases society of America and the society for healthcare epidemiology of America. Clin Infect Dis 2016; 62(10):e51–77.
34. CDC. Outpatient antibiotic prescriptions — United States, 2020. U.S. Department of Health and Human Services. 2022. Available at: https://www.cdc.gov/antibiotic-use/pdfs/Annual-Report-2020-H.pdf. Accessed 10/1/2022.
35. CDC. Core Elements of Hospital Antibiotic Stewardship Programs. US Department of Health and Human Services. 2022. Available at: https://www.cdc.gov/antibiotic-use/core-elements/hospital.html. Accessed 10/1/2022.
36. Cornelisse VJ, Williamson D, Zhang L, et al. Evidence for a new paradigm of gonorrhoea transmission: cross-sectional analysis of Neisseria gonorrhoeae infections by anatomical site in both partners in 60 male couples. Sex Transm Infect 2019;95(6):437–42.
37. Ross JDC, Brittain C, Cole M, et al. Gentamicin compared with ceftriaxone for the treatment of gonorrhoea (G-ToG): a randomised non-inferiority trial. Lancet 2019;393(10190):2511–20.
38. Unemo M. Current and future antimicrobial treatment of gonorrhoea - the rapidly evolving Neisseria gonorrhoeae continues to challenge. BMC Infect Dis 2015; 15:364.
39. Sena AC, Bachmann L, Johnston C, et al. Optimising treatments for sexually transmitted infections: surveillance, pharmacokinetics and pharmacodynamics, therapeutic strategies, and molecular resistance prediction. Lancet Infect Dis 2020;20(8):e181–91.
40. Theuretzbacher U, Barbee L, Connolly K, et al. Pharmacokinetic/pharmacodynamic considerations for new and current therapeutic drugs for uncomplicated

gonorrhoea-challenges and opportunities. Clin Microbiol Infect 2020;26(12): 1630–5.

41. Chen MY, McNulty A, Avery A, et al. Solithromycin versus ceftriaxone plus azithromycin for the treatment of uncomplicated genital gonorrhoea (SOLITAIRE-U): a randomised phase 3 non-inferiority trial. Lancet Infect Dis 2019;19(8): 833–42.

42. Farrell DJ, Sader HS, Rhomberg PR, et al. In Vitro Activity of Gepotidacin (GSK2140944) against Neisseria gonorrhoeae. Antimicrobial Agents Chemother 2017;61(3). https://doi.org/10.1128/aac.02047-16.

43. Jacobsson S, Golparian D, Alm RA, et al. High in vitro activity of the novel spiropyrimidinetrione AZD0914, a DNA gyrase inhibitor, against multidrug-resistant Neisseria gonorrhoeae isolates suggests a new effective option for oral treatment of gonorrhea. Antimicrobial Agents Chemother 2014;58(9):5585–8.

44. Taylor SN, Marrazzo J, Batteiger BE, et al. Single-dose zoliflodacin (ETX0914) for treatment of urogenital gonorrhea. N Engl J Med 2018;379(19):1835–45.

45. Taylor SN, Morris DH, Avery AK, et al. Gepotidacin for the treatment of uncomplicated urogenital gonorrhea: a phase 2, randomized, dose-ranging, single-oral dose evaluation. Clin Infect Dis 2018;67(4):504–12.

46. de Vries HJC, de Laat M, Jongen VW, et al. Efficacy of ertapenem, gentamicin, fosfomycin, and ceftriaxone for the treatment of anogenital gonorrhoea (NA-BOGO): a randomised, non-inferiority trial. Lancet Infect Dis 2022;22(5):706–17.

47. Jacobsson S, Paukner S, Golparian D, et al. In vitro activity of the novel pleuromutilin lefamulin (BC-3781) and effect of efflux pump inactivation on multidrug-resistant and extensively drug-resistant Neisseria gonorrhoeae. Antimicrobial Agents Chemother 2017;61(11). https://doi.org/10.1128/aac.01497-17.

48. Centers for Disease C, Prevention. Recommendations for the laboratory-based detection of Chlamydia trachomatis and Neisseria gonorrhoeae–2014. MMWR Recomm Rep (Morb Mortal Wkly Rep) 2014;63(RR-02):1–19.

49. Ota KV, Tamari IE, Smieja M, et al. Detection of Neisseria gonorrhoeae and chlamydia trachomatis in pharyngeal and rectal specimens using the BD probetec ET system, the gen-probe aptima combo 2 assay and culture. Sex Transm Infect 2009;85(3):182–6.

50. Serra-Pladevall J, Caballero E, Roig G, et al. Comparison between conventional culture and NAATs for the microbiological diagnosis in gonococcal infection. Diagn Microbiol Infect Dis 2015;83(4):341–3.

51. Bromhead C, Miller A, Jones M, et al. Comparison of the cobas 4800 CT/NG test with culture for detecting Neisseria gonorrhoeae in genital and nongenital specimens in a low-prevalence population in New Zealand. J Clin Microbiol 2013; 51(5):1505–9.

52. Bachmann LH, Johnson RE, Cheng H, et al. Nucleic acid amplification tests for diagnosis of Neisseria gonorrhoeae and chlamydia trachomatis rectal infections. J Clin Microbiol 2010;48(5):1827–32.

53. Chernesky MA, Jang DE. APTIMA transcription-mediated amplification assays for chlamydia trachomatis and Neisseria gonorrhoeae. Expert Rev Mol Diagn 2006;6(4):519–25.

54. Meyer T, Buder S. The laboratory diagnosis of Neisseria gonorrhoeae: current testing and future demands. Pathogens 2020;9(2). https://doi.org/10.3390/pathogens9020091.

55. Salow KR, Cohen AC, Bristow CC, et al. Comparing mail-in self-collected specimens sent via United States Postal Service versus clinic-collected specimens

for the detection of Chlamydia trachomatis and Neisseria gonorrhoeae in extra-genital sites. PLoS One 2017;12(12):e0189515.

56. Kettler H, White K, Hawkes SJ, Research UNWBWSPf, Training in Tropical D. Mapping the landscape of diagnostics for sexually transmitted infections : key findings and recommendations/Hannah Kettler, Karen White, Sarah Hawkes. Geneva: World Health Organization; 2004.

57. Asare K, Andine T, Naicker N, et al. Impact of point-of-care testing on the management of sexually transmitted infections in South Africa: Evidence from the HVTN702 HIV vaccine trial. Clin Infect Dis 2022. https://doi.org/10.1093/cid/ciac824.

58. Gaydos CA, Manabe YC, Melendez JH. A narrative review of where we are with point-of-care sexually transmitted infection testing in the United States. Sex Transm Dis 2021;48(8S):S71–7.

59. Kersh EN. Advances in sexually transmitted infection testing at home and in nonclinical settings close to the home. Sex Transm Dis 2022;49(11S Suppl 2):S12–4.

60. Doernberg SB, Komarow L, Tran TTT, et al. Simultaneous evaluation of diagnostic assays for pharyngeal and rectal Neisseria gonorrhoeae and chlamydia trachomatis using a master protocol. Clin Infect Dis 2020;71(9):2314–22.

61. Morris SR, Bristow CC, Wierzbicki MR, et al. Performance of a single-use, rapid, point-of-care PCR device for the detection of Neisseria gonorrhoeae, Chlamydia trachomatis, and Trichomonas vaginalis: a cross-sectional study. Lancet Infect Dis 2021;21(5):668–76.

62. Van Der Pol B, Taylor SN, Mena L, et al. Evaluation of the performance of a point-of-care test for chlamydia and gonorrhea. JAMA Netw Open 2020;3(5):e204819.

63. Dona V, Low N, Golparian D, et al. Recent advances in the development and use of molecular tests to predict antimicrobial resistance in Neisseria gonorrhoeae. Expert Rev Mol Diagn 2017;17(9):845–59.

64. Yahara K, Ma KC, Mortimer TD, et al. Emergence and evolution of antimicrobial resistance genes and mutations in Neisseria gonorrhoeae. Genome Med 2021; 13(1):51.

65. Xiu L, Yuan Q, Li Y, et al. Emergence of ceftriaxone-resistant Neisseria gonorrhoeae strains harbouring a novel mosaic penA gene in China. J Antimicrob Chemother 2020;75(4):907–10.

66. Hadad R, Golparian D, Velicko I, et al. First national genomic epidemiological study of Neisseria gonorrhoeae strains spreading across Sweden in 2016. Front Microbiol 2021;12:820998.

67. Nakayama S, Shimuta K, Furubayashi K, et al. New ceftriaxone- and multidrug-resistant Neisseria gonorrhoeae strain with a novel Mosaic penA gene isolated in Japan. Antimicrobial Agents Chemother 2016;60(7):4339–41.

68. Allan-Blitz LT, Adamson PC, Klausner JD. Resistance-guided therapy for Neisseria gonorrhoeae. Clin Infect Dis 2022. https://doi.org/10.1093/cid/ciac371.

69. Klausner JD, Bristow CC, Soge OO, et al. Resistance-guided treatment of gonorrhea: a prospective clinical study. Clin Infect Dis 2021;73(2):298–303.

70. Fifer H, Saunders J, Soni S, et al. 2018 UK national guideline for the management of infection with Neisseria gonorrhoeae. Int J STD AIDS 2020;31(1):4–15.

71. Hadad R, Cole MJ, Ebeyan S, et al. Evaluation of the SpeeDx ResistancePlus(R) GC and SpeeDx GC 23S 2611 (beta) molecular assays for prediction of antimicrobial resistance/susceptibility to ciprofloxacin and azithromycin in Neisseria gonorrhoeae. J Antimicrob Chemother 2021;76(1):84–90.

72. Abara WE, Llata EL, Schumacher C, et al. Extragenital gonorrhea and chlamydia positivity and the potential for missed extragenital gonorrhea with concurrent urethral chlamydia among men who have sex with men attending sexually

transmitted disease clinics-sexually transmitted disease surveillance network, 2015-2019. Sex Transm Dis 2020;47(6):361–8.

73. Farfour E, Dimi S, Chassany O, et al. Trends in asymptomatic STI among HIV-positive MSM and lessons for systematic screening. PLoS One 2021;16(6): e0250557.

74. Kent CK, Chaw JK, Wong W, et al. Prevalence of rectal, urethral, and pharyngeal chlamydia and gonorrhea detected in 2 clinical settings among men who have sex with men: San Francisco, California, 2003. Clin Infect Dis 2005;41(1):67–74.

75. Marcus JL, Bernstein KT, Kohn RP, et al. Infections missed by urethral-only screening for chlamydia or gonorrhea detection among men who have sex with men. Sex Transm Dis 2011;38(10):922–4.

76. USPSTF, Davidson KW, Barry MJ, et al. Screening for chlamydia and gonorrhea: US preventive services task force recommendation statement. JAMA 2021; 326(10):949–56.

77. Patton ME, Kidd S, Llata E, et al. Extragenital gonorrhea and chlamydia testing and infection among men who have sex with men–STD Surveillance Network, United States, 2010-2012. Clin Infect Dis 2014;58(11):1564–70.

78. Assaf RD, Cunningham NJ, Adamson PC, et al. High proportions of rectal and pharyngeal chlamydia and gonorrhoea cases among cisgender men are missed using current CDC screening recommendations. Sex Transm Infect 2022. https://doi.org/10.1136/sextrans-2021-055361.

79. Barbee LA, Dhanireddy S, Tat SA, et al. Barriers to bacterial sexually transmitted infection testing of HIV-infected men who have sex with men engaged in HIV primary care. Sex Transm Dis 2015;42(10):590–4.

80. Chapman KS, Gadkowski LB, Janelle J, et al. Automated sexual history and self-collection of extragenital chlamydia and gonorrhea improve detection of bacterial sexually transmitted infections in people with HIV. AIDS Patient Care STDS 2022;36(S2):104–10.

81. Lunny C, Taylor D, Hoang L, et al. Self-Collected versus clinician-collected sampling for chlamydia and gonorrhea screening: a systemic review and meta-analysis. PLoS One 2015;10(7):e0132776.

82. Moncada J, Schachter J, Liska S, et al. Evaluation of self-collected glans and rectal swabs from men who have sex with men for detection of Chlamydia trachomatis and Neisseria gonorrhoeae by use of nucleic acid amplification tests. J Clin Microbiol 2009;47(6):1657–62.

83. Wilson JD, Wallace HE, Loftus-Keeling M, et al. Swab-yourself Trial With Economic Monitoring and Testing for Infections Collectively (SYSTEMATIC): part 1. A diagnostic accuracy and cost-effectiveness study comparing clinician-taken vs self-taken rectal and pharyngeal samples for the diagnosis of gonorrhea and chlamydia. Clin Infect Dis 2021;73(9):e3172–80.

84. Sharma A, Gandhi M, Sallabank G, et al. Perceptions and experiences of returning self-collected specimens for HIV, bacterial STI and potential PrEP adherence testing among sexual minority men in the United States. AIDS Behav 2022. https://doi.org/10.1007/s10461-022-03846-8.

85. Aboud L, Xu Y, Chow EPF, et al. Diagnostic accuracy of pooling urine, anorectal, and oropharyngeal specimens for the detection of Chlamydia trachomatis and Neisseria gonorrhoeae: a systematic review and meta-analysis. BMC Med 2021;19(1):285.

86. Golden MR, Whittington WL, Handsfield HH, et al. Effect of expedited treatment of sex partners on recurrent or persistent gonorrhea or chlamydial infection. N Engl J Med 2005;352(7):676–85.

87. Kissinger P, Mohammed H, Richardson-Alston G, et al. Patient-delivered partner treatment for male urethritis: a randomized, controlled trial. Clin Infect Dis 2005; 41(5):623–9.
88. Gift TL, Kissinger P, Mohammed H, et al. The cost and cost-effectiveness of expedited partner therapy compared with standard partner referral for the treatment of chlamydia or gonorrhea. Sex Transm Dis 2011;38(11):1067–73.
89. Stenger MR, Kerani RP, Bauer HM, et al. Patient-reported expedited partner therapy for gonorrhea in the United States: findings of the STD surveillance network 2010-2012. Sex Transm Dis 2015;42(9):470–4.
90. Nelson T, Nandwani J, Johnson D. Gonorrhea and chlamydia cases are rising in the United States: expedited partner therapy might help. Sex Transm Dis 2022; 49(1):e1–3.
91. Clark JL, Segura ER, Oldenburg CE, et al. Expedited partner therapy (EPT) increases the frequency of partner notification among MSM in Lima, Peru: a pilot randomized controlled trial. BMC Med 2017;15(1):94.
92. Weiss KM, Jones JS, Katz DA, et al. Epidemiological impact of expedited partner therapy for men who have sex with men: a modeling study. Sex Transm Dis 2019;46(11):697–705.
93. Craig AP, Gray RT, Edwards JL, et al. The potential impact of vaccination on the prevalence of gonorrhea. Vaccine 2015;33(36):4520–5.
94. Hui BB, Padeniya TN, Rebuli N, et al. A gonococcal vaccine has the potential to rapidly reduce the incidence of Neisseria gonorrhoeae infection among urban men who have sex with men. J Infect Dis 2022;225(6):983–93.
95. Petousis-Harris H, Paynter J, Morgan J, et al. Effectiveness of a group B outer membrane vesicle meningococcal vaccine against gonorrhoea in New Zealand: a retrospective case-control study. Lancet 2017;390(10102):1603–10.
96. Abara WE, Bernstein KT, Lewis FMT, et al. Effectiveness of a serogroup B outer membrane vesicle meningococcal vaccine against gonorrhoea: a retrospective observational study. Lancet Infect Dis 2022;22(7):1021–9.
97. Wang B, Giles L, Andraweera P, et al. Effectiveness and impact of the 4CMenB vaccine against invasive serogroup B meningococcal disease and gonorrhoea in an infant, child, and adolescent programme: an observational cohort and case-control study. Lancet Infect Dis 2022;22(7):1011–20.
98. Bolan RK, Beymer MR, Weiss RE, et al. Doxycycline prophylaxis to reduce incident syphilis among HIV-infected men who have sex with men who continue to engage in high-risk sex: a randomized, controlled pilot study. Sex Transm Dis 2015;42(2):98–103.
99. Molina JM, Charreau I, Chidiac C, et al. Post-exposure prophylaxis with doxycycline to prevent sexually transmitted infections in men who have sex with men: an open-label randomised substudy of the ANRS IPERGAY trial. Lancet Infect Dis 2018;18(3):308–17.
100. Leutkemeyer A, Dombrowski J, Cohen S, et al. Doxycycline post-exposure prophylaxis for STI prevention among MSM and transgender women on HIV PrEP or living with HIV: high efficacy to reduce incident STI's in a randomized trial. 2022. https://programme.aids2022.org/Abstract/Abstract/?abstractid=13231. at AIDS 2022 in Montreal, Canada, July 29 to August 2, 2022.

Trichomoniasis

Olivia T. Van Gerwen, MD, MPH[a],*, Skye A. Opsteen[b],
Keonte J. Graves, MS[a], Christina A. Muzny, MD, MSPH[a]

KEYWORDS

- *Trichomonas vaginalis* • Trichomoniasis • Sexually transmitted infection
- Women's health • Vaginitis

KEY POINTS

- *T. vaginalis* is a prevalent, yet relatively understudied, sexually transmitted infection that is associated with significant adverse sexual and reproductive health outcomes for both men and women.
- *T. vaginalis* is most prevalent among women and Black individuals.
- Options for *T. vaginalis* diagnostics have grown in the last decade, with multiple point-of-care and highly sensitive and specific nucleic acid amplification tests now available.
- Treatment options for trichomoniasis are generally limited to 5-nitroimidazoles, including metronidazole, tinidazole, and secnidazole.
- Further studies are needed to determine the optimal treatment regimen among men.

INTRODUCTION

Approximately 20% of the US population has a sexually transmitted infection (STI) at any given time. The incidence of trichomoniasis, chlamydia, syphilis, and genital herpes has continually increased each year between 2010 and 2019.[1] Trichomoniasis, caused by the parasitic pathogen *T. vaginalis*, is the most common nonviral STI.[2] Unlike other common STIs such as chlamydia and gonorrhea, *T. vaginalis* is not a reportable disease in any location worldwide[3]; thus epidemiologic data related to this infection are from population and clinic-based studies. According to recent estimates, over 1 million people in the United States are infected with *T. vaginalis* each year.[4] Many individuals infected with *T. vaginalis* remain asymptomatic, facilitating its transmission.[5] In addition, almost 75% of male sexual partners of infected women can also be infected, demonstrating a high transmission rate.[6] *T. vaginalis* is associated with multiple adverse sexual and reproductive health outcomes in both women and men including increased rates of adverse birth outcomes (low birth weight, preterm birth, and pre-labor rupture of membranes) as well as increased risk of acquisition of human

[a] Division of Infectious Diseases, University of Alabama at Birmingham, 703 19th Street South, ZRB 218A, Birmingham, AL 35294, USA; [b] Heersink School of Medicine, University of Alabama at Birmingham, Birmingham, AL, USA
* Corresponding author.
E-mail address: oliviavangerwen@uabmc.edu
Twitter: @libbyvangerwen (O.T.V.G.)

Infect Dis Clin N Am 37 (2023) 245–265
https://doi.org/10.1016/j.idc.2023.02.001
0891-5520/23/© 2023 Elsevier Inc. All rights reserved.

id.theclinics.com

immunodeficiency virus (HIV) and other STIs, pelvic inflammatory disease (PID), infertility, and cervical cancer.[7-15] The most common clinical presentation among those with symptoms is vaginitis in women and urethritis in men. Although *T. vaginalis* is a common STI and can have detrimental effects, there are currently no routine screening recommendations for any population except women living with HIV.[16] In addition, the traditional diagnostic methods have low sensitivity, although multiple recent advances have been made in this area including the advent of highly sensitive and specific nucleic acid amplification tests (NAATs), including several that can be done on-demand or as point-of-care (POC) tests.[17-24] This review provides an update on the epidemiology, pathogenesis, and clinical significance of trichomoniasis as well as discusses the current approaches to diagnosis and treatment of this common STI.

EPIDEMIOLOGY

Based on data from the World Health Organization (WHO), the most recent prevalence estimates of trichomoniasis in women and men were 5.3% and 0.6%, respectively, with an estimated incidence of 156 million cases worldwide.[2] The most accurate US prevalence data in women and men ages 18 to 59 years come from the 2013 to 2014 cycle of the National Health and Nutrition Examination survey (NHANES), published in 2018.[25] *T. vaginalis* prevalence in this NHANES cohort was 1.8% among women and 0.5% among men, all of whom were screened using the Hologic Aptima *T. vaginalis* NAAT test on urine specimens.[25] In the NHANES cohort, *T. vaginalis* infection was associated with older age, lower educational level, lower socioeconomic status, and having multiple sexual partners.[25] Regarding older age and *T. vaginalis* infection, a recent systemic review of the literature also supports this association. Lindrose and colleagues investigated the prevalence and incidence of trichomoniasis among US adults ≥45 years. They found that the prevalence of *T. vaginalis* in this age group ranged from 0.2% to 21.4% among participants in the 20 articles included in their review, with several studies finding increased risk among older versus younger age groups.[26] The highest prevalence of *T. vaginalis* was seen among individuals seeking diagnostic testing for STIs. These data highlight the need for sexual health education and consideration of testing for *T. vaginalis* among older adults, if indicated.

T. vaginalis also disproportionately affects Black individuals. The prevalence of *T. vaginalis* among Black women and men in the US NHANES study was 6.8% compared with 0.4% among other racial and ethnic groups.[25] A recent review of *T. vaginalis* in Black Americans found compelling evidence that structural racism has generated and maintained the significant racial disparity regarding this STI among the Black community, arguing that current efforts to reduce its prevalence have failed globally, especially in the United States. This is compounded by a failure of strategies to control this infection including a lack of public awareness, noncompliance with prophylactic use of protective barrier methods, inconsistent STI testing, lack of a prophylactic *T. vaginalis* vaccine, and lack of mandatory national and global surveillance programs.[27] The investigators concluded that the critical strategies must be incorporated to reduce the negative burden of *T. vaginalis* infection on the Black community, including cultural competence training among health care providers, social workers, and sexual health educators as well as access to high-quality clinical services that serve minority communities, particularly focusing on Black women. Overall, multiple demographic and socioeconomic factors such as age, race, educational level, and income play a significant role in the epidemiology of trichomoniasis in the United States and globally.[27]

As it has traditionally been viewed as a benign infection in men, few studies have explored the epidemiology of trichomoniasis among this population.[28] As already noted, the prevalence of trichomoniasis is notably lower among men compared with women. In theory, however, prevalence should be similar between these two groups given that trichomoniasis is a highly transmissible STI. One explanation for this discrepancy is that spontaneous resolution of *T. vaginalis* infection may occur in some men, although the parasite and host factors influencing this phenomenon are not well understood.[29,30] The exact frequency at which this occurs is also not clear, but several small studies have reported spontaneous resolution in 36% to 69% of cases of *T. vaginalis* infection in men.[29–31]

Similar to women, a significant racial disparity regarding *T. vaginalis* infection also exists among men, with the US NHANES data finding Black men to be seven times more likely to be infected with *T. vaginalis* than White men.[32] This study also found higher rates of infection among men who smoked, had herpes simplex virus type-2 (HSV-2) infection, and reported high numbers of lifetime sexual partners.[32]

To date, most of the *T. vaginalis* research has focused on cisgender women. There is a need for further epidemiologic studies exploring the impact of trichomoniasis on gender diverse populations. A recent systematic review summarized HIV and STI prevalence among transgender individuals and found that there were no studies reporting the prevalence of trichomoniasis in this population.[33] Given the varied sexual identities and practices as well as diverse genital anatomy that is represented in this population, this is a clear gap in the literature which should be investigated further.

PATHOGENESIS

Humans are the only known hosts for *T. vaginalis*. The parasite is predominately spread through sexual contact from an infected to an uninfected person. *T. vaginalis* has a trophozoite stage where it actively grows and feeds in preparation for replication.[34] It subsequently undergoes replication through longitudinal binary fission in the lower genital tract of women (vaginal, urethra, and endocervix) and the urethra and prostate of men. The average incubation period is between 5 and 28 days; however, infection can persist over longer periods of time.[35] *T. vaginalis* does not exist in a cyst form and does not survive well in the environment, although it has been identified outside the human body in warm and wet locations (i.e., moist towels) for greater than 3 hours.[36]

T. vaginalis infects squamous epithelial cells of the human genital tract through membrane surface glycolipids and glycoproteins which attach to surface proteins on host genital epithelial cells.[37,38] This attachment, in combination with the release of proteases that contribute to cytoadherence, mucous membrane degradation, and cytotoxicity, elicits a host immune response.[39] This host immune response includes increased levels of cytokines including interleukin (IL)-1b, IL-6, IL-8, IL-17, IL-22, IL-23, regulated and normal T cell expressed and secreted protein, C–C motif chemokine ligand 2, interferon-β, macrophage inflammatory protein-3α, and tumor necrosis factor.[37,38,40] The same proteases used for cytoadherence and break down of mucous membranes can also be used to aid in the evasion of host immune defenses.[39]

T. vaginalis virus (TVV, a double-stranded RNA virus) and *Mycoplasma hominis* (bacterial pathogen) have also been known to infect *T. vaginalis*.[41] Some studies have reported associations between the presence of TVV in *T. vaginalis* and the inflammatory response in the human host, as well as increased susceptibility of *T. vaginalis* to metronidazole (MTZ), one of the 5-nitroimidazoles commonly used to treat this infection.[40] The presence of specific TVV subspecies (TVV1 and TVV2) was associated with severity of symptoms in one study.[42] In contrast, in a study of 355 US *T. vaginalis* isolates from women participating in a clinical trial, of which 40% were positive for TVV, there were no associations between TVV positivity and genital symptoms, repeat infections, or MTZ resistance, suggesting that TVV may be commensal to *T. vaginalis*.[43] In contrast, the presence of *M. hominis* in *T. vaginalis* has been associated with increased MTZ resistance and decreased levels of genes involved in resistance mechanisms.[44]

METHODS OF TRANSMISSION

Penile–vaginal sexual contact is the primary method in which *T. vaginalis* is transmitted, with partner studies in the 1950s and 1960s originally demonstrating this phenomenon.[36,45] Given its propensity to infect vaginal mucosal tissue, digital sexual activity involving the vagina, including mutual masturbation between women, can also transmit trichomoniasis.[46] Nonsexual transmission is uncommon, but several modes have been described. One study in Zambia among adolescent girls ages 13 to 16 years found that the overall prevalence of trichomoniasis among 397 self-reported virgins was 24.7%. In multivariate analyses in this study, borderline significant associations were found between trichomoniasis and the use of pit latrines or bushes instead of toilets as well as suboptimal bathing conditions including inconsistent soap use and shared bathing water.[47] Another proposed mechanism of nonsexual transmission is through the use of infected fomites such as shared sex toys and wet washcloths, the latter of which is supported by a study demonstrating transmission of trichomoniasis among one female–female sexual partnership using shared washcloths following receptive oral sex.[48] Iatrogenic transmission of trichomoniasis has also been described, though this is very rare and typically occurs in low-resource settings where adequate hand hygiene among practitioners is not always possible. For example, one case from the Gambia involved a traditional healer transmitting trichomoniasis to a female patient via an ungloved digital vaginal examination.[49]

CLINICAL SIGNIFICANCE
Women

Despite its reputation as a clinically minor infection, *T. vaginalis* can have a devastating impact on the sexual and reproductive health of women.[50] *T. vaginalis* has been associated with multiple adverse health outcomes including adverse birth outcomes (discussed in the section on trichomoniasis and pregnancy),[8] increased risk of HIV and other STI acquisition,[11–13] PID,[14] infertility,[15] and cervical cancer.[9] PID can manifest in a variety of ways, including endometritis, salpingitis, tubo-ovarian abscess, and pelvic peritonitis. In recent years, there are mounting data implicating *T vaginalis* as a potential pathogenic organism in PID,[14,51] especially among women coinfected with viral pathogens such as HIV and HSV-2.[10,52] If left untreated, PID can result in infertility, higher risk for ectopic pregnancy, and chronic pelvic pain.[53,54]

A recent systematic review by Zhang and colleagues summarized findings in support of a correlation between *T vaginalis* infection and infertility.[15] The proposed mechanisms for *T. vaginalis*-induced infertility in women include host immune system activation leading to uterine and fallopian tube epithelial cell damage and inflammation[55,56] as well as direct damage to oocytes and blockage of ovulation.[55,57]

Women with *T. vaginalis* infection are also at increased risk of cervical cancer, as was demonstrated by a 2018 meta-analysis including 7715 cases and 67,598 controls from 17 studies finding a significant association between these two entities.[9] The underlying pathophysiological explanation for this relationship is not well understood. This meta-analysis and other studies have proposed that this is due in part to increased coinfection rates with high-risk HPV types and *T. vaginalis* as well as an increased risk of HIV/STI acquisition.[9,58–62]

Men

Similar findings of increased risk of HIV/STI acquisition and infertility have been noted in T. vaginalis-infected men.[11,15,63,64] The proposed mechanism for infertility in men is impairment of sperm motility via attachment to sperm glycoproteins, which can induce phagocytosis[56] and/or interfere with horizontal sperm movement,[63] as well as direct damage and destruction of sperm cells.[55,64] T. vaginalis infection has also been associated with prostate cancer, but the studies reporting this relationship are not conclusive.[65–70] Some studies have proposed that T. vaginalis infection can induce prostate epithelial cell proliferation[66] and chronic inflammation,[71] and one study found that one-third of benign prostate hyperplasia (BPH) patients had a positive polymerase chain reaction test for T. vaginalis.[67] In addition, Sutcliffe and colleagues observed that serologic evidence of previous .T vaginalis infection was associated with an increased risk of prostate cancer.[71] However, others have observed no relationship between T. vaginalis and prostate cancer.[68,69] A more recent study by Yang and colleagues explored the association between trichomoniasis and BPH, prostate cancer, and bladder cancer and observed that trichomoniasis was associated with both BPH and prostate cancer.[70] In a meta-analysis of six studies, it was shown that the risk of prostate cancer was 1.17 fold higher in men with previous T. vaginalis exposure; however, this was not statistically significant.[68] The lack of adequate studies and/or heterogeneity concerns may have biased the authors' deductions about the impact of T. vaginalis on the outcome in this meta-analysis. Thus, whether T. vaginalis infection is a cause of prostate cancer remains controversial, and additional research on this topic is needed.

Extragenital sequelae have been rarely observed in men with trichomoniasis, such as rectal trichomoniasis and pharyngitis, but this is extremely uncommon and routine screening of these locations is not recommended.[72,73]

TRICHOMONIASIS AND PREGNANCY

As there is a considerable burden of trichomoniasis in women of childbearing potential,[2] the consequences of this STI in pregnant women are important to consider. Unfortunately, this STI has been understudied in pregnant women; thus, the epidemiologic data on incidence and prevalence estimates are limited. Recent WHO prevalence estimates on trichomoniasis do not report on the subset of pregnant women captured in the studies included in their systematic review.[2] Prevalence estimates of the burden of T. vaginalis infection among pregnant women in the United States are also limited as pregnant women were not represented in the recent NHANES study.[25] Thus, the available data are mainly from observational studies. One systematic review from 2016, which included only low- to middle-income countries, estimated a wide T. vaginalis prevalence range from 3.9% in Latin America to 24.6% in Southern Africa among pregnant women, after adjusting for age, test, and health care setting.[74] Among another study of 1821 US pregnant women living with HIV, T. vaginalis prevalence was estimated to be 14.5%; however, 30.3% of the women in this cohort were not tested for T. vaginalis.[75] Similarly, a 20% prevalence of T. vaginalis was noted in one South African cohort of pregnant women with HIV.[76] The high prevalence of T. vaginalis in both of these cohorts of pregnant women living with HIV underscores the importance of screening guideline adherence in this population of women.

Untreated trichomoniasis in pregnancy is not without consequence. A 2021 systematic review and meta-analysis, which included greater than 80,000 pregnant women and 19 studies worldwide, demonstrated significant associations between T. vaginalis and preterm delivery, pre-labor rupture of membranes, and delivery of low birth weight infants.[8] One potential pathophysiological mechanism of preterm delivery and pre-labor rupture of membranes in women with *T. vaginalis* relates to the postinfection maternal innate immune inflammatory response prompting these outcomes via early cervical ripening and dilation.[77] The mechanisms of low birth weight in the setting of *T. vaginalis* may be related to the infection inducing intrauterine inflammation that can impede placental blood flow.[78] Direct causal links between infection with *T. vaginalis* and these adverse birth outcomes are difficult to ascertain though, as some studies included in this systematic review and meta-analysis did not include data on coinfection with bacterial vaginosis (BV) and other STIs. Thus, it is unknown if coinfection confounds the effect of *T. vaginalis* on perinatal morbidity or if BV and/or other STIs could also be part of the causal pathway between trichomoniasis and adverse birth outcomes. Additional studies are needed to further clarify this important relationship.

CLINICAL PRESENTATION

Asymptomatic infection with *T. vaginalis* is common, more so among men than women. In men, *T. vaginalis* parasite burden is much lower compared with women.[28] Among symptomatic men, the most common presentation is urethritis, which includes dysuria and/or clear or mucopurulent urethral discharge.[28] As previously mentioned, spontaneous resolution of infection without treatment has been described in men,[29,30] but the exact frequency at which this occurs is unknown. If left untreated, however, some men can experience symptoms of prostatitis or epididymitis.[28,79,80] There have also been occasional case reports of rectal *T. vaginalis* infection leading to proctitis among men who have sex with men[81]; however, this is exceedingly rare and routine screening in this context is not recommended.[16]

Women with trichomoniasis are more frequently symptomatic than men. One US study found that women presenting with vaginal symptoms had higher rates of *T. vaginalis* infection (26%) compared with asymptomatic women who were screened for this infection (6.5%).[82] Most commonly, symptomatic women present with symptoms of vaginitis, including copious yellow-green frothy vaginal discharge, vaginal odor, and vulvovaginal irritation. Symptomatic women with *T vaginalis* may also note a wide range of additional symptoms including genital pruritus, dysuria, and dyspareunia. On physical examination, the characteristic discharge of trichomoniasis may be noted in the vaginal vault and, if the cervix is adequately visualized, may have a strawberry-like appearance ("colpitis macularis"); however, this is present in less than 5% of women.[83] As mentioned earlier, PID has been associated with trichomoniasis, so while it is not the most common presentation, *T. vaginalis* diagnostic testing should be performed in women presenting with PID.[51]

DIAGNOSIS

Table 1 details the current diagnostic testing options available for *T. vaginalis*. Traditionally, trichomoniasis has been diagnosed using POC methods, the most common of which is wet mount microscopy of vaginal secretions. After preparation of a wet mount slide, motile trichomonads can be visualized (**Fig. 1**A and B). The specificity of this finding is 100%, although the sensitivity is low at 44% to 68%.[84] This test should also be performed within 10 to 20 minutes of specimen collection to avoid the trichomonads losing viability, which increases the likelihood of a false-negative test. In addition, the requirement of a microscope and an experienced microscopist pose a challenge for diagnosing trichomoniasis in low-resource settings with this method. In recent years, other POC tests that do not require microscopy have become

Table 1
Diagnostic tests for *T. vaginalis*

Test	Population	Specimen Type	Sensitivity (Sens) and Specificity (Spec)	Time to Results	Complexity, Limitations, Other Comments
Wet mount microscopy[84]	Women	Women: vaginal secretions	Sens: 44%–68% Spec: 100%	<10 min (POC)	CLIA waived. Must be performed immediately after specimen collection Requires microscope and training
OSOM rapid test[84]	Symptomatic women	Women: vaginal secretions	Sens: 82%–95% Spec: 97%–100%	<10 min (POC)	CLIA waived. Detects antigen. No instrumentation needed.
InPouch *T vaginalis* culture system[87]	Men and women	Men: urethral specimens, urine sediment, and semen[a] Women: vaginal specimens	Men: Sens: 50%–80% Spec: 100% Women: Sens: 75%–96% Spec: 100%	5–7 d	Requires incubation at 37°C, microscope, and training. CLIA moderately complex test
Hologic Aptima NAAT[20]	Women	Women: endocervical, vaginal, urine, and pap smear specimens (preserved in PreservCyt Solutions)	Women: Sens: 88%–100% Spec 98%–100%	5.5 h	CLIA high complexity test. Requires Panther, Viper, or Tigris instrumentation.
Becton Dickinson ProbeTec Qx NAAT[21]	Women	Women: endocervical vaginal, and urine specimens	Sens: 98%–100% Spec: 98%–100%	<8 h	CLIA high complexity. Requires Viper system. Off market.
Becton Dickinson (BD) Max CT/GC/TV2 NAAT[23]	Men and women	Men: urine Women: vaginal specimens and urine	Men: Sens: 81.1%–100% Spec: 98.7%–100% Women Sens: 89.8%–99.7% Spec: 98.1%–99.5%	3.5 h	CLIA high complexity test. Requires BD Max system.

(continued on next page)

Table 1
(continued)

Test	Population	Specimen Type	Sensitivity (Sens) and Specificity (Spec)	Time to Results	Complexity, Limitations, Other Comments
Cepheid GeneXpert NAAT[18]	Men and women	Men: urine Women: endocervical and vaginal specimens, urine	Men: Sens: 97.2%–99.9% Spec: 97.2%–99.9% Women: Sens: 99.5%–100% Spec: 99.4%–99.9%	On demand results in 40–63 min	CLIA moderately complex.
Solana Trichomonas assay[88]	Women	Women: vaginal and urine specimens	Sens/Spec: > 98% for vaginal samples, > 92% for urine samples	~40 min	Not CLIA waived. Requires some instrumentation.
AmpliVue Trichomonas assay[19]	Women	Women: vaginal specimens	Sens: 90.7% Spec: 98.9%	~45 min	Not CLIA waived. Requires some instrumentation.
Roche cobas MG/TV NAAT[22]	Men and women	Men: penile-meatal specimens and urine Women: endocervical and vaginal specimens	Men: Sens: 77.2%–100% Spec: 97.2%–99.9% Women: Sens: 96.4%–100% Spec: 96.5%–98.8%	5 h	CLIA high complexity test. For use on Cobas 6800/ 8800 systems.
Visby GC/CT/TV NAAT[24]	Women	Women: vaginal specimens	Sens: 99.2% Spec: 96.9%	<30 min (POC)	CLIA waived. Requires electrical outlet.
Abbott Alinity m STI assay[89]	Women	Women: endocervical, vaginal, pap smear, and urine specimens		<2 h	CLIA high complexity.

Abbreviations: CLIA, clinical laboratory improvement amendments; CT, *Chlamydia trachomatis*; GC, *Neisseria gonorrhoeae*; MG, *Mycoplasma genitalium*; NAAT, nucleic acid amplification test; POC, point of care; STI, sexually transmitted infection; TV, *T vaginalis*.

[a] Inoculate the *T vaginalis* culture with multiple male specimens, if possible, to increase likelihood of a positive result.

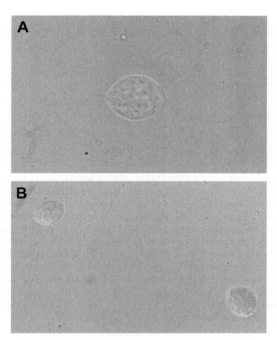

Fig. 1. (*A*) Wet mount microscopy showing a motile trichomonad with a flagellum. (*B*) Wet mount microscopy showing two motile trichomonads.

available. The OSOM rapid test (Sekisui Diagnostics, California) uses antibodies to detect protein antigens of *T. vaginalis* in vaginal secretion specimens. A positive test demonstrates the binding of antibodies to *T. vaginalis* antigens and results in a blue line on the test strip. However, the OSOM rapid test should mainly be used in symptomatic women or contacts to *T. vaginalis*. This test yields results in less than 10 minutes and has a sensitivity of 82% to 95% and specificity 97% to 100%, compared with wet mount and culture.[84]

For many years, before the advent of highly sensitive and specific NAATs, *T. vaginalis* culture was the gold standard for diagnosis (see **Fig. 1**). The InPouch *T. vaginalis* culture system (BioMed Diagnostics, White City, OR) is the most commonly used culture method and has a sensitivity of 44% to 81% and specificity of 100%.[84,85] Although this method has better sensitivity than wet mount and is highly specific, there are several challenges. First, the culture media should be inoculated with the genital specimen(s) within 1 hour of collection.[84] *T. vaginalis* culture can be performed on specimens from both women (vaginal swabs) and men (urethral swabs, urine sediment, semen; multiple specimens are recommended in men to increase yield).[84] Second, an inoculated InPouch culture system must be immediately incubated at 37°C and specimens must be read multiple times over several days, making this a Clinical Laboratory Improvement Amendments (CLIA) moderately complex test.[86,87] Culture is advantageous, however, as drug susceptibility testing to 5-nitroimidazole medications (**Fig. 2**) can be performed on positive specimens. This is especially useful in cases of persistent/resistant *T. vaginalis* infection.

A variety of molecular diagnostic tests have become available in the past decade for *T. vaginalis* diagnosis. The sensitivity of these molecular assays is far superior to wet mount microscopy and culture. Most recently, Visby has released an instrument-free

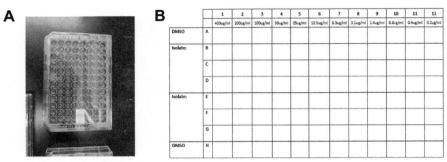

Fig. 2. *The 5-nitroimidazole drug susceptibility testing.* (*A*) 96-well plate used for 5-nitroimidazole drug susceptibility testing. (*B*) Graphical representation of a portion of the 96-well plate for the 5-nitroimidazole drug susceptibility testing. Rows A and H are DMSO control lanes, whereas lanes B–G contain the 5-nitroimdazoles tested for specific *T. vaginalis* isolates tested in triplicates. The 50 μL of media is initially added to each well. Next, 50 μL of drug/media is added to column 1 rows B–G, whereas 50 μL of DMSO/media are added to A and H and then serially diluted from left to right (column 1 [400 μg/mL] to column 12 [0.2 μg/mL]). The 150 μL of the *T. vaginalis* sample is added to each well from the lowest concentration to the highest (column 12 [0.2 μg/mL] to column 1 [400 μg/mL]). The plates are then incubated for 48 to 52 hours before being read on an inverted microscope. MLC is determined when no motile *T. vaginalis* is observed for all three wells with the same concentration. DMSO, dimethyl sulfoxide; MLC, minimum lethal concentration.

molecular assay which can be used at the POC and yields results in 25 minutes.[24] This test can be performed on self-collected vaginal specimens and uses a one-time use handheld cartridge.

Two molecular amplified assays are also available for additional POC *T. vaginalis* diagnostics: the Solana Trichomonas assay (Quidel, San Diego, CA)[88] and AmpliVue Trichomonas assay (Quidel, San Diego, CA).[19] The Solana Trichomonas assay qualitatively detects *T. vaginalis* with results on demand in less than 40 minutes. It is FDA-approved for use on female vaginal and urine specimens from asymptomatic and symptomatic women. This assay requires a testing instrument to run samples; therefore, an upfront investment is required, which could impact its cost-effectiveness in some settings. The AmpliVue Trichomonas assay works in a similar way to the Solana assay but can be performed using a small handheld cartridge instead of a testing platform. AmpliVue results are available within 45 to 50 minutes. Both assays are highly sensitive and specific. Finally, the Cepheid GeneXpert *T. vaginalis* NAAT assay can provide on-demand results in 40 to 63 minutes and can be performed on a small device that can fit on a benchtop in a clinic.[18]

In addition to POC and on-demand molecular diagnostic tests for *T. vaginalis*, there are several additional NAAT tests that require larger instruments for specimen analysis; thus, they are not able to be used at the POC. These include the Hologic Aptima *T vaginalis* NAAT assay, the Becton Dickinson (BD) ProbeTec Qx *T. vaginalis* NAAT assay, the BD Max CT/GC/TV2 NAAT assay, the Roche cobas MG/TV NAAT assay, and the Abbott Alinity m STI assay (including *T. vaginalis* NAAT testing).[18,20–23,89]

TREATMENT

The 5-nitroimidazole medications are the mainstay of treatment for trichomoniasis as they are the only class of antimicrobials with demonstrated in vitro anti-trichomonacidal activity.[90] This drug class includes medications such as MTZ, tinidazole (TDZ), and secnidazole (SEC). As detailed in the 2021 Centers for Disease Control and Prevention (CDC) STI treatment guidelines, the recommended treatment of uncomplicated urogenital trichomoniasis for both men and women is MTZ; however, for the first time, dosing and duration of treatment differ between genders.[16] For women, a 7-day course of oral MTZ 500 mg twice daily is now the recommended treatment regimen, as clinical trial data suggest that the single-dose oral 2-g MTZ treatment is suboptimal. This was shown in a multicenter randomized controlled trial (RCT) among women in the United States without HIV infection which directly compared the multidose oral MTZ regimen to the single-dose oral MTZ regimen. Those who received the multidose oral MTZ regimen were significantly less likely to retest positive for *T. vaginalis* at the 1 month test-of-cure (TOC) visit (11%) than women who received the single-dose therapy (19%); *P* < .0001.[91] The multidose oral MTZ regimen was also shown to be more highly efficacious among women living with HIV in an earlier RCT[92,93]; treatment of trichomoniasis among women with HIV has also been shown to reduce vaginal HIV-1 shedding.[7]

For men with *T. vaginalis*, the recommended treatment remains the single-dose oral 2-g MTZ. This is due to the lack of clinical trial data directly comparing oral single-dose MTZ and oral multidose MTZ regimens in men.

A single oral dose of 2-g TDZ is an alternative regimen for the treatment of uncomplicated trichomoniasis in women and men in the 2021 CDC STI Treatment Guidelines.[16] As the publication of those guidelines, new data have been published regarding a single dose of oral 2-g SEC being an additional option for treating trichomoniasis in women. SEC is a second-generation 5-nitroimidazole with a longer half-life (17–19 hours) than MTZ (7–8 hours) and TDZ (11–12 hours).[94] SEC is available in a granular formulation that must be administered to patients with a serving of either unsweetened apple sauce, pudding, or yogurt. A 2021 RCT including 147 women with trichomoniasis at 10 clinical sites across the United States demonstrated a microbiologic cure rate of 92.2% among women at the 6 to 12 day TOC receiving the single oral 2-g dose of SEC when compared with women receiving placebo (1.5%); *P* < .001.[95] SEC has since been FDA approved for *T. vaginalis* treatment in adolescent and adult women and men ages $\geq$ 12 years. Although not in the current CDC or ACOG guidelines, these data support SEC as an alternative treatment for trichomoniasis in both women and men.[95]

Current recommendations for the treatment of trichomoniasis in pregnant women are the same as those for nonpregnant women (i.e., multidose oral MTZ 500 mg twice daily for 7 days is the recommended treatment).[16] The mainstay of *T. vaginalis* treatment is MTZ, which crosses the placenta. Despite this fact, there are ample data to suggest that this medication poses minimal risk to the fetus in all trimesters of pregnancy and has no known teratogenic effects.[96,97] The 2021 CDC STI Treatment Guidelines recommend testing and treatment of all symptomatic pregnant women for *T. vaginalis*, in addition to counseling on partner treatment and condom use.[16] Data are limited regarding the use of TDZ in pregnancy, although animal data have demonstrated potential risks to a fetus.[98] Therefore, TDZ should be avoided for the treatment of *T. vaginalis* in pregnant women.[16,98] Limited data are available on the use of SEC in pregnant women; however, there is no evidence of adverse developmental outcomes in animal studies.[94]

For men, there have been no rigorous clinical trials directly comparing the efficacy of the multidose and single-dose oral MTZ regimens. Thus, the single-dose oral 2-g MTZ remains the recommended treatment regimen for *T. vaginalis* in men. There are data, however, suggesting that this single-dose regimen may be inadequate in men. One study found that treatment with the single-dose 2-g MTZ regimen in men resulted in only 77.1% microbiological efficacy.[99] Similar to recommendations for women, a single dose of oral 2-g TDZ is recommended as an alternative regimen.[16] TDZ has also been inadequately studied in men, but does have better absorption in the prostate and other male genital tissues compared with MTZ.[100,101] The few studies that have been conducted in men have demonstrated that TDZ may have similar efficacy to MTZ in the treatment of *T. vaginalis*, but these were small studies and more data are needed.[102,103] Similarly, there are few studies investigating the efficacy of SEC for the treatment of *T. vaginalis* in men, though these studies suggest that SEC may also be a good alternative to oral MTZ.[104–106] An RCT is needed to determine the optimal treatment regimen for men with trichomoniasis.

Persistent infection with trichomoniasis is not uncommon, especially given the proclivity of the parasite to reinfect a person if their partner was not treated. Thus, when treating patients for trichomoniasis, counseling on partner treatment and consistent condom use at the completion of therapy (discussed below) is essential. Once reinfection has been excluded in the setting of treatment failure, consideration should be given to antimicrobial resistance against 5-nitroimidazoles. Collection of a *T vaginalis* culture and performing 5-nitroimidazole resistance testing can be a helpful in managing these difficult cases (see **Fig. 2**). Resistance testing is currently available through the CDC and can be requested at the following website: https://www.cdc.gov/laboratory/specimen-submission/detail.html?CDCTestCode=CDC-10239 [16] as well as some local laboratories in the United States. While awaiting susceptibility testing results, clinicians can consider longer courses of treatment with higher doses than standard therapies with MTZ or TDZ.[16] Although the optimal regimen for treating resistant or persistent trichomoniasis infection has not be established, regimens such as MTZ or TDZ 2-g orally daily for 7 days have been used successfully in some cases. In the case that the 7-day MTZ or TDZ 2-g oral regimen fails, combining longer courses of high-dose oral TDZ 2 to 3 g daily in divided doses with intravaginal medications has also had successful results.[107,108] Two such regimens include (1) oral TDZ 1-g three times daily plus intravaginal paromomycin (4 g of 6.25% vaginal cream nightly, both for 14 days) or (2) oral TDZ 2 to 3 g daily in divided doses plus intravaginal TDZ 500 mg twice daily for 14 days.[109,110] It is important to note that both intravaginal paromomycin and intravaginal TDZ must be formulated at a compounding pharmacy. Topical use of intravaginal paromomycin cream can result in painful vulvar ulcers that are self-limited and resolve once treatment is discontinued. The use of lubricating jelly to the vulva before use has been successful in preventing the development of these ulcers in some women.[111]

Clinical data are limited regarding the efficacy in SEC as a treatment option for persistent or resistant trichomoniasis, but several studies suggest that SEC has better in vitro trichomonacidal activity compared with MTZ.[90,112] In one recent single-patient, investigator-initiated protocol, an extended 14-day course of 2-g oral SEC in combination with intravaginal boric acid 600 mg twice daily was successful in curing a case of persistent 5-nitroimidazole-resistant *T. vaginalis* infection.[113] Although there is little precedent for extended durations of oral SEC for persistent/resistant *T. vaginalis* infection, it was not considered excessively frequent based on its pharmacokinetics profile. The patient reported dysgeusia while on this treatment regimen, which resolved after therapy was completed. Additional in vivo data on clinical outcomes of multidose oral SEC treatment in the setting of 5-nitroimidazole resistance are needed.

Another difficult treatment scenario is trichomoniasis in the setting of 5-nitroimidazole hypersensitivity. Although MTZ hypersensitivity prevalence is reported to be approximately 0.15%,[114] patients often report a variety of intolerances (ie, nausea, vomiting) as "allergies" to providers. Therefore, obtaining a detailed allergy history is an essential first step in managing these patients to identify whether or not their prior history is truly consistent with a type 1, IgE-mediated hypersensitivity reaction.[115] If a true hypersensitivity reaction is deemed to be present, consultation with an allergist is recommended so that desensitization can be considered.[115] There are limited treatment options outside of the 5-nitroimidazole class for the treatment of trichomoniasis. For *T. vaginalis*-infected patients with serious allergies who are not candidates for desensitization, some successful treatment regimens containing drugs outside of the 5-nitroimidazole drug class have been reported. These include intravaginal boric acid 600 mg twice daily for at least 60 days[116–118] and intravaginal paromomycin 4 g of 6.25% vaginal cream nightly for 14 days.[110,111,119,120] As with intravaginal paromomycin and TDZ, intravaginal preparations of boric acid must be compounded.

After treatment, women who are sexually active should be retested for *T. vaginalis* between 3 weeks and 3 months due to a high reinfection rate. There are currently insufficient data to support retesting men after treatment.[58,121] If retesting by 3 months is not possible, women should be retested whenever they next seek medical care less than 12 months after treatment.[16]

PARTNER MANAGEMENT

Given high rates of asymptomatic infection as well as recurrence among men and women,[122,123] the appropriate management of sexual partners is essential in preventing transmission beyond the infected individual. It is currently recommended that all sexual partners of a person infected with *T. vaginalis* (both within the past 60 days and the last sexual partner, even if this was >60 days) be treated presumptively and that the infected individual avoid any further sexual activities until treatment has been completed and they are asymptomatic.[16] Although not permitted in all states, expedited partner therapy (EPT) could be an important tool in partner management for *T. vaginalis*. There have been multiple studies investigating EPT for trichomoniasis. One RCT demonstrated that partner treatment with single-dose oral 2-g TDZ resulted in a greater than fourfold reduction in repeat infections among *T. vaginalis*-infected index women.[124] Two other studies using single-dose 2-g oral MTZ for male partners of *T. vaginalis*-infected women found either no effect of EPT[125] or a borderline effect.[126] Although it is possible that the two studies using oral MTZ were either underpowered or did not use a correct control arm, it is also possible that oral TDZ (or SEC) could be a better treatment for men. Thus, further studies in this area are needed.

SUMMARY

Trichomoniasis has long been a neglected STI, a situation maintained by the erroneous perception that infection is inconsequential. However, recent evidence supports that this STI has the potential to effect significant adverse sexual and reproductive health outcomes for both women and men. Recent advances in diagnosis and treatment of *T vaginalis* offer the promise of controlling the high rates of infection, but more public health attention is needed to make a significant impact.

CLINICS CARE POINTS

- *T. vaginalis* in pregnancy has been associated with adverese birth outcomes such as preterm deliver, pre-labor rupture of membranes, and delivery of low birth weight infants.
- *T. vaginalis* nucleic acid amplification tests are the gold standard for diagnosis.

> • For women, a 7-day course of oral MTZ 500 mg twice daily is now the recommended treatment regimen. For men, the recommended treatment remains the single-dose oral 2-g MTZ.

FUNDING

This work was funded in part by the UAB Centers for Clinical and Translational Sciences TL1 grant (5TL1TR003106–04/Ruth L. Kirschstein National Research Service, United States Award to Author SAO) as well as the UAB Department of Medicine (2022 Frommeyer Fellowship in Investigative Medicine to Author OTVG).

DISCLOSURE

OTVG receives grant funding from the National Institutes of Health, United States, Gilead Sciences, United States, and Abbott Molecular, United States and has also served on scientific advisory boards for Scynexis; Christina A. Muzny, MD, MSPH has received research grant support from NIH, United States/NIAID, United States, Lupin Pharmaceuticals, United States, Abbott Molecular, United States, and Gilead Sciences, Inc.; is a consultant for BioNTech, Scynexis, and Cepheid, and has received honoraria from Visby, Elsevier, Abbott Molecular, Cepheid, Roche Diagnostics, and Lupin Pharmaceuticals. All other authors have no pertinent disclosures.

ACKNOWLEDGMENTS

None.

REFERENCES

1. Du M, Yan W, Jing W, et al. Increasing incidence rates of sexually transmitted infections from 2010 to 2019: an analysis of temporal trends by geographical regions and age groups from the 2019 Global Burden of Disease Study. BMC Infect Dis 2022;22(1):574.
2. Rowley J, Vander Hoorn S, Korenromp E, et al. Chlamydia, gonorrhoea, trichomoniasis and syphilis: global prevalence and incidence estimates, 2016. Bull World Health Organ 2019;97(8):548–562p.
3. Hoots BE, Peterman TA, Torrone EA, et al. A Trich-y question: should Trichomonas vaginalis infection be reportable? Sex Transm Dis 2013;40(2):113–6.
4. Kreisel KM, Spicknall IH, Gargano JW, et al. Sexually transmitted infections among us women and men: prevalence and incidence estimates, 2018. Sex Transm Dis 2021;48(4).
5. Sutton M, Sternberg M, Koumans EH, et al. The prevalence of Trichomonas vaginalis infection among reproductive-age women in the United States, 2001-2004. Clin Infect Dis 2007;45(10):1319–26.
6. Seña AC, Miller WC, Hobbs MM, et al. Trichomonas vaginalis infection in male sexual partners: implications for diagnosis, treatment, and prevention. Clin Infect Dis 2007;44(1):13–22.
7. Kissinger P, Amedee A, Clark RA, et al. Trichomonas vaginalis treatment reduces vaginal HIV-1 shedding. Sex Transm Dis 2009;36(1):11–6.
8. Van Gerwen OT, Craig-Kuhn MC, Jones AT, et al. Trichomoniasis and adverse birth outcomes: a systematic review and meta-analysis. Bjog 2021;128(12):1907–15.

9. Yang S, Zhao W, Wang H, et al. Trichomonas vaginalis infection-associated risk of cervical cancer: a meta-analysis. Eur J Obstet Gynecol Reprod Biol 2018; 228:166–73.

10. Cherpes TL, Wiesenfeld HC, Melan MA, et al. The associations between pelvic inflammatory disease, Trichomonas vaginalis infection, and positive herpes simplex virus type 2 serology. Sex Transm Dis 2006;33(12):747–52.

11. Masha SC, Cools P, Sanders EJ, et al. Trichomonas vaginalis and HIV infection acquisition: a systematic review and meta-analysis. Sex Transm Infect 2019; 95(1):36–42.

12. Barker EK, Malekinejad M, Merai R, et al. Risk of human immunodeficiency virus acquisition among high-risk heterosexuals with nonviral sexually transmitted infections: a systematic review and meta-analysis. Sex Transm Dis 2022;49(6): 383–97.

13. Ginocchio CC, Chapin K, Smith JS, et al. Prevalence of Trichomonas vaginalis and coinfection with Chlamydia trachomatis and Neisseria gonorrhoeae in the United States as determined by the Aptima Trichomonas vaginalis nucleic acid amplification assay. J Clin Microbiol 2012;50(8):2601–8.

14. Wiringa AE, Ness RB, Darville T, et al. em>Trichomonas vaginalis, endometritis and sequelae among women with clinically suspected pelvic inflammatory disease. Sex Transm Infections 2020;96(6):436–8.

15. Zhang Z, Li Y, Lu H, et al. A systematic review of the correlation between Trichomonas vaginalis infection and infertility. Acta Trop 2022;236:106693.

16. Workowski KA, Bachmann LH, Chan PA, et al. Sexually transmitted infections treatment guidelines, 2021. MMWR Recomm Rep 2021;70(4):1–187.

17. Gaydos CA, Manabe YC, Melendez JH. A narrative review of where we are with point-of-care STI testing in the United States. Sex Transm Dis 2021;48(8S): S71–7.

18. Schwebke JR, Gaydos CA, Davis T, et al. Clinical Evaluation of the Cepheid Xpert TV Assay for Detection of Trichomonas vaginalis with Prospectively Collected Specimens from Men and Women. J Clin Microbiol 2018;56(2).

19. Gaydos CA, Hobbs M, Marrazzo J, et al. Rapid Diagnosis of Trichomonas vaginalis by Testing Vaginal Swabs in an Isothermal Helicase-Dependent AmpliVue Assay. Sex Transm Dis 2016;43(6):369–73.

20. Schwebke JR, Hobbs MM, Taylor SN, et al. Molecular testing for Trichomonas vaginalis in women: results from a prospective U.S. clinical trial. J Clin Microbiol 2011;49(12):4106–11.

21. Van Der Pol B, Williams JA, Taylor SN, et al. Detection of Trichomonas vaginalis DNA by use of self-obtained vaginal swabs with the BD ProbeTec Qx assay on the BD Viper system. J Clin Microbiol 2014;52(3):885–9.

22. Van Der Pol B. A profile of the cobas® TV/MG test for the detection of Trichomonas vaginalis and Mycoplasma genitalium. Expert Rev Mol Diagn 2020;20(4): 381–6.

23. Van Der Pol B, Torres-Chavolla E, Kodsi S, et al. Clinical Performance of the BD CTGCTV2 Assay for the BD MAX System for Detection of Chlamydia trachomatis, Neisseria gonorrhoeae, and Trichomonas vaginalis Infections. Sex Transm Dis 2021;48(2):134–40.

24. Morris SR, Bristow CC, Wierzbicki MR, et al. Performance of a single-use, rapid, point-of-care PCR device for the detection of Neisseria gonorrhoeae, Chlamydia trachomatis, and Trichomonas vaginalis: a cross-sectional study. Lancet Infect Dis 2021;21(5):668–76.

25. Patel EU, Gaydos CA, Packman ZR, et al. Prevalence and Correlates of Tricho-monas vaginalis Infection Among Men and Women in the United States. Clin Infect Dis 2018;67(2):211–7.
26. Lindrose AR, Htet KZ, O'Connell S, et al. Burden of trichomoniasis among older adults in the United States: a systematic review. Sex Health 2022;19(3):151–6.
27. Bassey GB, Clarke AIL, Elhelu OK, et al. Trichomoniasis, a new look at a com-mon but neglected STI in African descendance population in the United States and the Black Diaspora. A review of its incidence, research prioritization, and the resulting health disparities. J Natl Med Assoc 2022;114(1):78–89.
28. Van Gerwen OT, Camino AF, Sharma J, et al. Epidemiology, Natural History, Diagnosis, and Treatment of Trichomonas vaginalis in Men. Clin Infect Dis 2021;73(6):1119–24.
29. Schwebke JR, Rompalo A, Taylor S, et al. Re-evaluating the treatment of nongonococcal urethritis: emphasizing emerging pathogens–a randomized clinical trial. Clin Infect Dis 2011;52(2):163–70.
30. Weston TE, Nicol CS. Natural history of trichomonal infection in males. Br J Vener Dis 1963;39(4):251–7.
31. Krieger JN, Verdon M, Siegel N, et al. Natural history of urogenital trichomoniasis in men. J Urol 1993;149(6):1455–8.
32. Daugherty M, Glynn K, Byler T. Prevalence of Trichomonas vaginalis Infection Among US Males, 2013–2016. Clin Infect Dis 2018;68(3):460–5.
33. Van Gerwen OT, Jani A, Long DM, et al. Prevalence of Sexually Transmitted In-fections and Human Immunodeficiency Virus in Transgender Persons: A Sys-tematic Review. Transgend Health 2020;5(2):90–103.
34. Pereira-Neves A, Ribeiro KC, Benchimol M. Pseudocysts in trichomonads–new insights. Protist 2003;154(3–4):313–29.
35. Tulchinsky TH, Varavikova EA. Communicable Diseases. The New Public Health. 2014:149–236. https://doi.org/10.1016/B978-0-12-415766-8.00004-5.
36. Burch TA, Rees CW, Reardon LV. Epidemiological studies on human trichomoni-asis. Am J Trop Med Hyg 1959;8(3):312–8.
37. Mercer F, Johnson PJ. Trichomonas vaginalis: Pathogenesis, Symbiont Interac-tions, and Host Cell Immune Responses. Trends Parasitol 2018;34(8):683–93.
38. Fichorova RN, Buck OR, Yamamoto HS, et al. The villain team-up or how Tricho-monas vaginalis and bacterial vaginosis alter innate immunity in concert. Sex Transm Infect 2013;89(6):460–6.
39. Menezes CB, Tasca T. Trichomoniasis immunity and the involvement of the pu-rinergic signaling. Biomed J 2016;39(4):234–43.
40. Fichorova RN, Lee Y, Yamamoto HS, et al. Endobiont viruses sensed by the hu-man host - beyond conventional antiparasitic therapy. PLoS One 2012;7(11): e48418.
41. Graves KJ, Ghosh AP, Kissinger PJ, et al. *Trichomonas vaginalis* virus: a review of the literature. Int J STD AIDS 2019. 956462418809767.
42. Graves KJ, Ghosh AP, Kissinger PJ, et al. Trichomonas vaginalis virus: a review of the literature. Int J STD AIDS 2019;30(5):496–504.
43. Graves KJ, Ghosh AP, Schmidt N, et al. Trichomonas vaginalis Virus Among Women With Trichomoniasis and Associations With Demographics, Clinical Out-comes, and Metronidazole Resistance. Clin Infect Dis 2019;69(12):2170–6.
44. Graves KJ, Novak J, Secor WE, et al. A systematic review of the literature on mechanisms of 5-nitroimidazole resistance in Trichomonas vaginalis. Parasi-tology 2020;147(13):1383–91.

45. Watt L, Jennison RF. Incidence of Trichomonas vaginalis in marital partners. Br J Vener Dis 1960;36(3):163–6.

46. Kellock D, O'Mahony CP. Sexually acquired metronidazole-resistant trichomoniasis in a lesbian couple. Genitourin Med 1996;72(1):60–1.

47. Crucitti T, Jespers V, Mulenga C, et al. Non-sexual transmission of Trichomonas vaginalis in adolescent girls attending school in Ndola, Zambia. PLoS One 2011; 6(1):e16310.

48. Muzny CA, Rivers CA, Mena LA, et al. Genotypic characterization of Trichomonas vaginalis isolates among women who have sex with women in sexual partnerships. Sex Transm Dis 2012;39(7):556–8.

49. Peterson K, Drame D. Iatrogenic transmission of Trichomonas vaginalis by a traditional healer. Sex Transm Infect 2010;86(5):353–4.

50. Van Gerwen OT, Muzny CA, Marrazzo JM. Sexually transmitted infections and female reproductive health. Nat Microbiol 2022;7(8):1116–26.

51. Mitchell CM, Anyalechi GE, Cohen CR, et al. Etiology and Diagnosis of Pelvic Inflammatory Disease: Looking Beyond Gonorrhea and Chlamydia. J Infect Dis 2021;224(12 Suppl 2):S29–35.

52. Moodley P, Wilkinson D, Connolly C, et al. Trichomonas vaginalis is associated with pelvic inflammatory disease in women infected with human immunodeficiency virus. Clin Infect Dis 2002;34(4):519–22.

53. McKee DL, Hu Z, Stahlman S. Incidence and sequelae of acute pelvic inflammatory disease among active component females. U.S. Armed Forces. Msmr 2018; 25(10):2–8.

54. Haggerty CL, Peipert JF, Weitzen S, et al. Predictors of Chronic Pelvic Pain in an Urban Population of Women With Symptoms and Signs of Pelvic Inflammatory Disease. Sex Transm Dis 2005;32(5):293–9.

55. Kranjcić-Zec I, Dzamić A, Mitrović S, et al. The role of parasites and fungi in secondary infertility. Med Pregl 2004;57(1–2):30–2.

56. Benchimol M, de Andrade Rosa I, da Silva Fontes R, et al. Trichomonas adhere and phagocytose sperm cells: adhesion seems to be a prominent stage during interaction. Parasitol Res 2008;102(4):597–604.

57. Casari E, Ferrario A, Morenghi E, et al. Gardnerella, Trichomonas vaginalis, Candida, Chlamydia trachomatis, *Mycoplasma hominis* and Ureaplasma urealyticum in the genital discharge of symptomatic fertile and asymptomatic infertile women. New Microbiol 2010;33(1):69–76.

58. Cu-Uvin S, Ko H, Jamieson DJ, et al. Prevalence, incidence, and persistence or recurrence of trichomoniasis among human immunodeficiency virus (HIV)-positive women and among HIV-negative women at high risk for HIV infection. Clin Infect Dis 2002;34(10):1406–11.

59. Yang M, Li L, Jiang C, et al. Co-infection with trichomonas vaginalis increases the risk of cervical intraepithelial neoplasia grade 2-3 among HPV16 positive female: a large population-based study. BMC Infect Dis 2020;20(1):642.

60. Lazenby GB, Taylor PT, Badman BS, et al. An association between Trichomonas vaginalis and high-risk human papillomavirus in rural Tanzanian women undergoing cervical cancer screening. Clin Ther 2014;36(1):38–45.

61. Zhang ZF, Begg CB. Is Trichomonas vaginalis a cause of cervical neoplasia? Results from a combined analysis of 24 studies. Int J Epidemiol 1994;23(4): 682–90.

62. Roeters AM, Boon ME, van Haaften M, et al. Inflammatory events as detected in cervical smears and squamous intraepithelial lesions. Diagn Cytopathol 2010; 38(2):85–93.

63. Jarecki-Black JC, Lushbaugh WB, Golosov L, et al. Trichomonas vaginalis: preliminary characterization of a sperm motility inhibiting factor. Ann Clin Lab Sci 1988;18(6):484–9.
64. Gopalkrishnan K, Hinduja IN, Kumar TC. Semen characteristics of asymptomatic males affected by Trichomonas vaginalis. J In Vitro Fert Embryo Transf 1990;7(3):165–7.
65. Sutcliffe S, Alderete JF, Till C, et al. Trichomonosis and subsequent risk of prostate cancer in the Prostate Cancer Prevention Trial. Int J Cancer 2009;124(9): 2082–7.
66. Kim SS, Kim JH, Han IH, et al. Inflammatory Responses in a Benign Prostatic Hyperplasia Epithelial Cell Line (BPH-1) Infected with Trichomonas vaginalis. Korean J Parasitol 2016;54(2):123–32.
67. Mitteregger D, Aberle SW, Makristathis A, et al. High detection rate of Trichomonas vaginalis in benign hyperplastic prostatic tissue. Med Microbiol Immunol 2012;201(1):113–6.
68. Najafi A, Chaechi Nosrati MR, Ghasemi E, et al. Is there association between Trichomonas vaginalis infection and prostate cancer risk?: A systematic review and meta-analysis. Microb Pathog 2019;137:103752.
69. Marous M, Huang WY, Rabkin CS, et al. Trichomonas vaginalis infection and risk of prostate cancer: associations by disease aggressiveness and race/ethnicity in the PLCO Trial. Cancer Causes Control 2017;28(8):889–98.
70. Yang HY, Su RY, Chung CH, et al. Association between trichomoniasis and prostate and bladder diseases: a population-based case-control study. Sci Rep 2022;12(1):15358.
71. Sutcliffe S, Giovannucci E, Alderete JF, et al. Plasma antibodies against Trichomonas vaginalis and subsequent risk of prostate cancer. Cancer Epidemiol Biomarkers Prev 2006;15(5):939–45.
72. Francis SC, Kent CK, Klausner JD, et al. Prevalence of rectal Trichomonas vaginalis and Mycoplasma genitalium in male patients at the San Francisco STD clinic, 2005-2006. Sex Transm Dis 2008;35(9):797–800.
73. Carter-Wicker K, Utuama O, Omole F. Can trichomoniasis cause pharyngitis? A case report. SAGE Open Med Case Rep 2016;4. 2050313x16682132.
74. Joseph Davey DL, Shull HI, Billings JD, et al. Prevalence of Curable Sexually Transmitted Infections in Pregnant Women in Low- and Middle-Income Countries From 2010 to 2015: A Systematic Review. Sex Transm Dis 2016;43(7).
75. Young MR, Broadwell C, Kacanek D, et al. Sexually Transmitted Infections in Pregnant People Living With Human Immunodeficiency Virus: Temporal Trends, Demographic Correlates, and Association With Preterm Birth. Clin Infect Dis 2022;75(12):2211–8.
76. Price CM, Peters RPH, Steyn J, et al. Prevalence and Detection of Trichomonas vaginalis in HIV-Infected Pregnant Women. Sex Transm Dis 2018;45(5):332–6.
77. Fichorova RN. Impact of T. vaginalis infection on innate immune responses and reproductive outcome. J Reprod Immunol 2009;83(1–2):185–9.
78. Silver BJ, Guy RJ, Kaldor JM, et al. Trichomonas vaginalis as a Cause of Perinatal Morbidity: A Systematic Review and Meta-Analysis. Sex Transm Dis 2014;41(6):369–76.
79. Papeš D, Pasini M, Jerončić A, et al. Detection of sexually transmitted pathogens in patients with chronic prostatitis/chronic pelvic pain: a prospective clinical study. Int J STD AIDS 2017;28(6):613–5.
80. Tsang SH, Peisch SF, Rowan B, et al. Association between Trichomonas vaginalis and prostate cancer mortality. Int J Cancer 2019;144(10):2377–80.

81. Hoffman CM, Fritz L, Radebe O, et al. Rectal Trichomonas vaginalis infection in South African men who have sex with men. Int J STD AIDS 2018;29(14):1444–7.

82. Meites E, Llata E, Braxton J, et al. Trichomonas vaginalis in selected U.S. sexually transmitted disease clinics: testing, screening, and prevalence. Sex Transm Dis 2013;40(11):865–9.

83. Wølner-Hanssen P, Krieger JN, Stevens CE, et al. Clinical manifestations of vaginal trichomoniasis. Jama 1989;261(4):571–6.

84. Hobbs MM, Seña AC. Modern diagnosis of Trichomonas vaginalis infection. Sex Transm Infect 2013;89(6):434–8.

85. Ohlemeyer CL, Hornberger LL, Lynch DA, et al. Diagnosis of Trichomonas vaginalis in adolescent females: InPouch TV culture versus wet-mount microscopy. J Adolesc Health 1998;22(3):205–8.

86. Rivers CA, Muzny CA, Schwebke JR. Diagnostic rates differ on the basis of the number of read days with the use of the InPouch culture system for Trichomonas vaginalis screening. J Clin Microbiol 2013;51(11):3875–6.

87. Nye MB, Schwebke JR, Body BA. Comparison of APTIMA Trichomonas vaginalis transcription-mediated amplification to wet mount microscopy, culture, and polymerase chain reaction for diagnosis of trichomoniasis in men and women. Am J Obstet Gynecol 2009;200(2):188.e181–7.

88. Gaydos CA, Schwebke J, Dombrowski J, et al. Clinical performance of the Solana® Point-of-Care Trichomonas Assay from clinician-collected vaginal swabs and urine specimens from symptomatic and asymptomatic women. Expert Rev Mol Diagn 2017;17(3):303–6.

89. Herrmann B, Malm K. Comparison between Abbott m2000 RealTime and Alinity m STI systems for detection of Chlamydia trachomatis, Neisseria gonorrhoeae, and Mycoplasma genitalium. Eur J Clin Microbiol Infect Dis 2021;40(10): 2217–20.

90. Mtshali A, Ngcapu S, Govender K, et al. In Vitro Effect of 5-Nitroimidazole Drugs against Trichomonas vaginalis Clinical Isolates. Microbiol Spectr 2022;10(4): e0091222.

91. Kissinger P, Muzny CA, Mena LA, et al. Single-dose versus 7-day-dose metronidazole for the treatment of trichomoniasis in women: an open-label, randomised controlled trial. Lancet Infect Dis 2018;18(11):1251–9.

92. Howe K, Kissinger PJ. Single-Dose Compared With Multidose Metronidazole for the Treatment of Trichomoniasis in Women: A Meta-Analysis. Sex Transm Dis 2017;44(1):29–34.

93. Kissinger P, Mena L, Levison J, et al. A randomized treatment trial: single versus 7-day dose of metronidazole for the treatment of Trichomonas vaginalis among HIV-infected women. J Acquir Immune Defic Syndr 2010;55(5):565–71.

94. Muzny CA, Van Gerwen OT, Legendre D. Secnidazole: a treatment for trichomoniasis in adolescents and adults. Expert Rev Anti Infect Ther 2022;20(8): 1067–76.

95. Muzny CA, Schwebke JR, Nyirjesy P, et al. Efficacy and Safety of Single Oral Dosing of Secnidazole for Trichomoniasis in Women: Results of a Phase 3, Randomized, Double-Blind, Placebo-Controlled, Delayed-Treatment Study. Clin Infect Dis 2021;73(6):e1282–9.

96. Mann JR, McDermott S, Zhou L, et al. Treatment of trichomoniasis in pregnancy and preterm birth: an observational study. J Womens Health (Larchmt) 2009; 18(4):493–7.

97. Sheehy O, Santos F, Ferreira E, et al. The use of metronidazole during pregnancy: a review of evidence. Curr Drug Saf 2015;10(2):170–9.

98. Tinidazole [package insert]. Atlanta, GA: Mission Pharmaceutical, Inc.; 2004.

99. Khrianin AA, Reshetnikov OV. [Clinical and microbiological efficacy of metronidazole and ornidazole in the treatment of urogenital trichomoniasis in men]. Antibiot Khimioter 2006;51(1):18–21.

100. Viitanen J, Haataja H, Männistö PT. Concentrations of metronidazole and tinidazole in male genital tissues. Antimicrob Agents Chemother 1985;28(6):812–4.

101. Lamp KC, Freeman CD, Klutman NE, et al. Pharmacokinetics and pharmacodynamics of the nitroimidazole antimicrobials. Clin Pharmacokinet 1999;36(5): 353–73.

102. Kawamura N. Metronidazole and tinidazole in a single large dose for treating urogenital infections with Trichomonas vaginalis in men. Br J Vener Dis 1978; 54(2):81–3.

103. Seña AC, Lensing S, Rompalo A, et al. Chlamydia trachomatis, Mycoplasma genitalium, and Trichomonas vaginalis infections in men with nongonococcal urethritis: predictors and persistence after therapy. J Infect Dis 2012;206(3): 357–65.

104. Ozbilgin A, Ozbel Y, Alkan MZ, et al. Trichomoniasis in non-gonococcic urethritis among male patients. J Egypt Soc Parasitol 1994;24(3):621–5.

105. Videau D, Niel G, Siboulet A, et al. A 5-nitroimidazole derivative with a long half-life. Br J Vener Dis 1978;54(2):77–80.

106. Siboulet A, Catalan F, Videau D, et al. La trichomonase urogénitale. Essais d'un imidazole à demi-vie longue: le secnidazole. Médecine et Maladies Infectieuses 1977;7(9):400–9.

107. Lossick JG, Muller M, Gorrell TE. In vitro drug susceptibility and doses of metronidazole required for cure in cases of refractory vaginal trichomoniasis. J Infect Dis 1986;153(5):948–55.

108. Bosserman EA, Helms DJ, Mosure DJ, et al. Utility of antimicrobial susceptibility testing in Trichomonas vaginalis-infected women with clinical treatment failure. Sex Transm Dis 2011;38(10):983–7.

109. Sobel JD, Nyirjesy P, Brown W. Tinidazole therapy for metronidazole-resistant vaginal trichomoniasis. Clin Infect Dis 2001;33(8):1341–6.

110. Nyirjesy P, Sobel JD, Weitz MV, et al. Difficult-to-treat trichomoniasis: results with paromomycin cream. Clin Infect Dis 1998;26(4):986–8.

111. Keating MA, Nyirjesy P. Trichomonas vaginalis Infection in a Tertiary Care Vaginitis Center. Sex Transm Dis 2015;42(9):482–5.

112. Ghosh AP, Aycock C, Schwebke JR. In Vitro Study of the Susceptibility of Clinical Isolates of Trichomonas vaginalis to Metronidazole and Secnidazole. Antimicrobial agents and chemotherapy 2018;62(4):e02329–17.

113. McNeil CJ, Williamson JC, Muzny CA. Successful Treatment of Persistent 5-Nitroimidazole-Resistant Trichomoniasis with an Extended Course of Oral Secnidazole Plus Intravaginal Boric Acid. Sexually Transmitted Diseases 2022. https://doi.org/10.1097/OLQ.0000000000001741. 9900.

114. Macy E, Romano A, Khan D. Practical Management of Antibiotic Hypersensitivity in 2017. J Allergy Clin Immunol Pract 2017;5(3):577–86.

115. Van Gerwen OT, Camino AF, Bourla LN, et al. Management of Trichomoniasis in the Setting of 5-Nitroimidazole Hypersensitivity. Sex Transm Dis 2021;48(8): e111–5.

116. Aggarwal A, Shier RM. Recalcitrant Trichomonas vaginalis infections successfully treated with vaginal acidification. J Obstet Gynaecol Can 2008;30(1):55–8.

117. Muzny C, Barnes A, Mena L. Symptomatic Trichomonas vaginalis infection in the setting of severe nitroimidazole allergy: successful treatment with boric acid. Sexual health 2012;9(4):389–91.

118. Backus KV, Muzny CA, Beauchamps LS. Trichomonas vaginalis Treated With Boric Acid in a Metronidazole Allergic Female. Sex Transm Dis 2017;44(2):120.

119. Helms DJ, Mosure DJ, Secor WE, et al. Management of trichomonas vaginalis in women with suspected metronidazole hypersensitivity. Am J Obstet Gynecol 2008;198(4). 370.e371-377.

120. Thomas R, Estcourt C, Metcalfe R. A case series-successful treatment of persistent Trichomonas vaginalis with paromomycin. Paper presented at: HIV MEDICINE2018.

121. Peterman TA, Tian LH, Metcalf CA, et al. High incidence of new sexually transmitted infections in the year following a sexually transmitted infection: a case for rescreening. Ann Intern Med 2006;145(8):564–72.

122. Meites E, Gaydos CA, Hobbs MM, et al. A Review of Evidence-Based Care of Symptomatic Trichomoniasis and Asymptomatic Trichomonas vaginalis Infections. Clin Infect Dis 2015;61(Suppl 8):S837–48.

123. Niccolai LM, Kopicko JJ, Kassie A, et al. Incidence and Predictors of Reinfection withTrichomonas vaginalisin HIV-infected Women. Sexually Transmitted Diseases 2000;27(5):284–8.

124. Lyng J, Christensen J. A double-blind study of the value of treatment with a single dose tinidazole of partners to females with trichomoniasis. Acta Obstet Gynecol Scand 1981;60(2):199–201.

125. Kissinger P, Schmidt N, Mohammed H, et al. Patient-delivered partner treatment for Trichomonas vaginalis infection: a randomized controlled trial. Sex Transm Dis 2006;33(7):445–50.

126. Schwebke JR, Desmond RA. A randomized controlled trial of partner notification methods for prevention of trichomoniasis in women. Sex Transm Dis 2010;37(6):392–6.

Update on the Epidemiology, Screening, and Management of *Chlamydia trachomatis* Infection

Jane S. Hocking, PhD[a],*, William M. Geisler, MD, MPH[b],
Fabian Y.S. Kong, PhD[a]

KEYWORDS

- *Chlamydia trachomatis* • Epidemiology • Natural history • Manifestations
- Screening • Diagnosis • Treatment

KEY POINTS

- *Chlamydia trachomatis* is the most frequently diagnosed bacterial sexually transmitted infection with infection occurring commonly at the genital and rectal anatomic sites in both women and men.
- Chlamydia rates remain high in young adults, in young racial and ethnic minority groups, and among men who have sex with men.
- Chlamydia infection is usually asymptomatic, and repeat infection is common, prompting recommendations to rescreen 3 months following treatment of infection.
- Chlamydia is an important cause of pelvic inflammatory disease in women, and clinicians should routinely consider the possibility of pelvic inflammatory disease and ask about pelvic inflammatory disease–associated symptoms when providing treatment for women diagnosed with a chlamydia infection.
- Appropriate and timely treatment and partner management are necessary to reduce transmission and the risk of complications, particularly among women.

INTRODUCTION

Chlamydia trachomatis infection ("chlamydia") is the most commonly diagnosed bacterial sexually transmitted infection (STI) globally with an estimated 130 million new cases each year.[1] As an STI, it can occur in the genitals (urethra or vagina/cervix), rectum, or pharynx. More than 1.5 million men and women in the United States are

---

[a] Melbourne School of Population and Global Health, University of Melbourne, 3/207 Bouverie Street, Carlton South, Melbourne, Victoria, Australia 3053; [b] Department of Medicine, University of Alabama at Birmingham, 703 19th Street South, ZRB 242, Birmingham, AL 35294, USA
* Corresponding author.
E-mail address: jhocking@unimelb.edu.au

Infect Dis Clin N Am 37 (2023) 267–288
https://doi.org/10.1016/j.idc.2023.02.007
0891-5520/23/© 2023 Elsevier Inc. All rights reserved.

diagnosed each year, representing the largest proportion of STIs reported to the Centers for Disease Control and Prevention (CDC) since 1994.[2] If left untreated in women, genital chlamydia can ascend into the upper genital tract causing pelvic inflammatory disease (PID), increasing their risk for ectopic pregnancy, infertility, and chronic pelvic pain.[3] In men, chlamydia can cause epididymitis and proctitis.[3] However, chlamydia is asymptomatic in more than 80% of cases in both men and women,[3,4] regardless of infection site (urogenital, rectal, or pharyngeal), and without screening, most infections will remain undetected. This has prompted several high-income countries to recommend regular chlamydia screening, particularly for young women.

This article provides an update on the epidemiology, natural history, and clinical manifestations of chlamydia in adults and discusses the current approaches to its management and control policy.

OVERVIEW OF *CHLAMYDIA TRACHOMATIS* MICROBIOLOGY

C trachomatis, the bacterium that causes chlamydia, is an obligate, intracellular, gram-negative bacteria that undergoes a biphasic developmental cycle consisting of infectious extracellular elementary bodies and noninfectious metabolically active intracellular reticulate bodies.[5] Currently, 19 serovars of *C trachomatis* are recognized (A, B/Ba, C, d/Da, E, F, G/Ga, H, I/Ia, J, K, L1, L2, L2a, and L3) according to specific epitopes of the major outer membrane protein (MOMP) encoded by the gene *ompA*.[6] Serovars A to C are associated with trachoma; D to K with urogenital, ocular, and rectal infections; and L1 to L3 with an invasive ulcerative infection called lymphogranuloma venereum (LGV).[5] Although most chlamydial infections are uncomplicated and mainly asymptomatic, infection associated with LGV is much more invasive and more likely to be symptomatic than other serovars.[5]

The most prevalent strains worldwide are serovars D, E, and F, accounting for ~70% of the urogenital serovars.[7] Although several studies have reported associations of specific serovars to particular risk groups (serovars G, D, J, and L2b with men who have sex with men [MSM] and E and F in heterosexual populations),[7–13] this is related to sexual behavior rather than specific serovar-tissue tropism. Bax and colleagues[7] also found differences in the dominant rectal serovars between MSM and women. Although this study was limited by small sample size, serovars G (40%) and E (28%) were the most prevalent rectal serovars among 25 rectal specimens from MSM, whereas serovars D (27.7%) and E (21.3%) were most prevalent among 47 rectal samples from women.

In practice, the serovar is only relevant for LGV, which is associated with symptoms and requires a longer course of treatment (see later discussion).

EPIDEMIOLOGY
Overall Pattern of Chlamydia Diagnoses

In 2016, the global prevalence estimate of chlamydia was 3.8% (95% CI: 3.3, 4.5) in women and 2.7% (95% CI: 1.9, 3.7) in men.[14] As chlamydia is largely asymptomatic at any infection site, chlamydia diagnosis data are likely to underestimate the true prevalence within a population. Furthermore, national surveillance data rarely report infection by site, so reported data will include infections at the urogenital, rectal, and pharyngeal site. Diagnosis rates have increased considerably over the last 20 years in most high-income countries, reaching a high of more than 1.8 million in the United States in 2019[2] (**Fig. 1**). These increases are in part due to increased testing (the more you test, the more you will find), but the increased use of more sensitive assays[15] and decreased condom use in recent years are also likely to be contributing.[16]

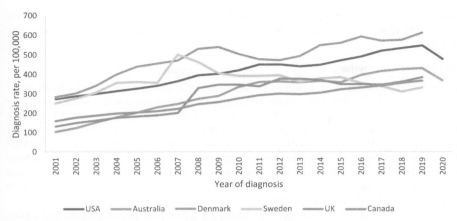

Fig. 1. Chlamydia diagnosis rates in high-income countries.

Chlamydia diagnosis rates declined in most high-income countries in 2020 reducing to 1.5 million in the United States, probably as a result of decreased testing during the COVID-19 pandemic.[15]

In most high-income countries, chlamydia diagnosis rates have tended to be higher in women than in men,[17–19] and this is indeed the case in the United States (**Fig. 2**).[2] However, in some high-income countries like Australia, for example, chlamydia diagnosis rates have increased considerably in men over the last 5 years particularly among those prescribed preexposure prophylaxis (PrEP) for HIV prevention, and now nearly 50% of diagnoses in Australia are among men.[17] As in most high-income countries, the majority (61%) of diagnoses in the United States are in those aged 15 to 24 years and 80% in those aged 15 to 29 years.[15]

There is considerable variation by ethnicity within most high-income countries. For example, rates in the United States are highest among black/African Americans (1086 per 100,000 in 2020) and American Indians/Alaskan Natives (613 per 100,000) and lowest among whites (179 per 100,000) and those of Asian ethnicity (88 per

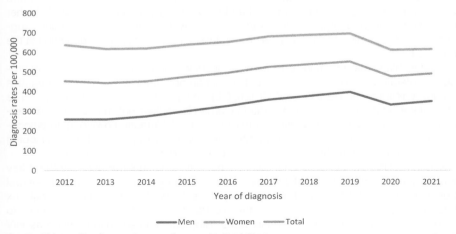

Fig. 2. Chlamydia diagnosis rates by sex, United States

100,000)[15]; in Australia, rates are considerably higher among Aboriginal and Torres Strait Islanders than among the non-Indigenous population (1162 vs 366 per 100,000).[17]

Urogenital Chlamydia

A systematic review of population-based chlamydia prevalence studies from high-income countries estimated a pooled average urogenital prevalence among sexually experienced women aged 18 to 26 years of 3.6% (95% CI: 2.4, 4.8) and 3.5% (95% CI: 1.9, 5.2) among similarly aged men.[20] Although young age is the predominant risk factor for chlamydial infection among women, other risk factors are well established and include having a new sexual partner, multiple partners, and/or a partner with an STI.[21] Past chlamydial infection is also an important risk factor for urogenital infection with repeat infection rates of up to 30% observed in young women within 3 to 12 months following diagnosis.[22–24]

Prevalence estimates of urogenital chlamydia among MSM are scarce, but clinic-based studies generally show that urogenital chlamydia positivity is lower than among women.[25,26] A respondent-driven sampling study among the general population in Canada estimated urogenital chlamydia prevalence to be 0.4% among MSM.[27] Urogenital infections with LGV are also rarely seen.[28]

Rectal Chlamydia

Unfortunately, most high-income countries do not report chlamydia diagnosis data by site of infection, so most information about extragenital chlamydia infections (rectal and pharyngeal) comes from clinic-based studies, which are often set in high-risk settings, such as STI clinics, and thus subject to selection bias. A systematic review of rectal chlamydia prevalence estimated a median rectal chlamydia prevalence of 9% among MSM, similar to that estimated among women (9%).[29]

Among women, up to 70% of rectal infections are associated with a concurrent urogenital infection.[30] Interestingly, anal sex is not associated with rectal chlamydia in women, raising the question of how rectal infection occurs.[30,31] It has been suggested that oral sex could cause rectal chlamydia by passage of the organism from the mouth to the rectum via the gastrointestinal tract, as has been observed in animals.[32] However, it is more likely that rectal chlamydia in women occurs via autoinoculation from an infected urogenital site. Evidence from longitudinal studies of women has found that women with concurrent urogenital and rectal chlamydia had significantly higher urogenital chlamydial organism loads than women with urogenital infection only, suggesting that high microbial load in the urogenital site may lead to autoinoculation at the rectal site.[33]

Rectal chlamydial infections do, however, occur in women without a concurrent urogenital infection, with one review estimating that among those women testing negative for urogenital infection, 2.2% (95% CI: 0.0, 5.2) were positive for rectal infection.[30] The clinical importance of rectal chlamydia in women is unclear but may be of considerable concern if it can act as a reservoir for repeat genital infection owing to autoinoculation from the rectum to the genital site, thereby increasing the risk of developing upper genital tract infection and its associated reproductive complications.[32,34]

Among MSM, condomless anal sex and number of sexual partners are the 2 key factors associated with rectal chlamydia. A systematic review of trends in sexual behavior among MSM in high-income countries found that condomless anal sex has been steadily increasing since the 1990s,[35] which may be contributing to increasing rectal chlamydia diagnosis rates. Biomedical interventions, such as HIV PrEP, have been highly successful in minimizing HIV transmission but have been associated with an increased incidence of STIs, including rectal chlamydia, potentially because of reduced condom use.[36] A recent systematic review and meta-analysis has shown that significant increases in rectal chlamydia (60% increase) are associated with PrEP.[36] Rectal chlamydia was also found to be highly prevalent among those initiating PrEP (8.5% rectal; 2.4% pharyngeal; 4.0% genital).[37]

Pharyngeal Chlamydia

The clinical significance of pharyngeal chlamydial infections remains unclear with most infections being asymptomatic. A systematic review has estimated the prevalence of pharyngeal chlamydia to be 1.7% among MSM, 1.7% among women, and 1.6% among men who have sex with women.[38]

Chlamydia and Human Immunodeficiency Virus Transmission

The evidence to support the role of chlamydia in HIV transmission or acquisition is limited and of lower quality. Urogenital chlamydia infections may be associated with HIV transmission. A meta-analysis of the effect of genital tract infections on HIV shedding reported that the odds of HIV shedding were increased by 80% (OR, 1.8; 95% CI: 1.1, 3.1) in the presence of chlamydia infection.[39] Treating chlamydia and/or gonorrhea in men with HIV was found to reduce HIV viral load, particularly in those not receiving antiretroviral treatment.[40,41] This suggests that treating chlamydia in men who practice vaginal or insertive anal sex could potentially reduce HIV viral shedding and reduce HIV (and chlamydia) transmission to sexual partners. However, much of this evidence is based on observational data and is subject to considerable bias and confounding.

An in vitro study examining the interaction between *C trachomatis* and HIV in endocervical cells provided good evidence that infection with chlamydia facilitated both the entry and the establishment of HIV infection across the epithelial cell membrane.[42]

Mathematical modeling suggests that 15.2% of new HIV infections among MSM could be attributable to chlamydia infection,[43] and a recent review found an increased risk of HIV seroconversion among MSM associated with chlamydia infection.[44] Once again, this evidence is based largely on observational studies and bias, and confounding cannot be excluded.

NATURAL HISTORY
Immunity to Chlamydia Infection

The host immune response can strongly affect their susceptibility to chlamydia infection, clearance of infection, and risk of upper genital tract pathogenesis.[45] Animal models of chlamydia infection provide strong evidence for immunity to reinfection, but immunity is short-term and partial only in the long-term; animals can be reinfected, but infections are usually of shorter duration and less intense than the primary infection.[46] Data from human studies suggest that some degree of protective immunity against chlamydia reinfection develops in some humans following infection, but it is also partial only.[47] Untreated infection that naturally clears might confer some immunity against further infection, but the duration of immunity is uncertain and likely to be short-term only.[48,49] The "arrested immunity" hypothesis suggests that antimicrobial treatment of chlamydia might reduce the immune response, and once treated, people become susceptible to infection more quickly, increasing their risk of chlamydia reinfection, with repeat chlamydia infections common.[50]

Duration of Infection

The majority (>80%)[3,4,51–53] of chlamydia infections at genital, rectal, and pharyngeal sites are asymptomatic with no clinical evidence of complications at the time of diagnosis. Estimates of duration of infection vary by infection site. A narrative review by Geisler[54] published in 2010 found that in studies of the duration of untreated, uncomplicated genital chlamydia infections, chlamydia clearance increased over time with about half of infections spontaneously clearing about 1 year after initial testing. Subsequent modeling studies have used available duration of infection data and estimate that the duration of infection is 1.36 years in women and 2.84 years in men.[55,56] These studies have also suggested that fewer infections become established in men than in women, but once established, they clear more slowly.

There have been fewer studies investigating the natural history of rectal chlamydia. A recent natural history study of rectal chlamydia among MSM in the United States reported a median duration of infection of about 13 weeks.[52] However, the outcome was censored in nearly 60% of participants with rectal chlamydia, mostly owing to treatment or reaching end of the study, so the actual duration of rectal chlamydia in the absence of treatment remains unknown. It is possible that the duration may be closer to that estimated from an analysis of prospective cohort studies, which suggested that rectal chlamydia may persist for as long as 578 days.[57] Two recent randomized controlled trials (RCTs) of chlamydia treatment found that nearly 20% of MSM participating in the trials cleared their rectal chlamydia in the time between initial positive test result and returning for treatment usually within 7 days.[58,59] It is uncertain whether these men had had an initial false positive test result or had an infection of short duration, or if the initial infection was identified near the end of its duration. There are few data available about duration of infection in women, but rectal chlamydia has been found to clear more frequently than genital infection (18.4% vs 6.8%) between the time of screening and treatment.[60]

There have also been few studies investigating the natural history of pharyngeal chlamydia infection, with studies often limited by a low incidence of infection among study participants and hence small sample size. A natural history cohort study of MSM in the United States by Khosropour and colleagues[51] reported a median duration of chlamydial infection ranging from 2 weeks if participants had at least 1 week of chlamydia-positive pharyngeal specimens to a more conservative estimate of 6 weeks if participants had at least 2 consecutive weeks of positive pharyngeal specimens. However, the outcome was censored in nearly 40% of participants because of treatment or reaching the end of the study, and it is possible that the duration maybe considerably longer. A modeling analysis using data from a cohort study suggested that the duration could be as long as 667 days.[57] Khosropour[51] also found that the median duration of infection was shorter for individuals with a history of chlamydia compared with those without a history of chlamydia (3.6 weeks vs 8.7 weeks), and in a secondary analysis, was shorter for individuals with concurrent rectal chlamydia. Further support to the study by Khosropour and colleagues comes from a study of STI clinic patients in the Netherlands that found a median duration of pharyngeal infection of 10 days.[61]

There are several limitations in published chlamydia natural history studies. First, with the exception of cohort studies with very regular follow-up, it is usually unclear when participants were initially infected, limiting the accuracy of estimates for the duration of infection. Second, in the absence of genomic sequencing or typing of the C trachomatis outer membrane protein A (OmpA) on both the initial and the subsequent chlamydia positive specimens to assess whether the subsequent infection is identical to the initial infection, it is difficult to reliably differentiate between persistent infection or a new infection. Geisler and colleagues[62] have previously estimated that about 5% of participants initially thought to have persistent chlamydia infection were subsequently found to have discordant OmpA types between initial diagnosis and follow-up, suggesting that they had acquired a new infection. Furthermore, studies of chlamydia duration have the inherent limitation that patients may clear infection and be reinfected during the follow-up period. Third, some participants may have been incidentally treated with antibiotics for another indication (eg, sinus infection) that may have cleared the chlamydial infection. Finally, modern diagnostic methods, such as nucleic acid amplification tests (NAAT), do not differentiate between viable and nonviable chlamydia nucleic acid, and given that it can take several weeks for chlamydia nucleic acids to clear after treatment, it is possible that some repeat positive diagnoses actually represent nonviable DNA or RNA rather than an active chlamydial infection.[63] Future studies using viability assays (see later discussion) will help give better estimates of duration of infection.

CLINICAL MANIFESTATIONS IN WOMEN

More than 80% of infections in women are asymptomatic,[3] but the most common clinical manifestations associated with chlamydia in women include cervicitis, urethritis, and PID.[3]

Among women, chlamydial infection in the genital tract initially infects the cervix and may cause cervicitis. There are 2 key diagnostic signs of cervicitis: a mucopurulent discharge and endocervical bleeding that is easily induced by genital passage of a cotton swab through the cervical os. Either or both signs may be present, and although cervicitis may be often asymptomatic, women might report an abnormal vaginal discharge and/or intermenstrual bleeding, particularly postcoital.[64]

Chlamydia can be associated with acute urethral syndrome in women, characterized by pain upon urination and a frequent and urgent need to urinate.[65,66] Although most cases (>90%) of chlamydia urethritis are associated with cervical infection in women,[65] failing to test for genital chlamydia in women presenting with a urinary tract infection can be a missed opportunity for chlamydia diagnosis and treatment.

The term PID encompasses a spectrum of inflammatory disorders of the female upper genital tract and can involve the endometrium (endometritis), fallopian tubes (salpingitis or tubo-ovarian abscess), and pelvic peritoneum.[64] It is a serious reproductive health issue, as it increases a woman's risk for ectopic pregnancy, infertility, and chronic pelvic pain.[67] Chlamydia is a well-established cause of PID and typically has an indolent clinical picture whereby much of the tubal damage occurs secondary to the immune response to infection, which is in contrast to PID caused by *Neisseria gonorrhoeae*, which presents with an acute inflammatory response leading to acute symptoms.[67] Studies estimate that about 20% of PID is attributable to chlamydial infection,[68,69] although modeling analyses suggest that the proportion attributable to chlamydia is likely to be higher in younger (16–24-years-old) than older women (25–44-years-old) at 35.3% versus 10.6%, respectively.[70]

Data linkage studies show that past chlamydial infection confers a higher risk of PID than no infection and that women experiencing repeated chlamydia are at higher risk of PID than women who had one infection.[71,72] A population-based study in Canada demonstrated that each repeat chlamydial infection increased the risk of PID by 20%, with a more than four-fold increased risk in younger women under 16 years, more than two-fold higher risk for women aged 16 to 19 years, and 1.5-fold increase in those aged 20 to 24 years compared with women over 30 years of age.[73]

Prompt diagnosis and treatment of PID are essential to minimize the risk of infertility or other sequelae. Diagnosis of PID is based on clinical history and examination, but with varying severity of symptoms and signs, it can be a challenging diagnosis to make.[67,74] There is no objective, noninvasive diagnostic test nor combination of signs and symptoms that are both sensitive and specific for a PID diagnosis.[64] Although laparoscopy is considered the gold standard, it is an invasive procedure that is generally limited to cases not responding to treatment.[64] Given the serious consequences of untreated PID, it is recommended that clinicians should have a low threshold for diagnosis once pregnancy is excluded. Overdiagnosis is preferable to underdiagnosis, as the risks of antibiotics are likely less than the potential long-term complications of a missed diagnosis or delayed treatment.[64] Younger women are particularly at risk, and a PID diagnosis should always be considered in assessment of women aged under 30 years presenting with recent onset lower abdominal pain.[67,74] Clinicians should also routinely consider the possibility of PID and ask about PID symptoms when providing treatment for women diagnosed with a chlamydial infection.

CLINICAL MANIFESTATIONS IN MEN

More than 80% of infections in men are asymptomatic,[4] but the most common clinical manifestations associated with chlamydia when they occur in men include urethritis and epididymitis or epididymo-orchitis. Chlamydia-associated urethritis in men is characterized by a thin, white, gray, or sometimes clear watery discharge and dysuria.[75]

Epididymitis and orchitis are inflammations of the epididymis and testes and can be subclassified as acute, subacute, or chronic based on symptom duration.[76] In acute epididymitis, symptoms are present for less than 6 weeks and are characterized by epididymal pain and swelling. Chronic epididymitis is characterized by pain, generally without swelling, that persists for more than 3 months. Orchitis usually occurs when the inflammation from the epididymis spreads to the adjacent testicle.[76] Acute chlamydia-associated epididymitis typically presents with unilateral pain and tenderness and swelling of the epididymitis felt on palpitation.[76] In men aged 14 to 35 years, epididymitis is most commonly caused by chlamydia or *N gonorrhoeae*.[76] There is little information available about the proportion of cases of chlamydia in men that leads to epididymitis but a retrospective cohort study of US Air Force men found that men previously testing positive for chlamydia were more likely to develop epididymitis during follow-up (hazard ratio = 1.38; 95% CI: 1.13–1.70).[77]

A direct association between prostatitis and urogenital chlamydia infections in men is poorly studied because prostatitis can be caused by multiple uropathogens.[78] Studies of the presence of chlamydia DNA or antibodies among men with chronic prostatitis are inconsistent.[79]

CLINICAL MANIFESTATIONS IN WOMEN AND MEN

STIs including chlamydia can cause proctitis presenting with inflammation of the rectum (ie, the distal 10–12 cm) that can be characterized by anorectal pain, tenesmus, and/or rectal discharge. Fecal leukocytes are common. Proctitis is more commonly associated with LGV chlamydia serovars than with non-LGV serovars.[64]

As mentioned above, chlamydia pharyngeal infection is usually asymptomatic, and although its clinical significance remains unclear, it may be clinically important particularly in women, if it can be transmitted to the genital site, increasing their risk of upper genital tract infection.[80]

Chlamydia conjunctivitis in adults can occur but is uncommon and usually is associated with autoinoculation from concurrent anogenital infection.[81] The conjunctivitis is clinically mild and may resemble viral conjunctivitis.

Lymphogranuloma Venereum Infection

Although most chlamydia infections at the epithelial surface are mainly asymptomatic, LGV infections are more systemically invasive. Urogenital LGV infections are much less common than anogenital infections[28] and can present initially with painless ulceration or ulcerations that are then followed by painful inguinal lymphadenopathy ("buboes").[82] Rectal infections are often associated with signs and symptoms of ulcerative proctitis.[83,84] Specifically, serovar L2b is more likely to be associated with pain and bleeding compared with other L2 serovars (L2/L2f).[85] However, increasing evidence suggests that LGV can be asymptomatic, with between 27% and 53% of Dutch[86-89] and German cases[90] and between 17% and 22% of UK cases[91-93] being asymptomatic on initial presentation in high-risk MSM. A meta-analysis investigating the association between LGV and HIV found that individuals with LGV were 8 times more likely to be HIV positive (OR, 8.2; 95% CI: 4.7, 14.3).[94]

DIAGNOSIS

NAATs are the most sensitive tests for detecting chlamydia and are the recommended chlamydia test.[64] For women, urogenital chlamydia can be diagnosed by testing vaginal or cervical swabs or first-void urine, and testing can be done on clinician- or patient-collected specimens. Patient-collected vaginal swabs have equivalent sensitivity and specificity to clinician-collected swabs for NAATs[95] and are highly acceptable to women.[96] For men, urogenital infection can be diagnosed by testing first-catch urine or a urethral swab.[64] Optimal urogenital specimen types for chlamydia screening by NAAT are urine for men and vaginal swabs for women.

Rectal and oropharyngeal swabs can be used for chlamydia testing when testing is indicated at those anatomic sites, and NAATs have been cleared by US Food and Drug Administration (FDA) to test these sites.[97] NAAT performance on self-collected rectal swabs is comparable to clinician-collected swabs and is acceptable to MSM.[98]

Point-of-care chlamydia tests can expedite time to results and treatment. A recent review identified at least one FDA-approved chlamydia point-of-care test that has excellent performance for chlamydia detection, the Cepheid GeneXpert.[21] There are several other promising point-of-care chlamydia tests based on NAATs under development that offer considerable hope for the future.[21] More recently, a lateral flow test for gonorrhea and chlamydia was FDA approved, but this approval was only for vaginal samples.[99]

Although NAATs are highly sensitive, they are unable to discriminate nucleic acid originating from viable or nonviable bacteria, and it can take 2 to 3 weeks to clear remnant nonviable chlamydial nucleic acids following treatment.[63,100] To distinguish between viable or nonviable nucleic acid, a Dutch team has developed a technique termed viability–polymerase chain reaction or "V-PCR," using a membrane-impermeable dye that can irreversibly inhibit amplification of any DNA that is free or within damaged cells[101]; this allows calculations of the proportion of DNA originating from viable (ie, membrane-intact) cells. Using this technique, Janssen and colleagues[101] found that in 76% (38/50) of genital samples, less than 10% of the chlamydial DNA originated from viable (ie, membrane-intact) cells, suggesting an overestimation of viable infections. Similar results were reported in a small study of 53 women with rectal chlamydia, in which 48% of infections had no viable chlamydia using V-PCR.[102] In the future, these V-PCR tests may play a role in further identifying true infections and avoiding unnecessary treatment for those with nonviable chlamydia.

If a person has LGV-associated symptoms (including genital or rectal ulcers, anal discharge, bleeding, tenesmus, lymphadenopathy) and is chlamydia NAAT–positive on testing, molecular PCR testing for *C trachomatis* LGV serovars should be considered to confirm LGV.[64]

SCREENING POLICY

As chlamydia is largely asymptomatic, screening is needed to detect and treat most infections. The US Preventive Services Task Force (USPSTF) recently updated its evidence report about screening for chlamydia infection concluding that based on the results from 4 RCTs of chlamydia screening interventions, screening for asymptomatic genital chlamydial infection was significantly associated with a lower risk of PID in young women.[103] As a result of this evidence, the United States continues to recommend annual chlamydia screening for sexually active women under 25 years of age and among older women if considered at increased risk (if they have a new partner, more than one sex partner, a sex partner with concurrent partners, or a sex partner who has an STI). As repeat infection rates of up to 30% are observed in young women within 3 to 12 months following diagnosis,[22–24] retesting is recommended about 3 months after treatment to detect repeat infections early enough to reduce the risk of PID.[64] The USPSTF concluded that there is insufficient evidence to support routine chlamydia screening in men who only have sex with women,[103] and screening among these men should only be considered in certain high chlamydia prevalence clinical settings, such as STI clinics (**Table 1**). They also found that screening on the basis of risk prediction was of limited accuracy beyond age, and testing for asymptomatic chlamydia was highly accurate at most anatomical sites, including urine and self-collected specimens.[103]

Although the United States continues to promote annual screening for young women, several countries are reassessing their chlamydia screening guidelines. The National Chlamydia Screening Programme (NCSP) in England has recently changed its aim to "focus on preventing adverse consequences of untreated chlamydia …rather than aiming to reduce prevalence."[104] As a result, they no longer offer testing to both women and men under 25 years, only to women. This change was introduced because after nearly 20 years of chlamydia screening policy in England, there has been no clear evidence that widespread testing has had an impact on prevalence and complications associated with chlamydia. Two RCTs of chlamydia test uptake among young women and men in the Netherlands[105] and Australia[106] did not find a reduction in the estimated prevalence of chlamydia associated with achievable levels of screening, and although chlamydia test uptake in the NCSP has been higher than the 16% to 20% achieved in the trials, the British National Surveys of Sexual Attitudes and Lifestyles has found no change in estimated population-based chlamydia prevalence over time.[104] It is unclear why these trials and the NCSP failed to observed a decline in population prevalence when mathematical models have suggested that prevalence should decline even with an annual testing rate of 20%.[107] A recent mathematical model investigated the NCSP results in more detail, concluding that partial immunity against reinfection and changes in differential screening coverage over time might have limited the reduction in chlamydia prevalence that would be expected for the level of screening coverage achieved in England.[108]

The Netherlands decided not to implement a screening program for women or men aged 15 to 29 years after the Chlamydia Screening Implementation Pilot of register-based screening,[105] and a recent expert consultation proposed a reduced role for chlamydia testing in people without symptoms.[109] In Australia, chlamydia policy now focuses on clinical management of people with diagnosed chlamydia, rather than on test uptake, to reduce transmission, and chlamydia testing is now

Table 1
United States chlamydia screening recommendations

Women	• Annual screening for sexually active women under 25 y of age
	• Annual screening for sexually active women 25 y of age and older if at increased risk
	• Retest approximately 3 mo after treatment
	• Rectal chlamydial testing can be considered in women based on reported sexual behaviors and exposure, through shared clinical decision between the patient and the provider
Pregnant women	• All pregnant women under 25 y of age at first perinatal visit
	• Pregnant women 25 y of age and older if at increased risk at first perinatal visit
	• Retest during the 3rd trimester for women under 25 y of age or at risk
	• Pregnant women with chlamydial infection should have a test of cure 4 wk after treatment and be retested within 3 mo
Men who have sex with women	• There is insufficient evidence for routine screening among heterosexual men who are at low risk for infection; however, screening young men can be considered in high chlamydia prevalence clinical settings (eg, adolescent clinics, correctional facilities, STI/sexual health clinic)
Men who have sex with men	• At least annually for sexually active MSM at anatomical sites of contact (urethra, rectum) regardless of condom use
	• Every 3–6 mo if at increased risk (ie, MSM on PrEP, with HIV infection, or if they or their sexual partners have multiple partners)
	• Oropharyngeal screening is not recommended
Transgender and gender diverse persons	• Screening recommendations should be adapted based on anatomy (ie, annual, routine screening for chlamydia in cisgender women <25-y-old should be extended to all transgender men and gender diverse people with a cervix. If over 25-y-old, persons with a cervix should be screened if at increased risk)
	• Consider screening at the rectal site based on reported sexual behaviors and exposure
Persons with HIV	• For sexually active individuals, screen at first HIV evaluation, and at least annually thereafter
	• More frequent screening might be appropriate depending on individual risk behaviors and the local epidemiology

(Data from Workowski KA, Bachmann LH, Chan PA, et al. Sexually Transmitted Infections Treatment Guidelines, 2021. MMWR Recomm Rep 2021;70(No. RR-4):1–187.)

recommended on request for a check for STIs, rather than every year, in women and men younger than 30 years.[104]

Although there have been calls to consider rectal chlamydia screening in women,[110] the ongoing uncertainty about its natural history and clinical significance in women has prompted many, including the USPSTF, to recommend against regular rectal chlamydia screening.[53,103,111,112]

Routine chlamydia screening at urogenital and extragenital sites continues to be recommended for MSM in guidelines in several high-income countries, particularly in those taking PrEP, largely because of concerns about the potential risk of HIV transmission and acquisition and the observed high rates of STIs.[103]

The USPSTF also concluded that the effectiveness of screening in men, including MSM, and during pregnancy, optimal screening interventions, and adverse effects of screening required further evaluation.[103]

MANAGEMENT
Treatment

Early treatment of chlamydia infection is vital to reduce ongoing transmission and minimize the risk of complications. Treatment of sexual partners within the last 60 days helps to prevent reinfection and spread to other partners. Treatment of pregnant women diagnosed with chlamydia reduces transmission to the baby during birth and may reduce risk for pregnancy complications (eg, preterm birth).

In response to growing concern about the efficacy of 1-g single-dose azithromycin[113,114] for chlamydia and the recent findings from 2 recent RCTs that provided conclusive evidence that doxycycline is significantly more efficacious for rectal chlamydia than azithromycin,[58,59] the CDC STIs Treatment Guidelines in the United States changed its chlamydia treatment recommendations to 7 days of doxycycline (100 mg twice daily) as the only first-line treatment for chlamydia at any anatomic site in nonpregnant persons, and azithromycin was relegated to alternative treatment except in pregnant women (**Table 2**).[64] A further RCT in women found that a 7-day course of doxycycline (100 mg twice daily) was significantly more efficacious of the treatment of rectal chlamydia that was concurrent with a genital infection.[115] For women, the change to doxycycline for urogenital infection should ensure that any concurrent rectal infections should also be effectively cured, minimizing the risk that an uncleared rectal infection could autoinoculate the genital site, causing a urogenital reinfection following initial treatment.

For pregnant women, azithromycin is still the treatment of choice, as doxycycline is contraindicated during the second and third trimesters of pregnancy because of risk for tooth discoloration.[64]

Patients should be advised to avoid sexual activity for 7 days after treatment initiation and not have any sexual contact with partners from the previous 6 months until they have also been tested and treated as appropriate. However, this can be

Table 2 Recommended chlamydia treatment in adolescents and adults	
Nonpregnant adolescents and adults	Doxycycline 100 mg orally 2 times/d for 7 d Alternative: Azithromycin 1 g orally in a single dose OR Levofloxacin 500 mg orally once daily for 7 d
Pregnant women	Azithromycin 1 g orally in a single dose Alternative: Amoxicillin 500 mg orally 3 times/d for 7 d
LGV	Doxycycline 100 mg orally 2 times/d for 21 d Alternative: Azithromycin 1 g orally once weekly for 3 wk[a] OR Erythromycin base 500 mg orally 4 times/d for 21 d

[a] Because this regimen has not been validated, a test of cure with C trachomatis NAAT 4 wk after completion of treatment can be considered.

(Data from Workowski KA, Bachmann LH, Chan PA, et al. Sexually Transmitted Infections Treatment Guidelines, 2021. MMWR Recomm Rep 2021;70(No. RR-4):1–187.)

challenging to enforce, with one study among MSM finding about 10% resumed condomless receptive anal sex with 7 days of receiving treatment.[116]

For those in whom LGV is diagnosed or suspected, a 21-day regimen of doxycycline (100 mg twice daily) is recommended.

Follow-up

Partner management

Most guidelines recommend testing and treatment of the sexual contacts of individuals diagnosed with chlamydia, and it is important for clinicians to discuss with the index case the reasons for notifying sexual partners that they may be at risk of chlamydia. In the United States, the CDC guidelines recommend that partners in the last 60 days should be contacted.[64] There are a number of strategies for partner management, and many patients will opt to inform their sexual partners themselves (patient-initiated referral). Online anonymous notification tools have been found to be effective at allowing people to send an anonymous SMS or email to sex partners informing them they have been exposed to an STI.[117] Provider-initiated referral may be appropriate in complex situations: for example, if there are concerns about partner violence.[118] Health department partner management services should be contacted directly for advice regarding partner notification in these situations.

Patient-delivered partner therapy (PDPT) is another strategy to reach partners for treatment and is the clinical practice of treating the sexual partners of patients diagnosed with chlamydia by providing prescriptions or medications to the patient to take to their partner or partners without the health care provider first evaluating the partner or partners. Compared with standard patient referral of partners, this approach to therapy has been associated with decreased rates of persistent or recurrent chlamydia and an increased percentage of partners receiving treatment.[119,120] PDPT is less appropriate among MSM because there is a high risk of sexual partners being coinfected with other STIs, including undiagnosed HIV, and it would limit the opportunity to discuss HIV PrEP in partners without HIV.

To avoid reinfection, sexual partners should be instructed to abstain from condomless sexual intercourse until they and their sex partners have been treated (ie, after completion of a 7-day regimen) and any symptoms have resolved.

Follow-up retesting

A test of cure at 4 weeks to detect treatment failure is not recommended for nonpregnant women treated for chlamydia unless there are concerns about treatment adherence, if symptoms persist, or if reinfection is suspected.[64] The time point of 4 weeks is chosen because it has been demonstrated that after treatment, chlamydia nucleic acid can continue to shed for 2 to 3 weeks, potentially generating a false positive NAAT test result.[63,100]

Repeat chlamydia infection is very common in women and men in the few months following treatment of infection, with most repeat infections likely to be due to reinfection from an untreated sexual partner or a new infected partner. As a result, guidelines in several high-income countries recommend retesting after treatment. The CDC Guidelines recommend that men and women treated for chlamydia should be retested at 3 months after treatment.[64]

Among pregnant women, a test-of-cure with an NAAT is recommended about 4 weeks after completing treatment to establish the infection has been cured during pregnancy because of the risk of pregnancy complications should the infection persist. Pregnant women at increased risk for chlamydia (those <25 years, those with a new sex partner, those with more than one partner, or those with a sex partner with an STI) should be rescreened for chlamydia during the third trimester to reduce the risk of pregnancy complications and chlamydia transmission to the newborn during delivery.[64]

VACCINE AND OTHER THERAPEUTIC AGENTS

Research on the development of human chlamydia vaccines is ongoing.[121] Recently, the results from a 3-armed, placebo-controlled trial assessing the safety and immunogenicity of a recombinant *C trachomatis* MOMP vaccine adjuvanted with 1 of 2 different adjuvants versus placebo saline were published.[122] Both adjuvants were well-tolerated, and immunoglobulin G (IgG) seroconversion occurred in 100% (15/15) of the participants receiving the MOMP vaccine versus none in the placebo group. Although the vaccine's efficacy in prevention of chlamydia infection is unknown at this time, progress such as this holds promise.

Other non-antibiotic interventions to treat chlamydia are in development, including new synthetic drugs, natural compounds, lipids, peptides, and cytokines.[123] Potential new drug therapies may include the use of novel compounds, such as the chlamydia HtrA inhibitor JT0146,[124] or capsaicin.[125] Furthermore, topical microbicides that target rectal transmission (including HIV) are also being explored as prophylaxis or treatment,[126] although a recent systematic review has questioned their efficacy in the prevention of STIs, including chlamydia, HIV, or syphilis,[127] and there is concern about the significant epithelial exfoliation observed with these products in animal studies.[128]

SUMMARY

Chlamydia continues to be the most commonly diagnosed bacterial STI regardless of global screening efforts, and if left untreated, it can cause significant complications, particularly in women. Younger women, individuals from certain racial/ethnic minorities, those with multiple sexual partners, and/or MSM are at increased risk of infection. Chlamydia NAATs are highly accurate for chlamydia detection and can be performed reliably on self-collected specimens, and the promise of new point-of-care and viability assays means testing will be become easier and more widely available and may also limit overtreatment for persons who do not have chlamydia. Recommended treatment of chlamydia is highly effective and readily available. Given the ongoing challenges in achieving sufficiently high enough test uptake to reduce transmission, we must continue to support further research into chlamydia vaccines if we are to reduce the burden of chlamydia and its complications in the population.

CLINICS CARE POINTS

- Chlamydia trachomatis disproportionately affects young adults, young racial and ethnic minority groups and men who have sex with men. Infection commonly occurs at the genital and rectal anatomic sites in both women and men.

- Doxycycline (100mg orally 2 times/d for 7 d) is the recommended treatment for non-pregnant persons and azithromycin (1 g orally in a single dose) for pregnant persons.

- Repeat chlamydia infection is common and rescreening 3 months after treatment for infection is recommended.

- Chlamydia can cause PID and clinicians should ask about PID associated symptoms when providing treatment for women diagnosed with chlamydia.

> • Partner management is necessary to reduce transmission and risk of complications particularly in women.

DISCLOSURE

J.S. Hocking reports receiving support from a National Health and Medical Research Council (NHMRC), Australia Senior Research Fellowship (GNT1136117). W.M. Geisler reports receiving research funding and honorarium from Hologic, United States and consulting fees from Sanofi. F.Y.S. Kong reports receiving funding from an NHMRC Ideas Grant (GNT1181057) and University of Melbourne's Faculty of Medicine, Dentistry & Health Sciences C.R. Roper Fellowship.

REFERENCES

1. World Health Organization. Global health sector strategy on sexually transmitted infections 2016-2021. Geneva: WHO; 2016.
2. Centers for Disease Control and Prevention. Table 1. Sexually Transmitted Diseases – Reported Cases and Rates of Reported Cases*, United States, 1941-2020. 2022. Available at: https://www.cdc.gov/std/statistics/2020/tables/1.htm. Accessed 04, December, 2022.
3. Peipert JF. Genital Chlamydial Infections. New Eng J Med 2003;349(25): 2424–30.
4. Sutton T, Martinko T, Hale S, et al. Prevalence and high rate of asymptomatic infection of *Chlamydia trachomatis* in male college reserve officer training corps cadets. Sex Trans Dis 2003;30:901–4.
5. Manavi K. A review on infection with *Chlamydia trachomatis*. Best Pract Res Clin Obstet Gynaeco 2006;20(6):941–51.
6. Lesiak-Markowicz I, Schötta A-M, Stockinger H, et al. *Chlamydia trachomatis* serovars in urogenital and ocular samples collected 2014–2017 from Austrian patients. Sci Rep 2019;9(1):18327.
7. Bax CJ, Quint KD, Peters RPH, et al. Analyses of multiple-site and concurrent *Chlamydia trachomatis* serovar infections, and serovar tissue tropism for urogenital versus rectal specimens in male and female patients. Sex Transm Inf 2011;87(6):503–7.
8. Quint KD, Bom RJ, Quint WGV, et al. Anal infections with concomitant *Chlamydia trachomatis* genotypes among men who have sex with men in Amsterdam, the Netherlands. BMC Inf Dis 2011;11:63.
9. Li J-H, Cai Y-M, Yin Y-P, et al. Prevalence of anorectal *Chlamydia trachomatis* infection and its genotype distribution among men who have sex with men in Shenzhen, China. Jap J Infect Dis 2011;64(2):143–6.
10. Klint M, Löfdahl M, Ek C, et al. Lymphogranuloma Venereum Prevalence in Sweden among Men Who Have Sex with Men and Characterization of *Chlamydia trachomatis* ompA Genotypes. J Clin Microbiol 2006;44(11):4066–71.
11. Geisler WM, Whittington WL, Suchland RJ, et al. Epidemiology of Anorectal Chlamydial and Gonococcal Infections Among Men Having Sex With Men in Seattle: Utilizing Serovar and Auxotype Strain Typing. Sex Trans Dis 2002;29(4): 189–95.
12. Christerson L, Bom RJM, Bruisten SM, et al. *Chlamydia trachomatis* strains show specific clustering for men who have sex with men compared to heterosexual

populations in Sweden, the Netherlands, and the United States. J Clin Microbiol 2012;50(11):3548–55.

13. Bom R, Christerson L, van der Loeff MFS, et al. Evaluation of high-resolution typing methods for *Chlamydia trachomatis* in samples from heterosexual couples. J Clin Microbiol 2011;49:2844–53.

14. Rowley J, Vander Hoorn S, Korenromp E, et al. Chlamydia, gonorrhoea, trichomoniasis and syphilis: global prevalence and incidence estimates, 2016. Bull World Health Organ 2019;97(8):548–562p.

15. Centers for Disease Control and Prevention. 2020 STD Surveillance Report - Chlamydia. 2022. Available at: https://www.cdc.gov/std/statistics/2020/overview.htm#Chlamydia. Accessed 09, December, 2022.

16. Katz DA, Copen CE, Haderxhanaj LT, et al. Changes in Sexual Behaviors with Opposite-Sex Partners and Sexually Transmitted Infection Outcomes Among Females and Males Ages 15-44 Years in the USA: National Survey of Family Growth, 2008-2019. Arch sex behav 2022;52(2):809–21.

17. King J, McManus H, Kwon A, et al. HIV, viral hepatitis and sexually transmissible infections in Australia: annual surveillance report 2022. Sydney: Kirby Institute; 2022.

18. European Centre for Disease Prevention and Control. Surveillance and disease data for chlamydia. 2022. Available at: https://www.ecdc.europa.eu/en/infectious-disease-topics/z-disease-list/chlamydia-infection/surveillance-and-disease-data. Accessed 30 November 2022.

19. Public Health Agency of Canada. Report on sexually transmitted infection surveillance in Canada, 2019. Ottawa: Public Health Agency of Canada; 2021.

20. Redmond SM, Alexander-Kisslig K, Woodhall SC, et al. Genital chlamydia prevalence in Europe and non-European high income countries: systematic review and meta-analysis. PLoS One 2015;10(1):e0115753.

21. Geisler WM, Hocking JS, Darville T, et al. Diagnosis and Management of Uncomplicated *Chlamydia trachomatis* Infections in Adolescents and Adults: Summary of Evidence Reviewed for the 2021 Centers for Disease Control and Prevention Sexually Transmitted Infections Treatment Guidelines. Clin Inf Dis 2022;74(Suppl_2):S112–s126.

22. Walker J, Fairley C, Bradshaw C, et al. *Chlamydia trachomatis* Incidence and Re-Infection among Young Women - Behavioural and Microbiological Characteristics. PLoS One 2012;7(5):e37778.

23. LaMontagne D, Baster K, Emmett L, et al. Incidence and reinfection rates of genital chlamydia infection among women aged 16 to 24 years attending general practice, family planning and genitourinary medicine clinics in England: a prospective cohort study by the Chlamydia Recall Study Advisory Group. Sex Transm Inf 2007;83:282–303.

24. Bowring A, Gouillou M, Guy R, et al. Missed opportunities–low levels of chlamydia retesting at Australian general practices, 2008-2009. Sex Transm Inf 2012;88(5):330–4.

25. Tabesh M, Fairley CK, Hocking JS, et al. Comparison of the patterns of chlamydia and gonorrhoea at the oropharynx, anorectum and urethra among men who have sex with men. Sex Transm Inf 2022;98(1):11–6.

26. van Liere GA, Hoebe CJ, Dukers-Muijrers NH. Evaluation of the anatomical site distribution of chlamydia and gonorrhoea in men who have sex with men and in high-risk women by routine testing: cross-sectional study revealing missed opportunities for treatment strategies. Sex Transm Inf 2014;90(1):58–60.

27. Harvey-Lavoie S, Apelian H, Labbé AC, et al. Community-Based Prevalence Estimates of *Chlamydia trachomatis* and Neisseria gonorrhoeae Infections Among Gay, Bisexual, and Other Men Who Have Sex With Men in Montréal, Canada. Sex Trans Dis 2021;48(12):939–44.

28. de Vrieze NHN, Versteeg B, Bruisten SM, et al. Low Prevalence of Urethral Lymphogranuloma Venereum Infections Among Men Who Have Sex With Men: A Prospective Observational Study, Sexually Transmitted Infection Clinic in Amsterdam, the Netherlands. Sex Trans Dis 2017;44(9):547–50.

29. Dewart CM, Bernstein KT, DeGroote NP, et al. Prevalence of Rectal Chlamydial and Gonococcal Infections: A Systematic Review. Sex Trans Dis 2018;45(5):287–93.

30. Chandra NL, Broad C, Folkard K, et al. Detection of *Chlamydia trachomatis* in rectal specimens in women and its association with anal intercourse: a systematic review and meta-analysis. Sex Transm Inf 2018;94(5):320–6.

31. Lau A, Kong FYS, Huston W, et al. Factors associated with anorectal *Chlamydia trachomatis* or *Neisseria gonorrhoeae* test positivity in women: a systematic review and meta-analysis. Sex Transm Inf 2019;95(5):361–7.

32. Rank RG, Yeruva L. Hidden in plain sight: chlamydial gastrointestinal infection and its relevance to persistence in human genital infection. Infect Immun 2014;82(4):1362–71.

33. Janssen KJH, Wolffs PFG, Hoebe C, et al. Determinants associated with viable genital or rectal *Chlamydia trachomatis* bacterial load (FemCure). Sex Transm Inf 2022;98(1):17–22.

34. Bavoil PM, Marques PX, Brotman R, et al. Does Active Oral Sex Contribute to Female Infertility? J Infect Dis 2017;216(8):932–5.

35. Hess KL, Crepaz N, Rose C, et al. Trends in Sexual Behavior Among Men Who have Sex with Men (MSM) in High-Income Countries, 1990-2013: A Systematic Review. AIDS Behav 2017;21(10):2811–34.

36. Traeger MW, Schroeder SE, Wright EJ, et al. Effects of Pre-exposure Prophylaxis for the Prevention of Human Immunodeficiency Virus Infection on Sexual Risk Behavior in Men Who Have Sex With Men: A Systematic Review and Meta-analysis. Clin Inf Dis 2018;67(5):676–86.

37. Ong JJ, Baggaley RC, Wi TE, et al. Global Epidemiologic Characteristics of Sexually Transmitted Infections Among Individuals Using Preexposure Prophylaxis for the Prevention of HIV Infection: A Systematic Review and Meta-analysis. JAMA Net Open 2019;2(12):e1917134.

38. Chan PA, Robinette A, Montgomery M, et al. Extragenital Infections Caused by *Chlamydia trachomatis* and *Neisseria gonorrhoeae*: A Review of the Literature. Infect Dis Obstet Gynecol 2016;2016:5758387.

39. Johnson LF, Lewis DA. The effect of genital tract infections on HIV-1 shedding in the genital tract: a systematic review and meta-analysis. Sex Trans Dis 2008;35(11):946–59.

40. Sadiq ST, Taylor S, Copas AJ, et al. The effects of urethritis on seminal plasma HIV-1 RNA loads in homosexual men not receiving antiretroviral therapy. Sex Transm Inf 2005;81(2):120–3.

41. Cohen MS, Hoffman IF, Royce RA, et al. Reduction of concentration of HIV-1 in semen after treatment of urethritis: implications for prevention of sexual transmission of HIV-1. AIDSCAP Malawi Research Group. Lancet 1997;349(9069):1868–73.

42. Buckner LR, Amedee AM, Albritton HL, et al. *Chlamydia trachomatis* infection of Endocervical Epithelial Cells Enhances Early HIV Transmission Events. PLoS One 2016;11(1):e0146663.
43. Xiridou M, Vriend HJ, Lugner AK, et al. Modelling the impact of chlamydia screening on the transmission of HIV among men who have sex with men. BMC Inf Dis 2013;13:436.
44. Malekinejad M, Barker EK, Merai R, et al. Risk of HIV Acquisition Among Men Who Have Sex With Men Infected With Bacterial Sexually Transmitted Infections: A Systematic Review and Meta-Analysis. Sex Trans Dis 2021;48(10):e138–48.
45. Darville T, Hiltke TJ. Pathogenesis of genital tract disease due to *Chlamydia trachomatis*. J Infect Dis 2010;201(Suppl 2):S114–25.
46. Rank RG, Whittum-Hudson JA. Protective immunity to chlamydial genital infection: evidence from animal studies. J Infect Dis 2010;201(Suppl 2):S168–77.
47. Batteiger BE, Xu F, Johnson RE, et al. Protective immunity to *Chlamydia trachomatis* genital infection: evidence from human studies. J Infect Dis 2010; 201(Suppl 2):S178–89.
48. Brunham RC. Immunity to Chlamydia trachomatis. J Infect Dis 2013;207(12): 1796–7.
49. Geisler WM, Lensing SY, Press CG, et al. Spontaneous resolution of genital *Chlamydia trachomatis* infection in women and protection from reinfection. J Infect Dis 2013;207(12):1850–6.
50. Brunham RC, Rekart ML. The arrested immunity hypothesis and the epidemiology of chlamydia control. Sex Trans Dis 2008;35(1):53–4.
51. Khosropour CM, Soge OO, Golden MR, et al. Incidence and Duration of Pharyngeal Chlamydia Among a Cohort of Men Who Have Sex With Men. Clin Inf Dis 2022;75(5):875–81.
52. Barbee LA, Khosropour CM, Soge OO, et al. The Natural History of Rectal Gonococcal and Chlamydial Infections: The ExGen Study. Clin Inf Dis 2022;74(9): 1549–56.
53. Lau A, Hocking JS, Kong FYS. Rectal chlamydia infections: implications for reinfection risk, screening, and treatment guidelines. Curr Opin Infect Dis 2022; 35(1):42–8.
54. Geisler WM. Duration of untreated, uncomplicated *Chlamydia trachomatis* genital infection and factors associated with chlamydia resolution: a review of human studies. J Infect Dis 2010;201(Suppl 2):S104–13.
55. Lewis J, Price MJ, Horner PJ, et al. Genital Chlamydia trachomatis Infections Clear More Slowly in Men Than Women, but Are Less Likely to Become Established. J Infect Dis 2017;216(2):237–44.
56. Price MJ, Ades AE, Soldan K, et al. The natural history of *Chlamydia trachomatis* infection in women: a multi-parameter evidence synthesis. Health Techn Assess 2016;20(22):1–250.
57. Chow EP, Camilleri S, Ward C, et al. Duration of gonorrhoea and chlamydia infection at the pharynx and rectum among men who have sex with men: a systematic review. Sex Health 2016;13(3):199–204.
58. Dombrowski JC, Wierzbicki MR, Newman LM, et al. Doxycycline Versus Azithromycin for the Treatment of Rectal Chlamydia in Men Who Have Sex With Men: A Randomized Controlled Trial. Clin Inf Dis 2021;73(5):824–31.
59. Lau A, Kong FYS, Fairley CK, et al. Azithromycin or Doxycycline for Asymptomatic Rectal Chlamydia trachomatis. New Eng J Med 2021;384(25):2418–27.
60. van Liere G, Hoebe C, Dirks JA, et al. Spontaneous clearance of urogenital, anorectal and oropharyngeal *Chlamydia trachomatis* and *Neisseria gonorrhoeae* in

women, MSM and heterosexual men visiting the STI clinic: a prospective cohort study. Sex Transm Inf 2019;95(7):505–10.

61. van Rooijen MS, van der Loeff MF, Morré SA, et al. Spontaneous pharyngeal *Chlamydia trachomatis* RNA clearance. A cross-sectional study followed by a cohort study of untreated STI clinic patients in Amsterdam, The Netherlands. Sex Transm Inf 2015;91(3):157–64.

62. Geisler W, Wang C, Morrison SG, et al. The Natural History of Untreated *Chlamydia trachomatis* Infection in the Interval Between Screening and Returning for Treatment. Sex Trans Dis 2008;35(2):119–23.

63. Renault CA, Israelski DM, Levy V, et al. Time to clearance of *Chlamydia trachomatis* ribosomal RNA in women treated for chlamydial infection. Sex Health 2011;8(1):69–73.

64. Workowski KA, Bachmann LH, Chan PA, et al. Sexually Transmitted Infections Treatment Guidelines, 2021. MMWR Recomm Rep (Morb Mortal Wkly Rep) 2021;70(4):1–187.

65. Gollow MM, Bucens MR, Sesnan K. Chlamydial infections of the urethra in women. Genitourin Med 1986;62(4):283.

66. Stamm WE, Wagner KF, Amsel R, et al. Causes of the acute urethral syndrome in women. The New Eng J Med 1980;303(8):409–15.

67. Ross J. Pelvic inflammatory disease. Medicine 2010;38(5):255–9.

68. Goller JL, De Livera AM, Fairley CK, et al. Population attributable fraction of pelvic inflammatory disease associated with chlamydia and gonorrhoea: a cross-sectional analysis of Australian sexual health clinic data. Sex Transm Inf 2016; 18(52195):2015–195.

69. Causer L, Liu B, Watts C, et al. Hospitalisations for pelvic inflammatory disease in young Aboriginal women living in remote Australia: the role of chlamydia and gonorrhoea. Sex Transm Inf 2022;98(6):445–7.

70. Price MJ, Ades AE, Welton NJ, et al. Proportion of Pelvic Inflammatory Disease Cases Caused by *Chlamydia trachomatis*: Consistent Picture From Different Methods. J Infect Dis 2016;214(4):617–24.

71. Reekie J, Donovan B, Guy R, et al. Risk of Pelvic Inflammatory Disease in Relation to Chlamydia and Gonorrhea Testing, Repeat Testing, and Positivity: A Population-Based Cohort Study. Clin Inf Dis 2018;66(3):437–43.

72. Davies B, Turner KM, Frolund M, et al. Risk of reproductive complications following chlamydia testing: a population-based retrospective cohort study in Denmark. Lancet Inf Dis 2016;8(16):30092–5.

73. Davies B, Ward H, Leung S, et al. Heterogeneity in risk of pelvic inflammatory diseases after chlamydia infection: a population-based study in Manitoba, Canada. J Infect Dis 2014;210(Suppl 2):S549–55.

74. Bateson D, Edmiston N. Pelvic inflammatory disease: Management of new onset low abdominal pain in young women. Med Today 2016;17(7):14–22.

75. Centers for Disease Control and Prevention. Chlamydia – CDC Detailed Fact Sheet. 2022. Available at: https://www.cdc.gov/std/chlamydia/stdfact-chlamydia-detailed.htm. Accessed 13 December 2022.

76. Trojian TH, Lishnak TS, Heiman D. Epididymitis and orchitis: an overview. Am Fam Phys 2009;79(7):583–7.

77. Trei JS, Canas LC, Gould PL. Reproductive tract complications associated with *Chlamydia trachomatis* infection in US Air Force males within 4 years of testing. Sex Trans Dis 2008;35(9):827–33.

78. Khan FU, Ihsan AU, Khan HU, et al. Comprehensive overview of prostatitis. Biomed Pharmacother 2017;94:1064–76.

79. Bielecki R, Ostaszewska-Puchalska I, Zdrodowska-Stefanow B, et al. The presence of *Chlamydia trachomatis* infection in men with chronic prostatitis. Cen European J Urol 2020;73(3):362–8.

80. Xu X, Chow EPF, Ong JJ, et al. *Chlamydia trachomatis* transmission between the oropharynx, urethra and anorectum in men who have sex with men: a mathematical model. BMC Med 2020;18(1):326.

81. Garland SM, Malatt A, Tabrizi S, et al. *Chlamydia trachomatis* conjunctivitis. Prevalence and association with genital tract infection. Med J Aust 1995; 162(7):363–6.

82. Haber R, Maatouk I, de Barbeyrac B, et al. Lymphogranuloma Venereum-Serovar L2b Presenting With Painful Genital Ulceration: An Emerging Clinical Presentation? Sex Trans Dis 2017;44(5):310–2.

83. de Vries H, Zingoni A, Kreuter A, et al. 2013 European guideline on the management of lymphogranuloma venereum. J Eur Acad Dermatol Venereol 2014; 29(1):1–6.

84. White JA. Manifestations and management of lymphogranuloma venereum. Curr Opin Inf Dis 2009;22(1):57–66.

85. Rodríguez-Domínguez M, Puerta T, Menéndez B, et al. Clinical and epidemiological characterization of a lymphogranuloma venereum outbreak in Madrid, Spain: co-circulation of two variants. Clin Microbiol Infect 2014;20(3):219–25.

86. Van der Bij AK, Spaargaren J, Morre SA, et al. Diagnostic and clinical implications of anorectal lymphogranuloma venereum in men who have sex with men: a retrospective case-control study. Clin Inf dis 2006;42(2):186–94.

87. Spaargaren J, Fennema HSA, Morre SA, et al. New lymphogranuloma venereum *Chlamydia trachomatis* variant, Amsterdam. Emerg Infect Dis 2005;11(7): 1090–2.

88. de Vrieze NHN, van Rooijen M, Schim van der Loeff MF, et al. Anorectal and inguinal lymphogranuloma venereum among men who have sex with men in Amsterdam, The Netherlands: trends over time, symptomatology and concurrent infections. Sex Transm Inf 2013;89(7):548–52.

89. Waalboer R, van der Snoek EM, van der Meijden WI, et al. Analysis of rectal *Chlamydia trachomatis* serovar distribution including L2 (lymphogranuloma venereum) at the Erasmus MC STI clinic, Rotterdam. Sex Transm Inf 2006;82(3): 207–11.

90. Haar K, Dudareva-Vizule S, Wisplinghoff H, et al. Lymphogranuloma venereum in men screened for pharyngeal and rectal infection, Germany. Emerg Infect Dis 2013;19(3):488–92.

91. Ward H, Martin I, Macdonald N, et al. Lymphogranuloma Venereum in the United Kingdom. Clin Inf Dis 2007;44(1):26–32.

92. Pallawela S, Dean G, French P, et al. Clinical presentation of Lymphogranuloma venereum in a multi-centre case-control study in the UK: LGV-net. HIV Med 2010;37. Conference.

93. Saxon CJ, Hughes G, Ison C. P3.138 Increasing Asymptomatic Lymphogranuloma Venereum Infection in the UK: Results from a National Case-Finding Study. Sex Transm Inf 2013;89(Suppl 1):A190–1.

94. Ronn MM, Ward H. The association between lymphogranuloma venereum and HIV among men who have sex with men: systematic review and meta-analysis. BMC Inf Dis 2011;11:70.

95. Knox J, Tabrizi SN, Miller P, et al. Evaluation of self-collected samples in contrast to practitioner-collected samples for detection of *Chlamydia trachomatis,*

Neisseria gonorrhoeae, and *Trichomonas vaginalis* by polymerase chain reaction among women living in remote areas. Sex Trans Dis 2002;29(11):647–54.

96. Doshi JS, Power J, Allen E. Acceptability of chlamydia screening using self-taken vaginal swabs. Int J STD AIDS 2008;19(8):507–9.

97. U.S Food and Drug Administration News Release. FDA clears first diagnostic tests for extragenital testing for chlamydia and gonorrhea. 2019. Available at: https://www.fda.gov/news-events/press-announcements/fda-clears-first-diagnostic-tests-extragenitaltesting-chlamydia-and-gonorrhea. Accessed March 19, 2023.

98. van der Helm JJ, Hoebe CJ, van Rooijen MS, et al. High performance and acceptability of self-collected rectal swabs for diagnosis of *Chlamydia trachomatis* and *Neisseria gonorrhoeae* in men who have sex with men and women. Sex Trans Dis 2009;36(8):493–7.

99. Dawkins M, Bishop L, Walker P, et al. Clinical Integration of a Highly Accurate Polymerase Chain Reaction Point-of-Care Test Can Inform Immediate Treatment Decisions for Chlamydia, Gonorrhea, and Trichomonas. Sex Transm Dis 2022; 49(4):262–7.

100. Wind CM, Schim van der Loeff MF, Unemo M, et al. Time to clearance of *Chlamydia trachomatis* RNA and DNA after treatment in patients coinfected with *Neisseria gonorrhoeae* - a prospective cohort study. BMC Inf Dis 2016; 16(1):554.

101. Janssen KJ, Hoebe CJ, Dukers-Muijrers NH, et al. Viability-PCR Shows That NAAT Detects a High Proportion of DNA from Non-Viable. Chlamydia trachomatis. PloS One 2016;11(11):e0165920.

102. Janssen KJH, Wolffs P, Lucchesi M, et al. Assessment of rectal Chlamydia trachomatis viable load in women by viability-PCR. Sex Transm Inf 2020; 96(2):85–8.

103. Cantor A, Dana T, Griffin JC, et al. Screening for Chlamydial and Gonococcal Infections: Updated Evidence Report and Systematic Review for the US Preventive Services Task Force. JAMA 2021;326(10):957–66.

104. Low N, Hocking JS, van Bergen J. The changing landscape of chlamydia control strategies. Lancet 2021;398(10309):1386–8.

105. van den Broek IVF, van Bergen JEAM, Brouwers EEHG, et al. Effectiveness of yearly, register based screening for chlamydia in the Netherlands: controlled trial with randomised stepped wedge implementation. BMJ 2012;345:e4316.

106. Hocking JS, Temple-Smith M, Guy R, et al. Population effectiveness of opportunistic chlamydia testing in primary care in Australia: a cluster-randomised controlled trial. Lancet 2018;392(10156):1413–22.

107. Regan D, Wilson D, Hocking J. Coverage is the key for effective screening of *Chlamydia trachomatis* in Australia. J Infect Dis 2008;198(3):349–58.

108. Smid J, Althaus CL, Low N. Discrepancies between observed data and predictions from mathematical modelling of the impact of screening interventions on *Chlamydia trachomatis* prevalence. Sci Rep 2019;9(1):7547.

109. van Bergen J, Hoenderboom BM, David S, et al. Where to go to in chlamydia control? From infection control towards infectious disease control. Sex Transm Inf 2021;97(7):501–6.

110. Andersson N, Boman J, Nylander E. Rectal chlamydia - should screening be recommended in women? Int J STD AIDS 2017;28(5):476–9.

111. Dukers-Muijrers N, Evers YJ, Hoebe C, et al. Controversies and evidence on Chlamydia testing and treatment in asymptomatic women and men who have sex with men: a narrative review. BMC Inf Dis 2022;22(1):255.

112. Khosropour CM, Dombrowski JC, Vojtech L, et al. Rectal *Chlamydia trachomatis* Infection: A Narrative Review of the State of the Science and Research Priorities. Sex Trans Dis 2021;48(12):e223–7.

113. Hocking JS, Kong F, Timms P, et al. Treatment for rectal chlamydia infection may be more complicated than we originally thought. J Antimicrob Chemother 2015; 70(4):961–4.

114. Kong FY, Hocking JS. Treatment challenges for urogenital and anorectal *Chlamydia trachomatis*. BMC Inf Dis 2015;15(1):293.

115. Peuchant O, Lhomme E, Martinet P, et al. Doxycycline versus azithromycin for the treatment of anorectal Chlamydia trachomatis infection in women concurrent with vaginal infection (CHLAZIDOXY study): a multicentre, open-label, randomised, controlled, superiority trial. Lancet Inf Dis 2022;22(8):1221–30.

116. Lau A, Kong FYS, Fairley CK, et al. Factors Associated With Early Resumption of Condomless Anal Sex Among Men Who Have Sex With Men After Rectal Chlamydia Treatment. Sex Trans Dis 2020;47(6):389–94.

117. Htaik K, Fairley CK, Bilardi JE, et al. Evaluation of the Online Partner Messaging Service for Sexually Transmitted Infections Let Them Know. Sex Trans Dis 2022; 49(1):12–4.

118. Coombe J, Goller J, Vaisey A, et al. New best practice guidance for general practice to reduce chlamydia-associated reproductive complications in women. Aust J Gen Pract 2021;50(1–2):50–4.

119. Golden MR, Kerani RP, Stenger M, et al. Uptake and population-level impact of expedited partner therapy (EPT) on *Chlamydia trachomatis* and *Neisseria gonorrhoeae*: the Washington State community-level randomized trial of EPT. PLoS Med 2015;12(1).

120. Golden MR, Whittington WL, Handsfield HH, et al. Effect of expedited treatment of sex partners on recurrent or persistent gonorrhoea or chlamydial infection. New Eng J Med 2005;352:676–85.

121. de la Maza LM, Zhong G, Brunham RC. Update on *Chlamydia trachomatis* Vaccinology. Clin Vaccine Immunol 2017;24(4).

122. Abraham S, Juel HB, Bang P, et al. Safety and immunogenicity of the chlamydia vaccine candidate CTH522 adjuvanted with CAF01 liposomes or aluminium hydroxide: a first-in-human, randomised, double-blind, placebo-controlled, phase 1 trial. Lancet Inf Dis 2019;19(10):1091–100.

123. Hou C, Jin Y, Wu H, et al. Alternative strategies for Chlamydia treatment: Promising non-antibiotic approaches. Front Microbiol 2022;13:987662.

124. Ong VA, Lawrence A, Timms P, et al. In vitro susceptibility of recent *Chlamydia trachomatis* clinical isolates to the CtHtrA inhibitor JO146. Microbes Infect 2015; 17(11–12):738–44.

125. Yamakawa K, Matsuo J, Okubo T, et al. Impact of capsaicin, an active component of chili pepper, on pathogenic chlamydial growth (*Chlamydia trachomatis* and *Chlamydia pneumoniae*) in immortal human epithelial HeLa cells. J Infect Chemother 2018;24(2):130–7.

126. Harrison PF, Rosenberg Z, Bowcut J. Topical microbicides for disease prevention: status and challenges. Clin Inf Dis 2003;36(10):1290–4.

127. Obiero J, Ogongo P, Mwethera PG, et al. Topical microbicides for preventing sexually transmitted infections. Cochran Database Syst Rev 2021;3(3): Cd007961.

128. Patton DL, Sweeney YT, Paul KJ. A summary of preclinical topical microbicide rectal safety and efficacy evaluations in a pigtailed macaque model. Sex Trans Dis 2009;36(6):350–6.

Sexually Transmitted Human Papillomavirus
Update in Epidemiology, Prevention, and Management

Rosalyn E. Plotzker, MD, MPH[a,b,*], Akanksha Vaidya, MD, MPH[a],
Utsav Pokharel, MD[c], Elizabeth A. Stier, MD[d]

KEYWORDS

- Human papillomavirus • Cervical cancer • Anal cancer • Anogenital warts
- Sexually transmitted infections

KEY POINTS

- Human papillomavirus (HPV) is the most common sexually transmitted infection worldwide.
- Low-risk HPV strains may cause anogenital warts, whereas high-risk HPV strains may cause cancers of the lower anogenital tract.
- HPV vaccination is an effective strategy to prevent HPV infection and its related diseases.
- Cervical cancer prevention screening programs use cervical high-risk HPV testing and/or cervical cytology.
- Anal cancer prevention screening programs using HPV testing and cytology exist for populations at risk for anal cancer; however guidelines are forthcoming.

INTRODUCTION

Human papillomavirus (HPV) is the most common sexually transmitted infection (STI) worldwide. In the United States, approximately 13 million new infections occur annually, half of which affect persons aged 15 to 24 years.[1] HPV is a double-stranded DNA virus with more than 200 distinct genotypes. Forty strains infect the anogenital area via direct skin-to-skin and/or mucosal contact. These 40 strains are further classified into low-risk

---

[a] California Prevention Training Center, University of California San Francisco, Bixby Center for Global Reproductive Health 490 Illinois Street, 10th Floor, San Francisco, CA 94143, USA; [b] Department of Epidemiology and Biostatistics, University of California San Francisco, Mission Hall: Global Health and Clinical Sciences, Box 0560 550 16th Street, San Francisco, CA 94143, USA; [c] California Emerging Infections Program, HPV Impact, 360 22nd Street #750, Oakland, CA 94612, USA; [d] Boston University School of Medicine, Boston Medical Center, 771 Albany Street, Dowling 4, Boston, MA 02118, USA
* Corresponding author.
E-mail address: Rosalyn.plotzker@ucsf.edu

Infect Dis Clin N Am 37 (2023) 289–310
https://doi.org/10.1016/j.idc.2023.02.008
0891-5520/23/© 2023 Elsevier Inc. All rights reserved.

id.theclinics.com

and high-risk (HR) types based on cancer association. Low-risk types are nononcogenic and responsible for anogenital warts (AGWs) and respiratory tract papillomas. HRHPV types are oncogenic, responsible for most lower genital tract, anal, and oropharyngeal cancers.[2–4] HPV is estimated to be responsible for greater than 99% of cervical, 90% of anal, 69% of vulvar, 75% of vaginal, 40% of penile, and 70% of oropharyngeal cancers.[5–11] Cervical cancer is the fourth most common cancer in women worldwide, with an estimated 604,000 new cases globally in 2020.[12] Most HPV-related diseases are preventable via vaccination, education, social mobilization, and screening and treatment programs.

EPIDEMIOLOGY OF HUMAN PAPILLOMAVIRUS AND HUMAN PAPILLOMAVIRUS–RELATED DISEASES
Human Papillomavirus

In the United States, from 2013 to 2016, the estimated case count of disease-associated HPV infections (ie, strains associated with either AGWs or HRHPV)—both new and persistent—among those 15 to 59 years old was 42.5 million. Approximately 9 million (21%) cases affected people 15 to 24 years old. With regard to new HPV infections, 13 million new cases occurred among those 15 to 59 years old in 2018.[1] Although high, these estimates represent a substantial decrease from a decade earlier. Before widespread HPV vaccine dissemination, the approximate US HPV case count from 2003 to 2006 was 79 million, with 14 million new cases annually.[13]

In the absence of vaccination, HPV is highly transmissible, typically occurring shortly after sexual debut. Before HPV vaccination availability, Winer and colleagues found that among female university students, the cumulative incidence of lower genital tract HPV infection was 39% at year 2 and 60% by year 5.[14] The 2-year cumulative incidence among unvaccinated men at the same university was 62.4%. HPV was also detected under the fingernails for 32% of male participants, approximately one-third of whom did not have HPV detected at any genital site.[15]

In the early years of vaccine introduction for male patients, the US 2013 to 2014 overall genital HPV infection prevalence for men aged 18 to 59 years was 45.2%, and HRHPV prevalence was 25.1%. Genital HPV infection followed a bimodal pattern with regard to age, with peak prevalence at 28 to 32 years and 58 to 59 years.[16]

For worldwide rates of HPV infection, a 2007 meta-analysis by De Sanjosé and colleagues estimated the global HPV case count among women was 291 million, about one-third of whom were infected with HPV16 and/or 18, the types most strongly associated with cancer.[17] Internationally, 69.4% of cervical cancers, 52% of precancerous high-grade cervical lesions, and 26% of low-grade cervical dysplasia have been associated with HPV types 16 or 18. These associations were consistent across continents and regions.[18] Yet, infection rates of types 16 and 18 in the setting of normal cervical cytology were higher in specific regions (eg, the Caribbean [15%], Eastern Europe [9.5%], and Australia/New Zealand [8.5%]) compared with the overall global prevalence (3.9%).[19] Overall HPV positivity in 2007 was estimated to be 10.4%, which also varied by region: 22.1%, 20.4%, and 11.3% positivity were estimated for Africa, Central America/Mexico, and North America, respectively, surpassing the global average.[17] More current data suggest modest decreases, from 10.4% overall in 2007 to 9.9% in 2019. The highest HPV prevalence in 2019 was in Oceania, inclusive of Australia and New Zealand, estimated to be 30.9%.[18]

Anogenital Warts

AGWs, also known as condyloma acuminatum, are common throughout the world. One systematic review of studies spanning 2001 to 2012 by Patel and colleagues found the median annual incidence of any AGW (new and recurrent) was 194.5 (range 160–289) per 100,000 person years (py). The median new-onset incident rates per 100,000 py for men and women were 137 (range 103–168) and 120.5 (range 76–191), respectively. Incidence peaked by age 24 years for women and between ages 25 to 29 years for men.[20] Between 2003 and 2010, declines occurred in AGW prevalence among US women ages 15 to 24 years, the group most likely to be affected by HPV vaccine introduction. By 2014, decreasing AGW prevalence was identified in young men as well.[16] In a meta-analysis of 65 studies published between 2014 and 2018 across 14 high-income countries, AGW diagnoses among women decreased 67%, 54%, and 31% for those 15 to 19 years, 20 to 24 years, and 25 to 29 years, respectively. Among men, AGW diagnoses decreased 48% and 32% for those 15 to 19 years and 20 to 24 years, respectively.[21]

Cervical Cancer

Cervical cancer is preceded by cervical intraepithelial neoplasia (CIN) grades 2 and 3 (CIN2, CIN3), also termed cervical high-grade squamous intraepithelial lesions (HSIL). It is the fourth most common cancer in women worldwide. In 2020, there were 604,127 cases of cervical cancer diagnosed and 341,831 cervical cancer deaths. The overall age-standardized incidence and mortality rates per 100,000 py were 13.3 and 7.3, respectively. Regional differences in incidence and mortality varied widely and were inversely related to the regional human development index (HDI). The collective incidence and mortality for very high HDI countries were 11.3 and 5.2, respectively, compared with 18.8 and 12.4 for low HDI countries' collective incidence and mortality, respectively.[12] By region, the highest rates for both incidence and mortality per 100,000 py were in Sub-Saharan Africa and Melanesia; Sub-Saharan African countries' incidence and mortality rates ranged 22.9 to 40.1 and 16.6 to 28.6, respectively, whereas in Melanesia, incidence and mortality were 28.2 and 18.6, respectively. In the United States, cervical cancer incidence rates per 100,000 py steadily declined from 9.7 in 1998 to 7.2 in 2019. Yet, regional differences exist, such that some states' incidence rates remain greater than 9.0 per 100,000 py, particularly in the southern and central United States.[22] Cervical cancer incidence per 100,000 py is also high among American Indian/Alaska Natives (10.1), Hispanic (10.0), and Black (9.0) populations. Despite vaccination and screening in the United States, cervical cancer incidence per 100,000 py continues to far outweigh incidences of other HPV-related anogenital cancers among women (eg, anal [2.5], vulvar [2.1], and vaginal [0.4]).[23]

Anal Cancer

Anal cancer in the general population is rare. In 2020, just more than 30,000 cases were diagnosed worldwide, affecting twice as many women as men. Half of male cases and nearly two-thirds of female cases were diagnosed in Europe and North America.[24] The 2020 worldwide age-standardized incidence and mortality rates per 100,000 py were 0.5 and 0.2, respectively; stratifying by gender, the incidence rates per 100,000 py were 0.5 for men and 0.6 for women. Interestingly, regionality differs from that of cervical cancer. While, similar to cervical cancer, higher rates of anal cancer are reported in Melanesia (1.7 incidence, 0.8 mortality per 100,000 py), the next highest anal cancer incidence rates are reported from very high HDI regions (West Europe, North America, Australia, New Zealand, and Northern Europe; incidence range 1.2–1.5 per 100,000 py). Yet, mortality rates are similar to the global average in these regions despite higher incidence, suggesting better access to diagnosis and treatment. In comparison, higher mortality rates exist in Middle, Eastern, and

Western African regions (range 0.6–0.9 per 100,000 py) despite lower incidence rates in these regions (0.8–1.1 per 100,000).[25]

Anal cancer incidence is higher among specific populations: those living with HIV (LWH) and other immunosuppression (eg, solid organ transplant recipients); men who have sex with men (MSM); and people with previous gynecologic lower genital tract dysplasia or cancer. Among those LWH anal cancer incidence per 100,000 py has been estimated to be 85, 32, and 22 for MSM, non-MSM men, and women respectively; risk increases with age, such that incidence among MSM LWH older than 60 years is approximately 107.5 per 100,000 py.[26]

PATHOPHYSIOLOGY

Person-to-person HPV transmission occurs through direct skin-to-skin or mucosal contact during vaginal, anal, or oral sex. Both asymptomatic and symptomatic individuals infected with HPV can transmit HPV. Risk factors include early age at sexual debut and an increased number of sexual partners.[27] After infection, HPV can spread from the primary site of infection to another site (eg, from genitals to anus via posttoilet wiping).[28] Most anogenital HPV infections resolve spontaneously. For instance, greater than 90% of cervical infections are cleared within 1 to 3 years.[29] However, resolution may vary by type. In an observational study of more than 11,000 women, representing more than 14,000 unique HRHPV infections, the risks of CIN3+ (inclusive of both CIN3 and cervical cancer) differed substantially by type, with HPV16 — approximately 1 of 4 infections — having a 7-year CIN3+ risk of 22%[30]; 90% of penile/scrotal infections resolve in around 2 years, with only a small fraction having chronic infection that can give rise to complications.[27,31] Anal HPV clearance rates vary depending on HPV type ranging from 14.6% to 62.5%, occurring in 6 months to a year.[32] In a meta-analysis on the impact of HIV co-infection for HPV incidence and clearance among people of all genders, overall HPV incidence and HRHPV incidence were approximately doubled, whereas clearance rates were halved.[33]

Illustrated in **Fig. 1**, HPV infects the basal epithelial cells of skin or squamous mucous membranes. HPV DNA replicates inside the basal cells as they differentiate and rise to the surface of the epithelium. Based on cancer association, HPV is grouped into low-risk (most commonly, HPV 6 and 11, others include 42, 43, and 44) and HR (most commonly, HPV16 and 18, others include types 31, 33, 34, 35, 39, 45, 51, 52, 56, 58, 59, 66, 68, and 70).[34] The difference between these strains is, in part, due to the capability of the HRHPV strains to inactivate tumor suppressor proteins p53 and pRB in host cells via oncoproteins E6 and E7, respectively.[3,35,36] HRHPV infection thus drives cell-cycle entry in the upper epithelium and simultaneously provokes uncontrolled cell proliferation in basal and parabasal cell layers. These cellular changes give rise to HSIL, which then may become invasive cancer.[3]

Consistent with this understanding, the Lower Anogenital Squamous Terminology (LAST) Standardization project for HPV-associated lesions recommended a 2-tiered nomenclature for squamous intraepithelial lesions (SIL). This terminology reflects the morphologic dichotomy of low-grade SIL (LSIL) versus HSIL. The terms HSIL and LSIL are used for all anogenital anatomic sites, although can be further described with "intraepithelial neoplasia" or IN-terminology such as CIN, anal IN (AIN), and vulvar IN (VIN), followed by grade (eg, CIN3).[37] Cervical HSIL corresponds to CIN3 as well as CIN2 when histologic p16 staining is positive. Anal HSIL similarly includes AIN grade 3 (AIN3), as well as grade 2 (AIN2) with p16 positivity.

Asymptomatic anogenital HPV infection is common and can occur in the setting of low-risk and HR strains.[38] When clinical manifestations arise, syndromes differ based

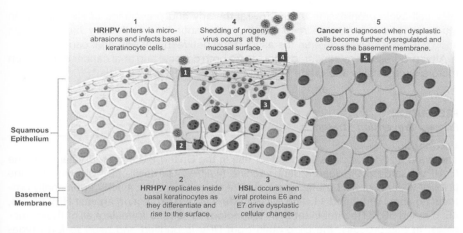

1 HRHPV enters via micro-abrasions and infects basal keratinocyte cells.

4 Shedding of progeny virus occurs at the mucosal surface.

5 **Cancer** is diagnosed when dysplastic cells become further dysregulated and cross the basement membrane.

Squamous Epithelium

2 HRHPV replicates inside basal keratinocytes as they differentiate and rise to the surface.

3 HSIL occurs when viral proteins E6 and E7 drive dysplastic cellular changes

Basement Membrane

Fig. 1. High-risk HPV life cycle and disease progression. High-risk HPV infects basal keratino-cytes, replicates within the keratinocytes, and eventually rises to the epithelial surface as keratinocytes differentiate (steps 1 and 2). Dysplastic changes in infected cells can occur due to oncogenic viral proteins E6 and E7, and these changes can give rise to HSIL (step 3), and further dysregulation in the cells can lead to cancer (step 5). (*Adapted from* K. Sax-ena S, Kumar S, Mati Goel M, Kaur A, LB Bhatt M. Recent Advances in Human Papillomavirus Infection and Management. Current Perspectives in Human Papillomavirus [Internet]. 2019 May 2; Available from: https://doi.org/10.5772/intechopen.81970.)

on genotype. AGWs are common lesions caused by low-risk HPV infection, about 90% of which are due to strains 6 or 11.[39,40] They are flat, papular, or pedunculated growths, commonly located around the vaginal introitus, on the vulva, under penile foreskin, on the penile shaft, and on the perianus. Warts can be found within the ano-genital tract (eg, cervix, vagina, vulva, urethra, perineum, perianal skin, anus, or scrotum). Intraanal warts can occur among those who have not had a history of anal sexual contact.[41] HPV-infected tissue can progress to AGW as quickly as 3 to 10 months after infection but can occur up to 47 months after initial infection.[42] Pa-tient- and provider-applied treatments are available, discussed in "Management." Warts are typically benign. They have the potential to resolve without treatment in around 6 months. However, around 30% of warts recur, even in the setting of treat-ment.[43] LSIL often reflects infection with low-risk HPV without AGW manifesta-tions.[44,45] LSIL can clear spontaneously in 60% of cases. In rare cases, cervical LSIL (CIN1) can progress to CIN3 (10% cases) and to cancer (around 1% cases).[46]

Although HRHPV strains 16 and 18 can be associated with LSIL and AGW, they are the most common strains associated with cancer and HSIL.[3,45] Compared with LSIL, a higher proportion of HSIL progress to cancer if left untreated (5% for CIN2, >12% for CIN3, 9%–13% for AIN3).[45,46] Although progression to cancer usually takes place over a prolonged period of 10 to 20 years, some anogenital cancers develop more rapidly, as quickly as 1 to 2 years, emphasizing the importance of timely detection and treat-ment of cancer precursors.[3]

Immune dysfunction is a key factor influencing progression to cancer. A risk ratio of 6.07 for cervical cancer has been calculated for those LWH. Similarly, a prior AIDS diagnosis was associated with a relative risk of 10.8 for anal cancer compared with populations not living with HIV. This increased risk is thought to be due to the immune dysregulation due to HIV, particularly CD4 and CD8 cell dysfunction, which may contribute to poor clearance of HPV, whereas HIV infection itself can also promote

HPV cell-cycle progression. Antiretroviral therapy and prevalence of HPV has been studied; however, immune reconstitution with antiretroviral therapy has not been shown to conclusively reverse the association between HIV and anal cancer.[47]

After progression to cancer, prognosis for both cervical and anal cancer depends on factors such as size and grade of the tumor and stage at diagnosis.[42,48,49]

PREVENTION
Primary Prevention Strategies

Vaccination
There are 3 HPV vaccines licensed for use in the United States: the 9-valent vaccine (9vHPV, Gardasil 9), quadrivalent vaccine (4vHPV, Gardasil), and bivalent vaccine (2vHPV, Cervarix). All 3 protect against HPV types 16 and 18. 4vHPV additionally protects against HPV 6 and 11, and 9vHPV offers added protection against HPV 31, 33, 45, 52, and 58.[50] Recombinant DNA technology is used to formulate all of these vaccines. In this process, the L1 protein from HPV is purified and used to form type-specific empty shells, called viruslike particles, that induce immunity.[51] Since late 2016, only Gardasil-9 (9vHPV) has been distributed in the United States.[52]

Multiple large clinical trials have shown HPV vaccines are efficacious, safe, and have good immunogenicity. The FUTURE I and II studies were phase 3 randomized controlled trials (RCTs) conducted exclusively among women to study the efficacy of the 4vHPV. In FUTURE I, among participants who had never had prior HPV infection (per protocol analysis/PPA), vaccine efficacy for the endpoints of vulvar, vaginal, perianal, and cervical disease was 100%.[53] In the intention-to-treat (ITT) analysis, which included women who had previously been infected with HPV, including strains covered by the vaccine, vaccination reduced the rate of vulvar/vaginal/perianal lesions by 34% and the rate of cervical lesions by 20%.[53] In FUTURE II, the primary composite endpoint was CIN2+ (CIN2, CIN3, adenocarcinoma in situ, or cervical cancer), related to HPV16 or 18. Vaccine efficacy was 98% in the PPA and 44% in the ITT (which included women with prior HPV infection).[54] Among men, an RCT conducted by Giuliano and colleagues found that vaccine efficacy for external genital lesions was 90.4% in the PPA and 60.2% in the ITT population.[55] A substudy found the efficacy against anal dysplasia was 77.5% in the per-protocol population and 50.3% in the intention to treat population.[56] Lastly, an RCT of the 9vHPV found the efficacy of the vaccine for prevention of high-grade cervical, vulvar, or vaginal disease was 96.7% for PPA and 42.5% in the ITT group.[57] Taken together, these trials showed that both the quadrivalent and 9-valent vaccines were efficacious, especially when given to those who had not been exposed to HPV. With regard to immunogenicity, the quadrivalent vaccine also seems to offer protection for prolonged periods of time, with one study showing protection for more than 12 years postvaccination.[58]

Although clinical trial data for the vaccines were promising, real-world data illustrate broader efficacy. One study conducted in Australia from 2004 to 2009 showed that after the implementation of HPV vaccination in young women in 2007, there was a 59% decrease in the number of genital wart diagnoses among women younger than 26 years.[59] Women not eligible for the vaccine (those older than 26 years or nonresidents) did not have a decline in genital warts. The study also found a decrease in genital warts among heterosexual men, an effect attributed to herd immunity.[59] In another Australian study, CIN2+ decreased significantly in women younger than 18 years after initiation of the HPV vaccination program.[60] In the United States, the Centers for Disease Control and Prevention (CDC) HPV IMPACT Monitoring Project collects data regarding CIN2+ across 5 sites. The proportion of HPV16 or 18 positive CIN2+ cases declined from 52.7% in 2008 to 44.1% in 2014 ($P < .001$). Declines were seen in both vaccinated and unvaccinated women, suggesting some herd immunity.[61] Additional analyses of HPV IMPACT 2008 to 2016 data further found declines of CIN2+ among women aged 18 to 19 years and 20 to 24 years and that the percentage of vaccine type HPV infections declined by 88% among women aged 14 to 19 years and 81% among those aged 20 to 24 years.[62,63] These real-world data are reassuring that HPV vaccines are highly efficacious.

The Advisory Committee on Immunization Practices (ACIP) currently recommends routine HPV vaccination at 11 to 12 years but can be given as early as 9 years old. Catch-up vaccination is recommended up to 26 years. ACIP guidelines recommend shared decision-making around vaccination for persons 27 to 45 years old and do not recommend it for adults beyond 45 years.[50]

Condom use and male circumcision

Condom use and male circumcision are 2 additional strategies for prevention of HPV and its related complications that have been studied. Regarding condom use, a meta-analysis of 20 studies in the prevaccine era found no clear evidence that condom use reduces the risk of HPV transmission itself; however, studies do suggest condoms may protect against AGW or CIN2+.[64] In this meta-analysis, 4 of 5 studies showed a decreased risk of cervical cancer (20%–80% decreased risk) and 4 of 6 showed a decreased risk of CIN2/3 (20%–70% decreased risk). However, the meta-analysis investigators note 2 significant limitations: (1) the studies were not designed to evaluate condom use specifically; (2) a temporal sequence was not established. To address temporality, a systematic review of longitudinal studies on the preventive effectiveness of male condoms was performed. Of 8 studies included, 4 showed condoms were effective at preventing HPV infection and were additionally associated with regression of cervical neoplasia; the other 4 trended toward a protective effect but did not reach statistical significance.[65] Another longitudinal study conducted exclusively in men found that among men with a high risk of HPV exposure (men with no steady sex partners), condom use was associated with a 50% decreased likelihood of becoming infected with HPV.[66] The results of these studies together suggest condoms may be an additional tool to protect somewhat against HPV infection and associated complications. However, HPV may be transmitted in the setting of consistent condom use.

Male circumcision has been studied via RCTs in Africa that showed that circumcised men, compared with those who are uncircumcised, have a lower prevalence of HPV infections.[67–69] A systematic review and meta-analysis looking at male circumcision and HPV infection found that circumcision was associated with a significantly reduced odds of HPV prevalence but not with acquisition of new HPV infections, HPV clearance, or genital warts.[70] Overall, more studies are needed to understand the efficacy of male circumcision as a strategy to prevent HPV transmission and downstream complications.

Secondary Prevention Strategies

Cervical cancer screening

Screening for cervical cancer and its precursors is part of a routine gynecologic examination that can be performed in both primary care and reproductive/sexual health settings. Screening tests help detect HSIL, allowing for timely treatment and cancer prevention. Cervical cytology, commonly known as the Pap test, identifies CIN. HRHPV genotype testing may be used as either a cotest or an alternative to cytologic screening. Cervical cancer screening recommendations are summarized in **Table 1**.

Table 1
Cervical cancer screening guidelines for those at average risk[a]

	American Cancer Society (2020)	US Preventive Services Task Force (2018)[b,c]
Age to start (years)	25	21
Screening approach, by age (* = preferred)	*Age 25 y and older* HRHPV testing, 5 y* *Alternatives*[d] Cytology 3 y Or HRHPV/cytology cotesting, 5 y	*Age 21–29*, cytology, 3 y *Age 30 y and older*, EITHER HRHPV testing, 5 y*[e] Or cytology, 3 y* *Alternative* HRHPV/cytology cotesting, 5 y
Criteria to discontinue screening[f]	Age 65 y or older And Adequate negative screening in the past 10 y And no history of CIN2+ for 25 y	Age 65 y or older And adequate prior screening history And not otherwise at high risk for cervical cancer

[a] Applies to people with a cervix, regardless of HPV vaccination status. These recommendations do not apply to high-risk populations, defined as those who are immunosuppressed (eg, living with HIV), had in-utero exposure to diethylstilbestrol, or those with a history of CIN2+. High-risk populations require more intensive or alternate screening.
[b] Endorsed by the American Society for Colposcopy and Cervical Pathology (ASCCP), the American College of Obstetricians and Gynecologists (ACOG), the Society of Gynecologic Oncology (SGO), and the Centers for Disease Control and Prevention (CDC).
[c] At the time this was prepared, an update of the US Preventive Services Task Force (USPSTF) Cervical Cancer Screening Guidance was in progress. Please refer to the USPSTF for the most current guidance: https://www.uspreventiveservicestaskforce.org/uspstf/recommendation/cervical-cancer-screening.
[d] If primary HRHPV testing not available.
[e] ACOG, ASCCP, and SGO advise that primary HRHPV testing every 5 years can be considered for average-risk patients aged 25–29 years based on its FDA-approved age for use and primary HRHPV testing's demonstrated efficacy in individuals aged 25 years and older.
[f] Those who have had a total hysterectomy with removal of the cervix do not require screening unless CIN2+ was diagnosed within the previous 20 years. However, those who have had supracervical hysterectomy, in which the cervix is not removed, should continue to have screening tests as indicated.

Cytology. Cytology as a cervical cancer screening technique was developed by Dr. and Mrs. Papanicolaou between 1925 and 1940.[71] This approach originated from a systematic study of aspirated vaginal specimens provided by volunteer female staff at the New York Women's Hospital, during which an asymptomatic malignancy was incidentally identified. A 1941 manuscript described the preparation and microscopic interpretation of aspirated vaginal specimen smears on glass slides to diagnose asymptomatic cervical cancer.[72] Pap screening was endorsed by the American Cancer Society (ACS) in 1957.[73] Surveillance data of countries where screening programs using cervical cytology are implemented have shown impressive declines in cervical cancer incidences, ranging from 50% up to 85%.[74]

Today, liquid-based cytology (LBC) accounts for greater than 90% of Pap tests in the United States.[75] Conventional Pap smears are limited by their broad range of sensitivity for HSIL (35%–87%) and suboptimal false-negative rate (14%–33%).[76,77] LBC is an alternative method of preparing cervical samples for cytological examination. Rather than being directly smeared onto a microscope slide, cervical cells are collected with a spatula, cytobrush, and/or cervical broom (described later) and rinsed into a vial with preservation solution. A suspension of cells from the sample are then used to produce a thin layer of cells on a slide. This technique decreases the rate of unsatisfactory smears by separating out obscuring inflammation or blood.[78] In one comparison study, just 0.13% of LBC slides were unsatisfactory, which was significantly lower than 0.89% of traditional smear Pap slide.[79] LBC has similar diagnostic accuracy for the detection of cervical HSIL compared with traditional cytology. An added advantage of LBC is that the residual material in the vial may be used for ancillary testing for HPV.[80]

Cervical cytology specimens are collected directly from the face of the cervix (ectocervix) and cervical canal (endocervix) to ideally include the cervical squamocolumnar junction (SCJ) where CIN is most likely to occur. Ectocervical specimens can be collected with a spatula followed by a second sample via endocervical brush. Alternatively, a broom can be used, where central and outer bristles simultaneously sample the endo- and ectocervix, respectively. Although more convenient, when compared with the spatula-brush combination, broom specimens have a higher frequency of (1) lacking endocervical cells, (2) unsatisfactory results, and (3) obscuring inflammation.[81] The broom can also be used routinely with an endocervical brush in nonpregnant patients, which can improve the likelihood of adequate endocervical sampling.

Both the conventional smear and LBC are read by cytopathologists and are subject to interobserver variability.[82] Automated slide interpretation systems used alongside manual interpretation have been shown to increase sensitivity to both HSIL and LSIL, as well as decrease unsatisfactory results.[83,84]

Human papillomavirus genotyping. In 1975, 50 years after the discovery of cervical cytology screening, Dr H. zur Hausen hypothesized HPV was the causative agent of cervical cancer.[85] By 1983, the first HPV genomic sequencing suggested a possible relationship with cervical cancer, which laid groundwork for scientific advances such as the first clinically available HPV test in 1988, the Food and Drug Administration (FDA) approval of an HPV test in 1995, and finally confirmation that HPV is associated with almost all cervical cancers in 1999.[86] Translating knowledge into practice, HPV testing evolved in the early 2000s with regard to the sophistication of its testing platforms, alongside its role in screening algorithms. In 2012, the US Preventive Services Task Force (USPSTF) included HPV testing in its screening guidance. Cervical HPV testing is FDA approved for people 25 years and older. Both the ACS and USPSTF include HPV testing every 5 years, with or without concomitant cytology (ie, cotesting), as a screening strategy for patients at average risk who are at least 25 (per ACS) or 30 (per USPSTF) years old (see **Table 1**). HRHPV with or without cytology detects more cases of CIN2 and CIN3. However, this can result in more diagnostic colposcopies for each case detected.[87]

Today, testing platforms identify at least 13 high-risk strains. Most, though not all, specify the presence or absence of strains 16, 18, and on occasion 45. Other non-16/non-18 types are usually not further defined. Specimens can be via physician-collected cervical testing (eg, cotesting with cytology, particularly with LBC where additional specimens need not be collected) or specially developed self-collection vaginal swabs.[88] Polymerase chain reaction assays are as sensitive on self- versus clinician-collected samples to detect CIN2+ or CIN3+, although signal amplification assays have shown less sensitivity on self-samples.[89] Although DNA is the primary target for such testing, a recent systematic review affirms that messenger RNA may be an equally accurate test, with similar sensitivity for CIN2/3 and slightly better specificity than DNA tests, and have suggested this approach could be acceptable for primary cervical cancer screening on clinician-collected cervical samples at intervals of around 5 years. However, the test was less sensitive on self-collected samples than clinician-collected samples.[90] Urine-based HRHPV screening is not routinely used; however, some research suggests it may be useful for resource-limited settings.[91]

Screening for anal cancer and dysplasia

Anal cancer is preceded by anal HSIL for years to decades, providing a window of time for screening for its precursor.[92] Similar to the uterine cervix, the anal canal develops embryologically as a fusion site of endodermal and ectodermal tissue, which progresses to form an SCJ. Therefore, the anal SCJ shares histologic and physiologic characteristics with the cervix. These similarities, in part, underly the rationale for anal cancer screening strategies that have been adapted from cervical cancer screening, namely cytology and HPV testing, as well as digital anorectal exam (DARE).

Anal cytology specimens are collected without visualization before DARE or anoscopy (anal canal visualization). A water-moistened polyester/dacron swab is inserted approximately 4 to 5 cm into the anal canal so that it is likely proximal to the SCJ and vigorously rotated against the wall of the anal canal as it is withdrawn to sweep cells for LBC. Cytology collection should be performed before the introduction of lubricant (eg, used for DARE) so as not to compromise cellular yield. This sample is commonly processed using LBC, which is preferred to the alternative of fixing with ethanol.[93] The utility of cytology is mixed. Among MSM LWH, anal cytology's sensitivity, specificity, and positive and negative predictive values to detect anal HSIL are 83%, 45%, 36%, and 88%, respectively.[94] In many clinical settings, abnormal anal cytology is considered an indication for further workup with high-resolution anoscopy (HRA) to visualize lesions and biopsy sites of potential HSIL. HRHPV testing as an alternative and as cotest has been explored for anal cancer screening. Thus far, its value remains inconclusive.[95,96]

For the general population, anal cancer screening is not recommended due to its rareness and therefore very high number needed to screen to prevent one case. However, screening is justifiable for populations at higher risk, especially in light of available treatment via ablation and known morbidity and mortality for those at risk in the absence of treatment. At the time this paper was prepared no formal national or international recommendations existed beyond the 2021 CDC recommendation to consider DARE to screen for early anal cancers for MSM.[41] However, the ANCHOR study, published in 2022, suggests that detection and treatment of anal HSIL is beneficial for PLWH. In the ANCHOR study, 4446 participants LWH aged 35 years or older with biopsy-proven anal HSIL were randomized to either a treatment or an active monitoring arm. Treatment of HSIL included ablation with follow-up every 3 to 6 months, whereas active monitoring followed HSIL lesions without intervention unless cancer occurred. Overall, 9 cases of anal cancer were diagnosed in the treatment group (173 per 100,000 py; 95% confidence interval [CI], 90–332) and 21 cases in the active monitoring group (402 per 100,000 py; 95% CI, 262–616). Treatment of known HSIL reduced the risk of anal cancer by 57%.[97] Although recent data demonstrate the benefit of HSIL detection and treatment in asymptomatic people LWH, evidence is lacking on the value of screening other at-risk groups (eg, MSM who are not immunocompromised, patients with histories of gynecologic cancers, and solid organ transplant recipients). There is similarly minimal consensus with regard to when to screen and how. The lack of national- or international-level guidance for whom, when, and how to screen likely contributes to heterogenous screening practices, limited uptake among providers, and limited awareness among patients considered at increased risk.[98]

MANAGEMENT
Anogenital Warts

AGWs can be asymptomatic. Patients who have AGWs in the vaginal or anal canal are often unaware of them because they are painless and not easily seen. However, some AGWs can cause pain, bleeding, or pruritis depending on their size and location.[41] AGWs can resolve spontaneously without any treatment in less than a year, but AGW treatment can be considered depending on symptom severity, size, patient preference, and provider experience. Many patients require multiple treatment sessions or a combination of therapies, rather than a single treatment, to completely eradicate AGWs. Therapies for AGW are classified as either patient applied or provider administered and are summarized in **Table 2**.

Patient-applied therapies

Patient-applied therapies include imiquimod cream, podofilox solution or gel, and sinecatechins ointment, and these can be applied to warts on the penis, groin, scrotum, vulva, perineum, and perianus.

Imiquimod induces production of interferon and other cytokines and thus enhances the immune system and prompts tumor growth inhibition.[99] A meta-analysis that included 3 RCTs of imiquimod found the clinical cure rate with imiquimod was around 56%.[100] Regarding side effects, case reports have seen associations between imiquimod cream and worsening of inflammatory or autoimmune skin diseases such as psoriasis or lichen planus.[101–103]

Podofilox or podophyllotoxin is an antimitotic drug that leads to wart necrosis. A meta-analysis that included 9 RCTs with podophyllotoxin found clinical cure rates were around 50%.[100] Side effects of podophyllotoxin include local erythema, swelling, pain, or pruritis.[104]

Sinecatechins (Polyphenon E) are extracted from green-tea, and the active products are catechins. The catechins can trigger the release of proinflammatory cytokines and can inhibit telomerase, thus triggering cell apoptosis and destruction of HPV-infected cells. A pooled analysis of studies involving this drug showed a 54% clearance rate.[105] Patients need to be aware that it can weaken condoms and diaphragms[104]; this also is ineffectual for immunocompromised individuals and those with HIV.[41] Side effects include pain, erythema, ulceration, or induration at the site of application.[104]

Among the patient-applied therapies, sinecatechins have the lowest rates of recurrence (6%–12%) followed by imiquimod (19%) and then podophyllotoxin (38%).[104]

Provider-administered therapies

Provider-administered therapies include cryotherapy with liquid nitrogen or cryoprobe, surgical removal (by tangential scissor excision, tangential shave excision, curettage, laser, or electrosurgery), trichloroacetic acid (TCA), or bichloroacetic acid (BCA) solution.

Cryotherapy is performed with direct application of nitrous oxide or liquid nitrogen (at a temperature of −196°C) to AGWs, which creates an area of necrosis below and around the wart. Overtreatment can result in scarring or wound complications, whereas undertreatment can result in low efficacy.[41] Clearance rates of 50% to 88% have been seen with cryotherapy, although clearance may require multiple treatments and is provider dependent.[106,107] Surgical therapy performed under either local or general anesthesia can address a high volume of disease at a single visit. However, recovery can be more painful, and larger excisions can lead to scarring. CO2 laser therapy emits a wavelength of about 10,000 nm laser that is absorbed by water and vaporizes HPV-infected keratinocytes. Overall clearance with this therapy ranges

Table 2
Management options of anogenital warts

Therapy Type	Recommended Treatment	Dose/Route	Notes
Patient-applied[a]	Imiquimod	3.75%: topically at bedtime nightly for up to 8 wk Or 5.00%: topically at bedtime 3 times per week, up to 16 wk	May weaken condoms and vaginal diaphragms Wash off 6–10 h after application
	Podofilox 0.5% solution or gel	Topically twice daily for 3 d, then no treatment for 4 d. Repeat for up to 4 cycles	Apply solution with cotton swab, gel with finger Contraindicated in pregnancy
	Sinecatechins 15% ointment	Topically 3 times per day for up to 16 wk	May weaken condoms and vaginal diaphragms Do not wash off. Not recommended for those who are immunosuppressed, living with HIV, and who have genital herpes
Provider-applied	Cryotherapy	Liquid nitrogen or cryoprobe, once up to every 1–2 wk	Local topical or injected anesthesia may be used for large surface areas
	TCA or BCA 80%–90%	Apply to warty tissue only, once up to every 1–2 wk	Not to be used on urethral meatus; TCA has low viscosity and must be applied carefully to avoid spreading to healthy skin
	Surgical removal/ablation	Tangential scissor excision, tangential shave excision, curettage, laser, or electrosurgery	

[a] Not recommended for urethral, vaginal, cervical, or anal AGWs.

from 23% to 52%.[106] However, a recent RCT study in China demonstrated a 100% clearance rate for small warts with 3 or less treatments; recurrence rate was 33%; this was a comparison study exploring 5-aminolevulinic acid photodynamic therapy (ALA PDT) versus CO2. ALA PDT was equivalent to CO2 in safety and efficacy, and recurrent rate was approximately 11%.[108]

TCA and BCA are provider-administered agents that chemically cauterize the skin/mucosa, destroying infected cells.[104] Only a few studies have examined the efficacy of TCA/BCA therapy. In one study comparing cryotherapy and TCA therapy for penile wart treatment found 81% resolution in the TCA group and 88% in the cryotherapy group.[109] It is important to note TCA solution has a low viscosity and can spread and damage adjacent tissues if not applied carefully. These treatments can be repeated weekly if needed.[41]

AGW recurrence is common and can occur with any treatment. Cryotherapy has a recurrence rate of 25% to 40%, TCA and BCA have recurrence rates of around 36%, whereas CO2 laser therapy recurrence rates of 33% have been reported.[108] In one study of anal warts, recurrence after surgical excision was 25%.[110]

Alternative therapies
Alternative regimens include podophyllin resin, intralesional interferon, photodynamic therapy, and topical cidofovir. These are not first-line recommended therapies and should only be considered when recommended regimens are either ineffective or contraindicated.[41]

Cervical and Anal Dysplasia

Cervical dysplasia
The 2019 Consensus Guidelines put forth by the American Society for Colposcopy and Cervical Pathology (ASCCP) define specific Clinical Action Thresholds (CATs) for management, based on the principal of equal management for equal risk.[111] CATs are based on estimates of a patient's immediate and 5-year risks for CIN3+, as percentage risk. Calculated risks factor in a patient's current and prior screening test results, plus characteristics such as age and immunosuppression. In updating guidance from the 2012 recommendations, the Consensus Guidance authors, Perkins and colleagues, note that (1) screening has shifted to being primarily HPV based, and (2) cytology is thought to be a marker for current CIN, whereas HPV subtypes denote risk for both current and future CIN. A patient's screening history is an important factor because past HPV history modifies the risk of developing CIN3+.[112] Thus, 2 patients with similar current screening results may differ in recommended management based on their prior HPV testing. Prior cytology results alone are less predictive in the development of CIN3+ and not used to modify management recommendations.[113]

Once calculated, a patient's estimated risk is used to assign them to 1 of 6 management categories. For those with an immediate CIN3+ risk of 4% or higher, management is stratified by immediate-risk magnitude: those with an immediate CIN3+ risk of 60% or more should receive expedited treatment; those between 25% and 59% should receive either expedited treatment or colposcopy with biopsies as needed; and those between 4% and 24% are indicated for colposcopy with biopsies to guide further management. Expedited treatment involves excision with preservation of the specimen for pathology; this is typically performed via loop electrosurgical excision procedure (LEEP).

For patients with an immediate CIN3+ risk less than 4%, colposcopy is not indicated. Surveillance with rescreening is recommended. In this case, repeat screening intervals are determined based on calculated 5-year risk. Patients whose 5-year

CIN3+ risk is 0.55% or higher are surveilled again in 1 year; 0.15% to 0.54% in 3 years; and less than 0.15%—equivalent to the 5-year risk in the general population without HRHPV—may be rescreened in 5 years.

Patients who are younger than 25 years, pregnant, and those who are immunosuppressed have different risk profiles and therefore different recommendations for screening and management of abnormal screening results. Younger patients are managed conservatively in light of a low cervical cancer risk due to age. Pregnant patients should not receive expedited treatment. For minimally abnormal results, clinical expert opinion recommends deferring colposcopy to the postpartum period.

CIN2+ recurrence after treatment can occur and may be predicted by HPV persistence postprocedure. One study of 178 patients who underwent LEEP for CIN2+ found HPV persistence with the same type among 3.1% 3 years postprocedure. In addition, 5.1% had residual or recurrent CIN2+ during the study period, emphasizing the importance of monitoring posttreatment.[114]

Anal dysplasia

Although there is not institutional guidance on treatment of anal dysplasia, expert opinion recommends treatment of HSIL in patients who are at increased risk of anal cancer, particularly people LWH. Treatment of LSIL alone is generally not recommended.[97] Treatment of anal HSIL can be topical or ablative. Topical therapy options include TCA, fluorouracil (FU), and imiquimod (also used for AGW treatment). Ablative modalities include infrared coagulation (IRC), electrocauterization, and less commonly argon plasma coagulation and radiofrequency ablation (RFA). Finally, HSIL can be excised surgically and can be guided by intraoperative HRA, which is particularly useful for lesions in the anal canal.

As with AGW, TCA is provider applied to chemically destroy infected cells. Lesions treated with TCA are usually smaller in volume. In a study that followed-up 56 cases of anal HSIL with TCA, about 61% had complete resolution, 23% partial, and 16% had persistent HSIL.[115] In another study, TCA resolved 79% of HSIL lesions; however, only 50% were resolved with a single treatment.[116] FU is a patient-applied therapy that can be administered to the intra- and perianus over several weeks, used in 5 day-on, 9 day-off cycles. Although exact regimens vary by study, FU has been shown to at least partially—and in some cases completely—resolve HSIL for 43% to 95% of cases. However, around 90% of patients experience side effects such as perianal irritation and bleeding.[117] Imiquimod can be applied in the same way that it is used for AGW treatment; HSIL clearance is just less than 50%.[117] One RCT by Richel and colleagues compared the efficacies of imiquimod, FU, and electrocautery among 148 MSM LWH, 57% of whom had biopsy-proven HSIL. Among those with HSIL who were included in the PPA, the complete response rates for imiquimod, FU, and electrocautery were 21%, 21%, and 53%, respectively; an additional 25%, 21%, and 16% had partial response, respectively.[118]

Ablative therapies destroy HSIL by burning off lesions, most commonly via IRC or electrocauterization such as hyfrecation. Although far less commonly used, RFA is the only FDA-approved method for anal HSIL treatment. In a small study of patients who received RFA treatment, 29% had recurrence within 1 year, 19% had persistence at 3 months, and 2.9% had persistence at 12 months.[119]

IRC is approved for treatment of hemorrhoids and AGW and destroys tissue using infrared light as a heat source to burn tissue to a depth of about 1.5 mm. Electrocautery may be preferable for larger keratotic lesions. Both modalities have been shown to be efficacious; however, anal HSIL recurrence and new lesions in untreated areas (metachronous lesions) are commonly seen, suggesting that continued monitoring and iterative treatments may be needed to avert anal cancer.[120]

SUMMARY

HPV is a common, highly transmissible STI. Although most infections clear spontaneously within a few years, persistent low-risk strain infections cause most cases of AGWs, whereas persistent HR strains—particularly types 16 and 18—underly the vast majority of cervical cancer, as well as the less common anal, vulvar, vaginal, and penile cancers. Immunosuppression including HIV coinfection increases the risk of HPV-related diseases. Immunization in combination with screening campaigns for cervical cancer and anal cancer for at-risk populations show promise for prevention, as indicated by significant epidemiologic declines following screening implementation and more so in the postvaccination era. However, global efforts are needed to bolster cervical screening and vaccine availability in regions where HPV-related disease burden remains high—particularly in Sub-Saharan Africa and Melanesia. Moreover, as our understanding of anal cancer continues to evolve, research and advocacy are needed to develop anal cancer screening strategies for anal cancer prevention for populations at high risk.

DISCLOSURE

All contributing authors confirm they have no conflicts of interest.

REFERENCES

1. Lewis RM, Laprise J-F, Gargano JW, et al. Estimated prevalence and incidence of disease-associated human papillomavirus types among 15-to 59-year-olds in the United States. Sex Transm Dis 2021;48(4):273–7.

2. Forman D, de Martel C, Lacey CJ, et al. Global burden of human papillomavirus and related diseases. Vaccine 2012;30:F12–23.

3. Doorbar J, Egawa N, Griffin H, et al. Human papillomavirus molecular biology and disease association. Rev Med Virol 2015;25:2–23.

4. zur Hausen H. Papillomaviruses in the causation of human cancers—a brief historical account. Virology 2009;384(2):260–5.

5. Lin C, Franceschi S, Clifford GM. Human papillomavirus types from infection to cancer in the anus, according to sex and HIV status: a systematic review and meta-analysis. Lancet Infect Dis 2018;18(2):198–206.

6. Gargano JW, Wilkinson EJ, Unger ER, et al. Prevalence of human papillomavirus types in invasive vulvar cancers and vulvar intraepithelial neoplasia 3 in the United States before vaccine introduction. J Low Genit Tract Dis 2012;16(4):471–9.

7. Sinno AK, Saraiya M, Thompson TD, et al. Human papillomavirus genotype prevalence in invasive vaginal cancer from a registry-based population. Obstet Gynecol 2014;123(4):817.

8. Parkin DM, Bray F. The burden of HPV-related cancers. Vaccine 2006;24:S11–25.

9. Chaturvedi AK, Engels EA, Pfeiffer RM, et al. Human papillomavirus and rising oropharyngeal cancer incidence in the United States. J Clin Oncol 2011;29(32):4294.

10. Saraiya M, Unger ER, Thompson TD, et al. US assessment of HPV types in cancers: implications for current and 9-valent HPV vaccines. Journal of the National Cancer Institute 2015;107(6):djv086.

11. Walboomers JM, Jacobs MV, Manos MM, et al. Human papillomavirus is a necessary cause of invasive cervical cancer worldwide. J Pathol 1999; 189(1):12–9.

12. Sung H, Ferlay J, Siegel RL, et al. Global Cancer Statistics 2020: GLOBOCAN Estimates of Incidence and Mortality Worldwide for 36 Cancers in 185 Countries. A Cancer Journal for Clinicians 2021;71(3):209–49.

13. Satterwhite CL, Torrone E, Meites E, et al. Sexually transmitted infections among US women and men. Sex Transm Dis 2013;40(3):187–93.

14. Winer RL, Lee S-K, Hughes JP, et al. Genital human papillomavirus infection: incidence and risk factors in a cohort of female university students. Am J Epidemiol 2003;157(3):218–26.

15. Partridge JM, Hughes JP, Feng Q, et al. Genital human papillomavirus infection in men: incidence and risk factors in a cohort of university students. JID (J Infect Dis) 2007;196(8):1128–36.

16. Hall E, Wodi AP, Hamborsky J, et al. Epidemiology and prevention of vaccine-preventable diseases. Centers for Disease Control and Prevention Public Health Foundation 2021;4:2022.

17. De Sanjosé S, Diaz M, Castellsagué X, et al. Worldwide prevalence and genotype distribution of cervical human papillomavirus DNA in women with normal cytology: a meta-analysis. Lancet Infect Dis 2007;7(7):453–9.

18. Kombe Kombe AJ, Li B, Zahid A, et al. Epidemiology and burden of human papillomavirus and related diseases, molecular pathogenesis, and vaccine evaluation. Front Public Health 2021;8:552028.

19. Bruni L, Albero G, Serrano B, et al. Human papillomavirus and Related diseases in the world—summary Report 22 october 2021. Barcelona, Spain: ICO HPV Information Centre; 2021.

20. Patel H, Wagner M, Singhal P, et al. Systematic review of the incidence and prevalence of genital warts. BMC Infect Dis 2013;13(1):1–14.

21. Drolet M, Bénard É, Pérez N, et al. Population-level impact and herd effects following the introduction of human papillomavirus vaccination programmes: updated systematic review and meta-analysis. Lancet 2019;394(10197): 497–509.

22. U.S. Cancer Statistics Working Group. U.S. Cancer Statistics Data Visualizations Tool, based on 2021 submission data (1999-2019): U.S. Department of Health and Human Services, Centers for Disease Control and Prevention and National Cancer Institute; https://www.cdc.gov/cancer/dataviz, released in November 2022.

23. Centers for Disease Control and Prevention. Cancers associated with human papillomavirus, United States—2013–2017. USCS data brief, no 18. Atlanta, GA: Centers for Disease Control and Prevention, US Department of Health and Human Services; 2020.

24. Deshmukh AA, Damgacioglu H, Georges D, et al. Global burden of HPV-attributable squamous cell carcinoma of the anus in 2020, according to sex and HIV status: a worldwide analysis. Int J Cancer 2022;152(3):417–28.

25. International Agency for Research on Cancer, World Health Organization. Anus: Source Globocan. 2020. Available at: https://gco.iarc.fr/today/data/factsheets/cancers/10-Anus-fact-sheet.pdf. Accessed December. 12, 2022.

26. Clifford GM, Georges D, Shiels MS, et al. A meta-analysis of anal cancer incidence by risk group: Toward a unified anal cancer risk scale. Int J Cancer 2021;148(1):38–47.

27. Castellsagué X. Natural history and epidemiology of HPV infection and cervical cancer. Gynecol Oncol 2008;110(3):S4–7.
28. Simpson S Jr, Blomfield P, Cornall A, et al. Front-to-back & dabbing wiping behaviour post-toilet associated with anal neoplasia & HR-HPV carriage in women with previous HPV-mediated gynaecological neoplasia. Cancer Epidemiology 2016;42:124–32.
29. Burd EM. Human papillomavirus and cervical cancer. Clin Microbiol Rev 2003; 16(1):1–17.
30. Demarco M, Hyun N, Carter-Pokras O, et al. A study of type-specific HPV natural history and implications for contemporary cervical cancer screening programs. EClinicalMedicine 2020;22:100293.
31. Giuliano AR, Lee J-H, Fulp W, et al. Incidence and clearance of genital human papillomavirus infection in men (HIM): a cohort study. Lancet 2011;377(9769): 932–40.
32. Machalek DA, Poynten M, Jin F, et al. Anal human papillomavirus infection and associated neoplastic lesions in men who have sex with men: a systematic review and meta-analysis. The lancet oncology 2012;13(5):487–500.
33. Looker KJ, Rönn MM, Brock PM, et al. Evidence of synergistic relationships between HIV and Human Papillomavirus (HPV): systematic reviews and meta-analyses of longitudinal studies of HPV acquisition and clearance by HIV status, and of HIV acquisition by HPV status. J Int AIDS Soc 2018;21(6):e25110.
34. Muñoz N, Bosch FX, De Sanjosé S, et al. Epidemiologic classification of human papillomavirus types associated with cervical cancer. N Engl J Med 2003; 348(6):518–27.
35. Tomaić V. Functional roles of E6 and E7 oncoproteins in HPV-induced malignancies at diverse anatomical sites. Cancers 2016;8(10):95.
36. Münger K, Scheffner M, Huibregtse J, et al. Interactions of HPV E6 and E7 oncoproteins with tumour suppressor gene products. Cancer Surv 1992;12: 197–217.
37. Darragh TM, Colgan TJ, Cox JT, et al. The lower anogenital squamous terminology standardization project for HPV-associated lesions: background and consensus recommendations from the College of American Pathologists and the American Society for Colposcopy and Cervical Pathology. Arch Pathol Lab Med 2012;136(10):1266–97.
38. Kerkar SC, Latta S, Salvi V, et al. Human papillomavirus infection in asymptomatic population. Sexual & Reproductive Healthcare 2011;2(1):7–11.
39. Steben M, Duarte-Franco E. Human papillomavirus infection: epidemiology and pathophysiology. Gynecol Oncol 2007;107(2):S2–5.
40. Brown DR, Schroeder JM, Bryan JT, et al. Detection of multiple human papillomavirus types in Condylomata acuminata lesions from otherwise healthy and immunosuppressed patients. J Clin Microbiol 1999;37(10):3316–22.
41. Workowski KA, Bachmann LH, Chan PA, et al. Sexually transmitted infections treatment guidelines, 2021. MMWR Recomm Rep 2021;70(4):1.
42. Dunne EF, Park IU. HPV and HPV-associated diseases. Infectious Disease Clinics 2013;27(4):765–78.
43. Beutner K, Friedman-Kien A, Artman N, et al. Patient-applied podofilox for treatment of genital warts. Lancet 1989;333(8642):831–4.
44. Lungu O, Sun XW, Felix J, et al. Relationship of human papillomavirus type to grade of cervical intraepithelial neoplasia. JAMA 1992;267(18):2493–6.
45. Siddharthan RV, Lanciault C, Tsikitis VL. Anal intraepithelial neoplasia: diagnosis, screening, and treatment. Ann Gastroenterol 2019;32(3):257.

46. Ostör A. Natural history of cervical intraepithelial neoplasia: a critical review. Int J Gynecol Pathol 1993;12(2):186–92.

47. Pérez-González A, Cachay E, Ocampo A, et al. Update on the Epidemiological Features and Clinical Implications of Human Papillomavirus Infection (HPV) and Human Immunodeficiency Virus (HIV) Coinfection. Microorganisms 2022;10(5): 1047.

48. Theophanous S, Samuel R, Lilley J, et al. Prognostic factors for patients with anal cancer treated with conformal radiotherapy—a systematic review. BMC Cancer 2022;22(1):1–12.

49. Hu C, Cao J, Zeng L, et al. Prognostic factors for squamous cervical carcinoma identified by competing-risks analysis: A study based on the SEER database. Medicine 2022;101(39):e30901.

50. Meites E, Szilagyi PG, Chesson HW, et al. Human papillomavirus vaccination for adults: updated recommendations of the Advisory Committee on Immunization Practices. MMWR Morb Mortal Wkly Rep 2019 Aug 16;68(32):698–702.

51. De Oliveira CM, Fregnani JHT, Villa LL. HPV vaccine: updates and highlights. Acta Cytol 2019;63(2):159–68.

52. Centers for Disease Control and Prevention. HPV Vaccination: What Everyone Should Know. 2022. Available at: https://www.cdc.gov/vaccines/vpd/hpv/ public/index.html. Accessed November. 1, 2022.

53. Garland SM, Hernandez-Avila M, Wheeler CM, et al. Quadrivalent vaccine against human papillomavirus to prevent anogenital diseases. N Engl J Med 2007;356(19):1928–43.

54. Group FIS. Quadrivalent vaccine against human papillomavirus to prevent high-grade cervical lesions. N Engl J Med 2007;356(19):1915–27.

55. Giuliano AR, Palefsky JM, Goldstone S, et al. Efficacy of quadrivalent HPV vaccine against HPV Infection and disease in males. N Engl J Med 2011;364(5): 401–11.

56. Palefsky JM, Giuliano AR, Goldstone S, et al. HPV vaccine against anal HPV infection and anal intraepithelial neoplasia. N Engl J Med 2011;365(17): 1576–85.

57. Joura EA, Giuliano AR, Iversen O-E, et al. A 9-valent HPV vaccine against infection and intraepithelial neoplasia in women. N Engl J Med 2015;372(8):711–23.

58. Kjaer SK, Nygård M, Sundström K, et al. Final analysis of a 14-year long-term follow-up study of the effectiveness and immunogenicity of the quadrivalent human papillomavirus vaccine in women from four nordic countries. EClinicalMedicine 2020;23:100401.

59. Donovan B, Franklin N, Guy R, et al. Quadrivalent human papillomavirus vaccination and trends in genital warts in Australia: analysis of national sentinel surveillance data. Lancet Infect Dis 2011;11(1):39–44.

60. Brotherton JM, Fridman M, May CL, et al. Early effect of the HPV vaccination programme on cervical abnormalities in Victoria, Australia: an ecological study. Lancet 2011;377(9783):2085–92.

61. McClung NM, Gargano JW, Bennett NM, et al. Trends in human papillomavirus vaccine types 16 and 18 in cervical precancers, 2008–2014. Cancer Epidemiol Biomarkers Prev 2019;28(3):602–9.

62. McClung NM, Gargano JW, Park IU, et al. Estimated number of cases of high-grade cervical lesions diagnosed among women—United States, 2008 and 2016. MMWR Morb Mortal Wkly Rep 2019;68(15):337.

63. Rosenblum HG, Lewis RM, Gargano JW, et al. Declines in prevalence of human papillomavirus vaccine-type infection among females after introduction of

vaccine—United States, 2003–2018. MMWR Morb Mortal Wkly Rep 2021; 70(12):415.

64. Manhart LE, Koutsky LA. Do condoms prevent genital HPV infection, external genital warts, or cervical neoplasia? A meta-analysis. Sex Transm Dis 2002; 29(11):725–35.

65. Lam JUH, Rebolj M, Dugue P-A, et al. Condom use in prevention of Human Papillomavirus infections and cervical neoplasia: systematic review of longitudinal studies. J Med Screen 2014;21(1):38–50.

66. Hariri S, Warner L. Condom use and human papillomavirus in men, 208. The Journal of infectious diseases, 208(3), 367–369.

67. Auvert B, Sobngwi-Tambekou J, Cutler E, et al. Effect of male circumcision on the prevalence of high-risk human papillomavirus in young men: results of a randomized controlled trial conducted in Orange Farm, South Africa. Journal of infectious diseases 2009;199(1):14–9.

68. Tarnaud C, Lissouba P, Cutler E, et al. Association of low-risk human papillomavirus infection with male circumcision in young men: results from a longitudinal study conducted in Orange Farm (South Africa). Infect Dis Obstet Gynecol 2011;2011.

69. Tobian AA, Serwadda D, Quinn TC, et al. Male circumcision for the prevention of HSV-2 and HPV infections and syphilis. N Engl J Med 2009;360(13):1298–309.

70. Albero G, Castellsague X, Giuliano AR, et al. Male circumcision and genital human papillomavirus: a systematic review and meta-analysis. Sex Transm Dis 2012;39(2):104–13.

71. Vilos GA. The history of the Papanicolaou smear and the odyssey of George and Andromache Papanicolaou. Obstet Gynecol 1998;91(3):479–83.

72. Papanicolaou GN, Traut HF. The diagnostic value of vaginal smears in carcinoma of the uterus. Am J Obstet Gynecol 1941;42(2):193–206.

73. Breslow L, Wilner D, Agran L. A history of cancer control in the US with emphasis on the period 1946-1971. Los Angeles: University of California at Los Angeles School of Public Health; 1977.

74. Benedet J, Anderson G, Matisic J. A comprehensive program for cervical cancer detection and management. Am J Obstet Gynecol 1992;166(4):1254–9.

75. Gibb RK, Martens MG. The impact of liquid-based cytology in decreasing the incidence of cervical cancer. Reviews in Obstetrics and Gynecology 2011; 4(Suppl 1):S2.

76. American College of Obstetricians and Gynecologists. ACOG Practice Bulletin No. 99: management of abnormal cervical cytology and histology. Obstet Gynecol 2008;112:1419–44.

77. Hartmann KE, Hall SA, Nanda K, et al. Screening for Cervical Cancer. Agency for Healthcare Research and Quality (US), Rockville (MD); 2002. PMID: 20722121.

78. Ronco G, Cuzick J, Pierotti P, et al. Accuracy of liquid based versus conventional cytology: overall results of new technologies for cervical cancer screening: randomised controlled trial. BMJ 2007;335(7609):28.

79. Beerman H, Van Dorst E, Kuenen-Boumeester V, et al. Superior performance of liquid-based versus conventional cytology in a population-based cervical cancer screening program. Gynecol Oncol 2009;112(3):572–6.

80. Siebers AG, Klinkhamer PJ, Grefte JM, et al. Comparison of liquid-based cytology with conventional cytology for detection of cervical cancer precursors: a randomized controlled trial. JAMA 2009;302(16):1757–64.

81. Marchand L, Mundt M, Klein G, et al. Optimal collection technique and devices for a quality pap smear. WMJ-MADISON 2005;104(6):51.
82. Stoler MH, Schiffman M. Interobserver reproducibility of cervical cytologic and histologic interpretations: realistic estimates from the ASCUS-LSIL Triage Study. JAMA 2001;285(11):1500–5.
83. Lozano R. Comparison of computer-assisted and manual screening of cervical cytology. Gynecol Oncol 2007;104(1):134–8.
84. Davey E, d'Assuncao J, Irwig L, et al. Accuracy of reading liquid based cytology slides using the ThinPrep Imager compared with conventional cytology: prospective study. BMJ 2007;335(7609):31.
85. Gissmann L, Pfister H, Zur Hausen H. Human papilloma viruses (HPV): characterization of four different isolates. Virology 1977;76(2):569–80.
86. Saraiya M, Steben M, Watson M, et al. Evolution of cervical cancer screening and prevention in United States and Canada: implications for public health practitioners and clinicians. Prev Med 2013;57(5):426–33.
87. Curry SJ, Krist AH, Owens DK, et al. Screening for cervical cancer: US Preventive Services Task Force recommendation statement. JAMA 2018;320(7):674–86.
88. Hawkes D, Keung MH, Huang Y, et al. Self-collection for cervical screening programs: from research to reality. Cancers 2020;12(4):1053.
89. Arbyn M, Verdoodt F, Snijders PJ, et al. Accuracy of human papillomavirus testing on self-collected versus clinician-collected samples: a meta-analysis. Lancet Oncol 2014;15(2):172–83.
90. Arbyn M, Simon M, de Sanjosé S, et al. Accuracy and effectiveness of HPV mRNA testing in cervical cancer screening: a systematic review and meta-analysis. Lancet Oncol 2022;23(7):950–60.
91. Daponte A, Michail G, Daponte A-I, et al. Urine HPV in the Context of Genital and Cervical Cancer Screening—An Update of Current Literature. Cancers 2021;13(7):1640.
92. Kreuter A, Potthoff A, Brockmeyer N, et al. Anal carcinoma in human immunodeficiency virus-positive men: results of a prospective study from Germany. Br J Dermatol 2010;162(6):1269–77.
93. Palefsky JM, Holly EA, Ralston ML, et al. Anal squamous intraepithelial lesions in HIV-positive and HIV-negative homosexual and bisexual men: prevalence and risk factors. JAIDS 1998;17(4):320–6.
94. Dias Gonçalves Lima F, Viset JD, Leeflang MM, et al. The accuracy of anal swab–based tests to detect high-grade anal intraepithelial neoplasia in HIV-infected patients: A systematic review and meta-analysis. Paper presented at: Open Forum Infect Dis, 2019.6(5):ofz191.
95. Burgos J, Hernández-Losa J, Landolfi S, et al. The role of oncogenic human papillomavirus determination for diagnosis of high-grade anal intraepithelial neoplasia in HIV-infected MSM. AIDS 2017;31(16):2227–33.
96. Clarke MA, Cheung LC, Lorey T, et al. 5-year prospective evaluation of cytology, human papillomavirus testing, and biomarkers for detection of anal precancer in human immunodeficiency virus–positive men who have sex with men. Clin Infect Dis 2019;69(4):631–8.
97. Palefsky JM, Lee JY, Jay N, et al. Treatment of anal high-grade squamous intraepithelial lesions to prevent anal cancer. N Engl J Med 2022;386(24):2273–82.
98. Plotzker RE, Barnell GM, Wiley DJ, et al. Provider preferences for anal cancer prevention screening: Results of the International Anal Neoplasia Society survey. Tumour Virus Research 2022;13:200235.

99. Yuan J, Ni G, Wang T, et al. Genital warts treatment: Beyond imiquimod. Hum Vaccines Immunother 2018;14(7):1815–9.
100. Yan J, Chen S-L, Wang H-N, et al. Meta-analysis of 5% imiquimod and 0.5% po-dophyllotoxin in the treatment of condylomata acuminata. Dermatology 2006; 213(3):218–23.
101. Patel U, Mark N, Machler B, et al. Imiquimod 5% cream induced psoriasis: a case report, summary of the literature and mechanism. Br J Dermatol 2011; 164(3):670–2.
102. Domingues E, Chaney KC, Scharf MJ, et al. Imiquimod reactivation of lichen pla-nus. Cutis 2012;89(6):276–7.
103. Kumar B, Narang T. Local and systemic adverse effects to topical imiquimod due to systemic immune stimulation. Sex Transm Infect 2011;87(5):432.
104. Kollipara R, Ekhlassi E, Downing C, et al. Advancements in pharmacotherapy for noncancerous manifestations of HPV. J Clin Med 2015;4(5):832–46.
105. Hoy SM. Polyphenon E 10% ointment. Am J Clin Dermatol 2012;13(4):275–81.
106. Vender R, Bourcier M, Bhatia N, et al. Therapeutic options for external genital warts. J Cutan Med Surg 2013;17(6_suppl):S61–7.
107. Reyna-Rodríguez IL, Chavez-Alvarez S, Garza-Rodríguez V, et al. Cryotherapy plus low-dose oral isotretinoin vs cryotherapy only for the treatment of anogen-ital warts: a randomized clinical trial. Arch Dermatol Res 2021;313(10):815–27.
108. Tu P, Zhang H, Zheng H, et al. 5-Aminolevulinic photodynamic therapy versus carbon dioxide laser therapy for small genital warts: A multicenter, randomized, open-label trial. J Am Acad Dermatol 2021;84(3):779–81.
109. Godley M, Bradbeer C, Gellan M, et al. Cryotherapy compared with trichloro-acetic acid in treating genital warts. Sex Transm Infect 1987;63(6):390–2.
110. D'Ambrogio A, Yerly S, Sahli R, et al. Human papilloma virus type and recur-rence rate after surgical clearance of anal condylomata acuminata. Sexually Transmitted Diseases 2009;36:536–40.
111. Perkins RB, Guido RS, Castle PE, et al. 2019 ASCCP risk-based management consensus guidelines for abnormal cervical cancer screening tests and cancer precursors. J Low Genit Tract Dis 2020;24(2):102.
112. Castle PE, Kinney WK, Xue X, et al. Effect of several negative rounds of human papillomavirus and cytology co-testing on safety against cervical cancer: an observational cohort study. Ann Intern Med 2018;168(1):20–9.
113. Schiffman M, Kinney WK, Cheung LC, et al. Relative performance of HPV and cytology components of cotesting in cervical screening. JNCI: Journal of the National Cancer Institute 2018;110(5):501–8.
114. Söderlund-Strand A, Kjellberg L, Dillner J. Human papillomavirus type-specific persistence and recurrence after treatment for cervical dysplasia. J Med Virol 2014;86(4):634–41.
115. Burgos J, Martin-Castillo M, Landolfi S, et al. Brief report: effectiveness of tri-chloroacetic acid vs. electrocautery ablation for the treatment of anal high-grade squamous intraepithelial lesion in HIV-infected patients. Journal of Ac-quired Immune Deficiency Syndromes 2018;79(5):612–6.
116. Cranston RD, Baker JR, Liu Y, et al. Topical application of trichloroacetic acid is efficacious for the treatment of internal anal high-grade squamous intraepithelial lesions in HIV-positive men. Sex Transm Dis 2014;41(7):420–6.
117. Megill C, Wilkin T. Topical therapies for the treatment of anal high-grade squa-mous intraepithelial lesions. Paper presented at: Semin Colon Rectal Surg:2017.28(2):86-90.

118. Richel O, de Vries HJ, van Noesel CJ, et al. Comparison of imiquimod, topical fluorouracil, and electrocautery for the treatment of anal intraepithelial neoplasia in HIV-positive men who have sex with men: an open-label, randomised controlled trial. Lancet Oncol 2013;14(4):346–53.
119. Goldstone RN, Hasan SR, Goldstone SE. Brief report: radiofrequency ablation therapy for anal intraepithelial neoplasia: results from a single-center prospective pilot study in HIV+ participants. J Acquir Immune Defic Syndr 2017; 76(4):e93–7.
120. Goldstone SE, Lensing SY, Stier EA, et al. A randomized clinical trial of infrared coagulation ablation versus active monitoring of intra-anal high-grade dysplasia in adults with human immunodeficiency virus infection: an AIDS malignancy consortium trial. Clin Infect Dis 2019;68(7):1204–12.

Update in Epidemiology and Management of *Mycoplasma genitalium* Infections

Gwendolyn E. Wood, PhD[a],*, Catriona S. Bradshaw, MD, PhD[b,c],
Lisa E. Manhart, PhD, MPH[d]

KEYWORDS

- *Mycoplasma genitalium* • Urethritis • Pelvic inflammatory disease
- Antimicrobial resistance

KEY POINTS

- *M genitalium* (MG) is a frequent cause of STI syndromes including urethritis and perhaps proctitis in men; and cervicitis, pelvic inflammatory disease, infertility, and ectopic pregnancy in women.
- Diagnosis requires sensitive nucleic acid amplification tests (NAAT) accompanied with macrolide resistance marker detection (where available).
- Antibiotic resistance is common. More than 50% of strains in the United States are macrolide resistant and 10% or more carry markers of potential fluoroquinolone resistance. Optimal management involves the use of resistance assays and individualized therapy based on the resistance profile.

INTRODUCTION

Mycoplasma genitalium (MG) is a sexually transmitted bacterial pathogen whose role in reproductive tract disease has, until recently, been underappreciated in the United States. It is receiving increasing attention because of the Food and Drug Administration (FDA) approval of diagnostic tests in 2019 and the rapid expansion of antimicrobial resistance.

BIOLOGY AND PATHOGENESIS

MG cells are tiny (<0.5 μm), lack a cell wall, and cannot be diagnosed by microscopy. MG grows slowly and depends on its human host, or complex growth medium in vitro,

[a] Division of Infectious Diseases, University of Washington, Center for AIDS and STD, Box 359779, 325 9th Avenue, Seattle, WA 98104, USA; [b] Melbourne Sexual Health Centre, Alfred Health, Melbourne, VIC, Australia; [c] Central Clinical School, Nursing and Health Sciences, Monash University, Melbourne, VIC, Australia; [d] Department of Epidemiology, University of Washington, Center for AIDS and STD, Box 359931, 325 9th Avenue, Seattle, WA 98104, USA
* Corresponding author.
E-mail address: gwenwood@uw.edu

Infect Dis Clin N Am 37 (2023) 311–333
https://doi.org/10.1016/j.idc.2023.02.009
0891-5520/23/© 2023 Elsevier Inc. All rights reserved.

for nutrients because it has lost many biosynthetic capabilities through extensive genome reduction. Although many mycoplasmas lack a defined cell shape, the tip organelle, which functions in adherence to cell surfaces and gliding motility, gives MG a distinct flask shape. The MgpB/MgpC adhesin proteins are located on the tip organelle and are the primary targets of antibodies in infected patients[1–3]; however, antigenic and phase variation of these proteins probably allow immune evasion[4–7] enabling persistence in the genital tract.[4–9] The fact that nearly 5% of the highly reduced MG genome is dedicated to variation of MgpB and MgpC suggests it is essential to survival in the human host.[4,7] An immunoglobulin binding protein postulated to block the biologic activity of antibodies against MG may also function in immune evasion.[10] Because no toxins have been identified, tissue damage seems to be mediated by proinflammatory lipoproteins.[11] In vitro studies have demonstrated that MG lipoproteins induce cytokine secretion by human genital tract epithelial cells[12,13] and immune cells[14,15] via engagement of toll-like receptors.[16] Production of reactive metabolic products may also contribute to tissue damage[17] because adherence of MG to human fallopian tube explants induces distention and loss of ciliated cells.[18] MG forms biofilms[19] and may occupy an intracellular niche,[20–22] both of which could reduce clearance by the immune system and antibiotic efficacy.

Animal Models

Numerous animal studies have confirmed the pathogenicity of MG. In hormone-treated mice, MG rapidly ascended to the upper reproductive tract, persisted for several weeks, and induced hydrosalpinx[23] in approximately 60% suggesting that the uterus may be the preferred site of infection.[23] Studies in nonhuman primates confirmed the pathogenesis of MG for the lower[24–26] and upper genital tract.[27] Direct inoculation of MG into the oviducts of grivet monkeys and marmosets induced moderate to severe endosalpingitis, infiltration of inflammatory cells into the tubal epithelium and lumen, and mucosal adhesions. No vaginal discharge or polymorphonuclear leukocytes (PMNs) were detected despite ongoing pathology in the fallopian tubes. The ability of MG to ascend to the upper reproductive tract was demonstrated in pig-tailed macaques where MG persisted in the lower genital tract for at least 18 weeks and invaded the upper reproductive tract, including the fallopian tubes.[6,28,29] Cervicovaginal organism load decreased after MG-specific cervical antibody appeared. However, cervical antibodies waned, and MG was detectable for an additional 10 to 15 weeks indicating that antibodies alone cannot provide sterilizing immunity. MG was frequently undetectable in vaginal swabs late in infection even though high organism loads were present in the endometrium and fallopian tubes[29] suggesting that sampling the vagina or cervix may not detect female upper reproductive tract infections in all cases.

EPIDEMIOLOGY
Prevalence

In a meta-analysis of studies published from 1991 to 2016, the general population prevalence of MG among persons ages 16 to 44 years was 1.3% (95% confidence interval [CI], 1.0%–1.8%) in high-income countries with a somewhat higher prevalence of 3.9% (95% CI, 2.2%–6.7%) in countries with lower human development indices.[30] Prevalence was higher among people at high risk, ranging from 3.2% among men who have sex with men (MSM) to 15.9% among female sex workers in lower-income countries.[30] The global prevalence among pregnant women was 0.9% (95% CI, 0.6%–1.4%), similar to women in general (1.4%; 95% CI, 0.8%–2.4%). However, more recent studies reported MG prevalence in US pregnant people of 5.7%[31] to 8.0%[32] and 13.5% (95% CI, 4.0–27.2) in a meta-analysis of pregnant people in sub-Saharan Africa, similar to *Chlamydia trachomatis* (CT) (10.8%) and higher than *Neisseria gonorrhoeae* (GC) (3.3%).[33] Prevalence among men and women at high-risk in a large multicenter study in the United States varied by sex and type of health care facility. Among women, prevalence was lowest in family medicine and obstetrics/gynecology clinics (4.8%); ranged from 10% to 13% in family planning, sexually transmitted infection (STI), and public health clinics; and was highest in women attending emergency clinics (16.7%). Among men, MG was most frequently detected at STI clinics (16.7%).[34,35]

Risk Factors

Risk factors for MG infection are similar to those for most STI. In population-based studies, MG was more common among Black people, those greater than 30 years, and those with lower education.[36,37] Lower socioeconomic status, as measured by poverty level or neighborhood indices, has been variably associated with MG.[36,37] MG is generally not associated with sex; prevalence is similar in males and females in most settings.[34,36,37] Consistent with sexual transmission, persons reporting more sex partners and younger age at sexual debut are at higher risk of MG infection.[36] Inconsistent condom use was associated with higher MG prevalence in Natsal-3, but not among Ugandan men with urethritis,[38] nor among adolescents and young adults in the general population,[39] or young women seeking gynecologic care.[40]

Strain Typing

Strain typing among partners first confirmed that MG is sexually transmitted[41] and since has been used to define sexual networks.[42,43] Given the difficulties in culturing MG strains, strain typing depends on molecular methods (polymerase chain reaction [PCR] amplification and sequencing) most often targeting a semiconserved region in the *mgpB* gene, with more than 300 strain types described.[42] Additional discriminatory power is achieved by assessing short tandem repeats (AGT/AAT) in the MG_309 gene, which is a valuable tool in populations with few circulating *mgpB* types, allowing one to distinguish persistent infection from reinfection in individual patients.[42,44,45] A recent study applied both methods and identified three strain type clusters differentiated by gender, male sexual practices, and geographic location.[42] Despite this utility, strain type cannot inform treatment because macrolide and fluoroquinolone resistance–associated mutations have not been associated with particular strain types.[42,44,46] Similarly, strain type has not been associated with specific clinical signs and symptoms but data are limited in this regard.[42,45] However, whole-genome sequencing of 28 MG strains demonstrated greater than 99% conservation of gene content suggesting that clinical outcomes are not attributable to different virulence genes.[47]

NATURAL HISTORY OF *MYCOPLASMA GENITALIUM* INFECTION

The natural history of MG infection is incompletely understood because of the limited number of longitudinal studies. MG has a lower organism load than other STI pathogens, which may reduce its transmissibility, and its slow growth rate may result in longer incubation periods before symptom onset[48]; however, no studies have formally investigated this. Overall, concordant infection occurs in 27% to 50% of sexual partnerships involving an MG-positive individual.[49,50] Among Australian sexual health clinic patients, concordant MG infection was detected in 48% of women, 42% of MSM, and 31% of heterosexual men with MG-positive partners.[51]

Persistence

Like most mycoplasmas, MG can cause chronic infections. In one study of US men, urethral infections persisted for a median of 143 days (range, 21–228) in the absence of effective treatment. Symptoms resolved after azithromycin in some men with macrolide-resistant infections even though MG persisted for another 89 to 186 days.[52] In contrast, spontaneous clearance of asymptomatic MG infection occurred in 30% of HIV-infected MSM with normal CD4 T-cell levels.[53] MG infections in women can persist for months to years without effective treatment.[49] Among Kenyan women, MG persisted for greater than 7 months in 21% and several were infected for greater than 3 years. Importantly, this study demonstrated that a single strain type was present through 10 to 21 months of follow-up suggesting persistent infection rather than reinfection.[54] The median time to clear MG from the lower genital tract was 3.9 months in a separate population of Kenyan women[55] and MG persisted for 3 months in 45% and for 12 months in 7% of MG-infected Ugandan women.[56] Among young women in London, 26% were MG-positive after 12 to 21 months[57] similar to a US study where 21% had persistent MG spanning 12 months.[58] The true duration of MG infection is challenging to determine. Unreported incidental antibiotic usage in longitudinal studies and suboptimal detection methods result in underestimates of duration,[49,59] whereas unmeasured reinfections likely inflate estimates of duration.

REPRODUCTIVE TRACT SYNDROMES
Men

Urethritis

First isolated from men with urethritis, MG is now recognized as the cause of 15% to 30% of symptomatic nongonococcal urethritis (NGU) in men.[60–62] It is also responsible for up to 40% of cases of persistent or recurrent NGU because standard doxycycline empiric therapy has poor efficacy against MG and azithromycin treatment failures are increasingly common.[48,61] Similar to other bacterial etiologies, symptoms of MG-associated urethritis include urethral discharge, dysuria, and urethral pruritis. In a large US multisite clinical study,[34] MG prevalence was higher in symptomatic than asymptomatic men (odds ratio [OR], 1.42; 1.02–1.99), but the only individual symptom associated with MG was urethral discharge (OR, 2.77; 1.94–3.94). Clinician-observed abnormal urethral discharge and swollen inguinal lymph nodes were also significantly associated with MG (OR, 2.97 [1.42–5.77] and OR, 2.34 [2.14–4.13], respectively). Nevertheless, overall clinical signs are not demonstrably different from those observed in men with CT- and *Trichomonas vaginalis* (TV)-urethritis[63]; therefore, definitive diagnosis of MG depends on highly sensitive nucleic acid amplification tests (NAAT).

Rectal infection and proctitis

MG was more frequently detected in rectal than urethral samples in several studies of MSM[64–66] but data regarding proctitis are limited and inconsistent. Among MSM attending a sexual health clinic, 7% were MG-positive in the rectum versus 2.7% in urethral specimens, but there was no significant association with proctitis.[65] A subsequent study reported a significant association, detecting MG in 9.4% of MSM with proctitis but in only 5.1% of asymptomatic MSM.[67] Two case series of proctitis in MSM found that MG was common: MG was present in 12%[68] and was the sole pathogen detected in 17%, similar to CT prevalence (21%).[69] Supporting an association with proctitis, a systematic review and meta-analysis of 25 studies found significantly higher MG prevalence in the rectum in symptomatic than asymptomatic MSM (16.1% vs 7.5%; $P = .039$).[70] Rectal symptoms may depend on organism load because significantly more MG genomes were detected in men with proctitis than asymptomatic men.[68] Current Centers for Disease Control and Prevention (CDC) guidelines suggest testing for MG if proctitis symptoms persist after standard treatment with ceftriaxone plus doxycycline.[61] British, Australian, and European guidelines suggest testing for MG after excluding other agents (GC, CT, syphilis, herpes).[71,72]

Women

The consequences of MG infection in women are less well defined than in men. Like other reproductive tract pathogens, MG infections in women are usually asymptomatic and serious upper tract sequelae may manifest long after initial infection. Despite frequent asymptomatic infection, MG infection among women presenting for clinical care was more common in symptomatic than asymptomatic women (OR, 1.53; 1.09–2.14). MG was detected in 14.6% reporting abnormal vaginal odor and 13.0% reporting abnormal vaginal discharge.[34] However, similar to men, differentiating between MG and other pathogens based on clinical signs and symptoms is not reliable and NAAT is preferred.

Female urethritis

The few studies on MG and female urethritis have demonstrated associations, but data regarding MG and the symptom of dysuria are inconsistent. MG was associated with a two-fold increased risk of female urethritis when defined as greater than 4 polymorphonuclear leukocytes per high power field (PMN/HPF) on microscopic examination[73,74] or approximately three-fold increased risk when defined by dysuria or urgency.[75] In a small study of women attending an emergency department, 24% of women presenting with dysuria had MG[76] but there was no association in a larger study of 1318 women (OR, 1.12; 0.56–2.25).[77]

Cervicitis

Although studies are complicated by the lack of standard diagnostic criteria and varying sensitivities of diagnostic tests, MG is implicated in 10% to 30% of clinical cervicitis cases.[78] A 2015 meta-analysis identified a significant association between MG and cervicitis (pooled OR, 1.7; 1.35–2.04).[79] Proinflammatory cytokines and leukocytes were elevated in cervical secretions of women with chronic MG infection and leukocytic infiltrates in cervical curettage specimens from MG-positive women were eliminated after clearance of MG.[80] More recently, MG was significantly associated with diagnoses of mucopurulent cervicitis among greater than 1300 Australian women attending a sexual health clinic (adjusted OR, 4.38; 1.69–11.33; $P = .002$), despite similar prevalence in symptomatic and asymptomatic women.[77]

Pelvic inflammatory disease

Pelvic inflammatory disease (PID) is a syndrome comprising endometritis, salpingitis, tubo-ovarian abscess, and peritonitis that can lead to infertility. Although pelvic pain is a common symptom of PID, many cases are asymptomatic, and therefore untreated. Early evidence linking MG infection to PID came from serologic studies demonstrating increased antibody titer to MG after onset of disease.[81] Since then, several studies have demonstrated MG prevalence of 6% to 33% in women with PID.[82] Mathematical modeling[83] and cross-sectional studies[84,85] estimate that 5% to 10% of women with MG infection will develop PID (as compared with ~14% of CT infections). Although MG infections may induce milder symptoms,[61,82,86] severe disease attributable to MG has been reported, including perihepatitis in a woman hospitalized with MG-associated PID[87] and an MG-positive patient with moderate to severe adhesions who suffered pelvic pain for more than a year.[88] Among young adults in the United

States, 17% to 19% of mild to moderate PID was attributable to MG, and this remained unchanged 3 months after standard PID treatment regimens, which have poor efficacy against MG.[89,90] In one study, MG infection was strongly associated with postabortal PID (OR, 6.29; 1.56–25.2)[91]; consequently the European guidelines advise practitioners to consider MG testing before termination of pregnancy.[71]

MG has specifically been associated with endometritis and salpingitis in several studies. Detection of MG in the endometrium was associated with a 13.4-fold increased risk of histologically confirmed endometritis in the PID Evaluation and Clinical Health (PEACH) trial.[89] MG infection was also associated with endometritis in women attending urban outpatient clinics in Pittsburgh (adjusted relative risk, 2.0; 1.1–3.7).[92]

Infertility

Consistent with its ability to invade the upper reproductive tract and induce inflammation, MG has been associated with tubal factor infertility in women. Two early studies that accounted for CT infection linked tubal factor infertility with serologic evidence of MG infection.[2] One of these[93] further linked strong MG-specific IgG responses with tubal factor infertility. A meta-analysis of studies published through 2014 demonstrated a nonsignificant approximately 2.4-fold increased risk of infertility associated with MG,[79] but a subsequent meta-analysis that excluded serologic studies reported a significant association.[94] Of two additional serologic studies, also controlling for antibodies to CT, one reported a nonsignificant increased risk of infertility[95] and one identified significantly more infertility among MG-seropositive women.[96] The latter also reported a significantly longer time to pregnancy (hazard ratio, 0.76; 0.58–0.99) among MG-seropositive versus MG-seronegative women.[96] Studies that detect MG by NAAT are hampered by low prevalence and are challenging to interpret because the time between MG infection and infertility diagnosis may be lengthy. Larger studies with adequate statistical power are needed to definitively determine the association between MG and infertility.

Ectopic pregnancy

Although the ability of MG to damage fallopian tube tissue in vitro suggests biologic plausibility,[18] few studies have examined MG infection and ectopic pregnancy and results are inconsistent. MG was detected by PCR in tubal specimens from women with ectopic pregnancy significantly more often than women undergoing hysterectomy or tubal ligation (OR, 2.3; 1.1–8.6; $P = .03$).[97] In contrast, using multiplex PCR there was a nonsignificant association with ectopic pregnancy (OR, 1.5; 0.7–19) relative to women undergoing hysterectomies[98]; MG infection was accompanied by increased interleukin-6, consistent with in vitro experiments described previously.[12,13] In contrast, using a first-generation serologic assay, MG seropositivity was similar in women with ectopic pregnancy (18%) and healthy pregnant women (15%).[99]

Preterm birth

Comprehensive reviews published in 2015[79] and 2022[100] concluded that MG is significantly associated with increased risk of preterm birth (OR, 1.89 [1.25–2.85] and OR, 2.34 [1.17–4.71], respectively). However, those same meta-analyses differed in their conclusions about the association with spontaneous abortion, with one reporting a significant association (OR, 1.82; 1.10–3.03)[79] and one reporting no association.[100] Most studies have major limitations including small sample size, testing for MG infection months prior to preterm birth, use of suboptimal specimen types (eg, female urine), and using MG NAATs with unreported sensitivities. Given the absence of definitive causal evidence on pregnancy complications, screening asymptomatic pregnant women for MG is not recommended.

Rectal Mycoplasma genitalium in women

As in men, MG also infects the female rectum.[101–103] Among high-risk women attending a Seattle sexual health clinic, 65% with MG were positive in vaginal and rectal specimens, despite most participants denying anal sex.[101] In fact, rectal-only MG was more common than vaginal-only MG (23% vs 15%).[101] MG was detected in rectal specimens from 2.7% of South African women visiting a primary health clinic,[104] and in 4.3% of women attending a sexual health clinic in New Orleans, but there was no association between rectal infection and reported anal intercourse in the latter.[102] No studies have investigated MG and female proctitis. The consequences of asymptomatic rectal MG infection in women are unclear, although the possibility that vaginal inoculation from the rectum could lead to reproductive tract outcomes has been suggested.[101]

COINFECTIONS

Similar to coinfection with GC and CT,[105] MG is often present with other STI pathogens, likely because of similar risk behaviors. In recent studies of male urethritis, MG monoinfection occurred in 38% to 47% of men, whereas approximately one-quarter were infected with GC and MG (25.8% in Ugandan men with urethral discharge syndrome[38]; 21.2% among US men with urethritis[62]). Approximately 11.8% of symptomatic and asymptomatic MG-infected men attending a US sexual health clinic were coinfected with CT.[106] In contrast, there was no association between CT and MG in the general population in the United Kingdom, despite higher odds of high-risk human papillomavirus infection in MG-infected males and females.[36] Approximately 13% of Ugandan men with MG were coinfected with syphilis,[38] but few other reports have measured this. Coinfection also occurs in extragenital sites. In a case series of Australian MSM, MG was detected in 13% with rectal CT and 14% with rectal GC.[107] Despite these coinfections, the association between MG and reproductive tract syndromes is strengthened rather than weakened in most multivariable analyses that account for CT and/or GC infection, supporting an independent role of MG.[79]

Mycoplasma genitalium and Bacterial Vaginosis

Women with bacterial vaginosis (BV) are at increased risk for acquisition of STIs,[108] including MG, and adverse reproductive tract sequelae.[109] Several studies suggest a link between MG infection and BV. Kenyan women who exchange sex for money with BV had a 3.5-fold increased risk of acquiring MG infection compared with women without BV.[110] Similarly, the odds of detecting MG in women with BV at routine gynecology visits were nearly three-fold higher than in women with normal vaginal microbiota (adjusted OR, 2.88; 1.19–7.16).[111] In a large cohort of 1139 women with asymptomatic BV, the incidence of MG was high (36.6 per 100 person years; 95% CI, 32.4–41.3) and 20.6% had MG infections persisting up to 12 months.[58] The addition of metronidazole to standard therapy for PID resulted in less cervical MG infection 30-days posttreatment (4% vs 14%; $P < .05$),[112] and the incidence of new MG infections was 44% lower in women randomized to periodic presumptive treatment for vaginal infections that included metronidazole to target BV than in women who did not receive periodic presumptive treatment (IRR, 0.66; 0.38–1.15), although this was not statistically significant.[108]

Mycoplasma genitalium and HIV Acquisition

As with other genital tract pathogens, MG is associated with HIV, with a two-fold increased odds of infection (summary OR, 2.01; 1.44–2.79).[113] This risk was higher among MSM in China where risk of HIV infection was 3.2-fold higher for men with than without MG.[114] A meta-analysis demonstrated that MG-infected women were approximately three-fold more likely to acquire HIV (relative risk, 3.10; 1.63–5.92) than women without MG and this effect was greater for MG than any other nonviral STI.[115] People infected with HIV and MG may also have a higher likelihood of transmitting HIV to partners. High MG cervical load was associated with a three-fold increase in the likelihood of HIV viral shedding in one study,[116] but this has not been consistently reported.[117,118]

Other Infrequent Sites of Mycoplasma genitalium Infection

MG has been infrequently detected in the oropharynx with prevalence of approximately 1% in MSM and less than 0.2% in female sex workers.[119,120] Published evidence suggests that the pharynx does not contribute significantly to transmission of MG[107] and testing for oral MG is not recommended.[61]

Although uncommon, MG-associated arthritis has been reported. Reactive arthritis occurred in an HLA-B27-positive man with MG PCR-positive urethritis[121] and MG DNA was detected in the joints of two men with arthritis, one of whom developed arthritis 1 week after urethritis.[122] MG was reportedly isolated from the synovial fluid of an *Mycoplasma pneumoniae*–infected patient[123]; however, this was later attributed to laboratory contamination.[47] The association with arthritis is supported by animal studies detecting MG DNA in the joints of vaginally inoculated mice.[23] Other human mycoplasmas including *M pneumoniae*[124] and *Ureaplasma parvum*[125] are associated with reactive arthritis in rare cases, and mycoplasmas are well-known causes of arthritis in agricultural animals, emphasizing the biologic plausibility of MG-associated arthritis.

Insufficient evidence exists regarding MG as a cause of prostatitis or epididymitis, although the European guidelines suggest MG testing in cases of epididymo-orchitis.[71] A single study reported an association between MG infection and balanoposthitis among men with acute NGU[126] but no further evidence has emerged.

One case report describes conjunctivitis attributable to autoinoculation from urethral MG[127] and MG was detected in the conjunctiva of approximately 10% of neonates born to women with genital MG infection. Therefore, European guidelines suggest that infants should be monitored for conjunctivitis and respiratory infection.[128]

MANAGEMENT OF PATIENTS WITH SUSPECTED *MYCOPLASMA GENITALIUM* INFECTION

CDC guidelines recommend testing for MG only in men with recurrent or persistent NGU, and in women with recurrent cervicitis. MG testing should also be considered for women with PID. Men with proctitis should be tested for MG if standard treatments are ineffective. This differs from recommendations in British, European, and Australian guidelines where testing is recommended for: (1) NGU in men (acute or chronic), (2) signs and symptoms of cervicitis including postcoital bleeding, (3) signs and symptoms suggestive of PID, and (4) current sexual partners of persons infected with MG. It may be considered in people with epididymo-orchitis, and sexually acquired proctitis.

Diagnosis

Testing should use a sensitive, FDA-approved NAAT test. Currently, three assays are available in the United States: Hologic Aptima Mycoplasma genitalium, Roche cobas TV/MG, and Abbott Alinity m STI. In general, first void urine is the preferred specimen type for men (urethral swabs may also be used); vaginal swabs (clinician or self-collected) are preferred for testing women. Other specimen types (eg, meatal swabs, endocervical swabs, or female urine) are also acceptable but may be less sensitive.[35] No test is FDA-approved to detect MG in rectal swabs; however, research-use-only tests are available in some centers. Because MG organism load is low compared with other STI pathogens test sensitivity is important. The value of increased assay sensitivity was demonstrated by a recent study reporting that a laboratory-developed quantitative PCR-based assay was 64.5% sensitive compared with the TMA-based assay, and that 54% of individuals missed by quantitative PCR were symptomatic and thus candidates for treatment.[129]

Where available, diagnostic testing should be accompanied by detection of 23S rRNA macrolide resistance mutations (MRM) to guide treatment. Detection of any of the single-nucleotide polymorphisms (SNPs) associated with macrolide resistance is highly predictive of azithromycin failure. Several tests that detect MG and MRM are available outside the United States. Within the United States, such tests are currently only available at research centers.

Although macrolide resistance and treatment failure are clearly associated with specific 23S rRNA SNPs, the molecular basis for moxifloxacin resistance has been more difficult to define. Mutations in *parC* affecting serine at position 83 (eg, S83I, S83R; *M genitalium* numbering) and aspartic acid at position 87 (eg, D87N, D87Y), are associated with moxifloxacin failure[130–133] and increased moxifloxacin minimal inhibitory concentrations (MICs).[47,134] The strongest candidate for resistance is the *parC* S83I variation, which is also the most common *parC* mutation; approximately 60% of cases carrying this mutation fail moxifloxacin treatment.[130,132,133] Conversely the presence of wild-type *parC* S83 is associated with a greater than 96% probability of moxifloxacin cure. Other *parC* changes are less common and less strongly associated with moxifloxacin failure.[133] Data regarding the importance of *gyrA* mutations are more limited. Mutations in *gyrA* affecting M95 or D99 commonly coexist with a *parC* S83I mutation and further increase the probability of moxifloxacin failure and high moxifloxacin MICs.[132] In the United States, quinolone resistance-associated mutations are detected by PCR and sequencing that is available only in specialized research centers. Although some commercial quinolone resistance-associated mutations detection assays are available internationally, many include uncommon targets that have not been definitively associated with moxifloxacin failure. Given the limited treatments for MG, any clinically useful quinolone resistance-associated mutations assay must contain *parC* ± *gyrA* targets to be highly predictive of moxifloxacin treatment outcomes.

Culture has no practical use in diagnosing MG. Growth of MG from clinical specimens requires weeks to months of coculture with mammalian cell lines and few laboratories in the United States[135,136] and worldwide[137] have demonstrated this capability. No commercial serologic assays are approved for diagnosing MG infections. Serologic tests are complicated by cross reactivity of antibodies to *M pneumoniae*, a common respiratory pathogen, although second- and third-generation research serologic assays are more specific.

Treatment

Treating MG infections is challenging because of poor efficacy of recommended therapy for lower genital tract syndromes and inherent and acquired antimicrobial resistance. Doxycycline is only 30% to 45% effective[138] and resistance to macrolides has increased in recent decades. Globally macrolide resistance was greater than 50% in 2016 to 2017.[139] It is high in Canada (63.6%),[140] and among men with urethritis attending US sexual health clinics (64.4%),[62] and is often higher in MSM than men who have sex with women (89.7% vs 50% in Australia).[141] Moxifloxacin is the recommended alternative for macrolide-resistant strains, but resistance to fluoroquinolones is also increasing. Globally, fluoroquinolone resistance-associated mutations were found in 7.7% of MG-positive specimens in 2016 to 2017[139] with higher rates in the Western Pacific. Alarmingly, a recent study in China found that 88% of MG strains infecting men with symptomatic urethritis had macrolide and quinolone resistance-associated mutations.[142] Among HIV-positive MSM in Alabama, S83R and S83I mutations were detected in 27% and 40% of urogenital and rectal specimens, respectively, and markers of dual resistance to macrolides and quinolones were detected in 20% to 30%.[143]

Resistance-guided therapy using assays to detect MRM is the recommended strategy in most countries.[144,145] In this strategy (**Fig. 1**), patients with symptomatic infection are treated empirically with doxycycline (100 mg twice daily for 7 days) while awaiting NAAT results for MG and MRM. Patients are then treated either with azithromycin (1 g on day 1 followed by 500 mg daily for 3 days) if macrolide sensitive or moxifloxacin (400 mg once daily for 7 days) if macrolide resistant. Current sexual partners should be treated with the same regimen. US, British, Australian, and European

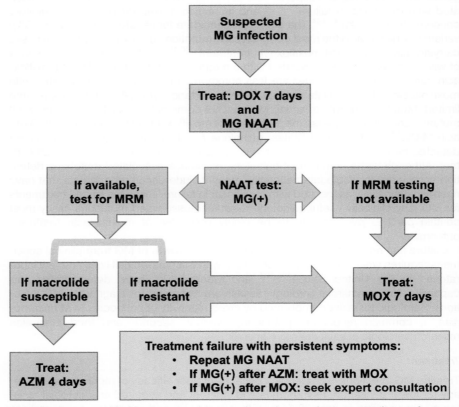

Fig. 1. Resistance-guided treatment of uncomplicated *Mycoplasma genitalium* infections. AZM, azithromycin (1 g initial dose, then 3 days, 500 mg qd); DOX, doxycycline (7 days, 100 mg bid); MOX, moxifloxacin (7 days, 400 mg qd).

guidelines recommend 14 days of moxifloxacin for PID, although this is based on observational data rather than randomized controlled trials.[86]

Doxycycline monotherapy is the recommended first-line treatment of urethritis and cervicitis but cures only 30% to 40% of MG infections.[138] The reasons for this partial efficacy are not clear but drug concentrations in genital sites may be lower than MICs for many strains.[135,146] Studies assessing longer doxycycline therapy report conflicting results. Two weeks of doxycycline in patients with macrolide-resistant MG resulted in 58.9% cure.[147] However, treatment with 7 days of doxycycline followed by dual treatment with doxycycline + azithromycin or doxycycline + moxifloxacin was associated with more side effects and was not more effective than sequential monotherapy implying that the extended doxycycline was of little value.[130]

Doxycycline postexposure prophylaxis (DoxyPEP) has received recent attention as a strategy to reduce the incidence of bacterial STIs. DoxyPEP (200-mg single dose taken within 24–72 hours of unprotected sex) was highly effective in preventing incident CT and syphilis infection in MSM,[148,149] but there was no impact on the acquisition of MG infection in one trial.[150] Results are pending from a second trial and additional data are needed.

The increasing role of doxycycline in treatment and prevention of bacterial STIs raises concerns about the development of resistance. The *tetM* resistance determinant identified in other genital tract mycoplasmas has not been reported in MG. SNPs in the 16S rRNA gene associated with tetracycline resistance in other organisms (including mycoplasmas) have been detected in MG but the significance is uncertain. Although 16S rRNA SNPs were detected in MG infecting 52 patients before and after doxycycline treatment, none were associated with treatment efficacy or changes in organism load.[151] Furthermore, they found no association between MICs and 16S rRNA SNPs among published strains. Le Roy and coworkers[152] attempted to induce doxycycline resistance in vitro by 30 serial passages in subinhibitory concentrations; however, no mutants with increased doxycycline MICs or 16S rRNA SNPs were isolated. Two clinical isolates from immunocompromised individuals demonstrated doxycycline MICs greater than or equal to eight, but *tetM* was not detected.[136] Future studies assessing the association between DoxyPEP, possible doxycycline resistance-associated mutations, and in vitro susceptibility will be important to perform.

Despite the low efficacy of doxycycline, it is an important component of resistance-guided therapy because it reduces organism load approximately 100-fold, improving cure rates for a subsequent antibiotic.[145] Additionally, macrolide resistance develops in only 3.8% of patients treated sequentially with doxycycline and azithromycin,[145] whereas a single 1-g dose of azithromycin selects for macrolide resistance in 10% to 12% of MG infections.[48,135] Of note, specimens with low organism load may erroneously be classified as macrolide-susceptible because detection of MRM is less sensitive than detection of MG.[144,145] Furthermore, macrolide-sensitive and -resistant MG may exist simultaneously in individual patients. Wild-type and multiple MRM alleles could be detected among different specimen types (urine, vaginal, ectocervical, and endocervical) collected at the same time in 11.7% of women in a recent study.[153] Vaginal swab specimens were the most sensitive (96.3%) for detecting MRM. Where possible, it may be prudent to pool specimen types from individual patients to be certain MRM are detected.

Management of Treatment Failures

Treatment of MG infections failing first- and second-line therapies is extremely challenging. MG is inherently resistant to many classes of antibiotics including β-lactams, cephalosporins, and glycopeptides (no peptidoglycan); sulfonamides (no folic acid synthesis); rifampins (*rpoB* mutation common to all Mollicutes[154]); aminoglycosides[155] (except spectinomycin[156]); and colistins (no outer membrane/LPS).

Alternative therapies available in the United States include an extended course of minocycline (100 mg twice daily for 14 days), which was 71% effective in a recent study of 35 patients[157] and confirmed in 123 patients with 68% cured (personal communication, C. Bradshaw). Omadacycline and lefamulin, available in the United States, have in vitro activity but treatment efficacy has not been described.[136,158,159]

Several antibiotics available outside the United States were effective in patients with prior treatment failure. Pristinamycin was 75% effective,[157,160] and sitafloxacin in combination with doxycycline for 7 days was greater than 90% effective in patients who had failed multiple prior drugs in Australia and Japan.[144,161] Solithromycin cured MG infections in six of seven patients,[162] but it was not FDA-approved because of concerns about hepatotoxicity. Gepotidacin and zoliflodacin have in vitro activity against MG[158,163] but neither has been assessed against MG in patients or approved by the FDA.

Treatment During Pregnancy

Treating MG infections in pregnancy is especially challenging. For symptomatic infection, azithromycin is considered safe during pregnancy in people with macrolide-sensitive MG, but doxycycline and minocycline are teratogenic and should not be used. Moxifloxacin is a Pregnancy Category C drug and should not be used in pregnant persons unless the benefits of treating MG are clear. In the Australian and European guidelines, pristinamycin, which is considered safe in pregnancy, may be considered in symptomatic people after specialist consultation. Because the magnitude of risk associated with MG infection during pregnancy is uncertain, symptomatic pregnant people with macrolide-resistant infections should be counseled on the potential harms of treatment and encouraged to delay therapy until after delivery. Given the uncertain implications of MG infection during pregnancy and the challenges associated with treatment, asymptomatic pregnant people should not be screened for MG.

Test of Cure

International guidelines differ on recommendations for tests of cure and the CDC explicitly counsels against them in asymptomatic people.[61] If clinician judgment suggests a test of cure is important, this should be done at least 14 days after completion of antimicrobial therapy to avoid false-positives (caused by residual nucleic acid) and false-negatives (caused by low organism load).

Screening

Given the lack of rigorous data on consequences of asymptomatic infection and the need to limit antimicrobial pressure, asymptomatic people should not be screened for MG. Although the role of MG in female upper reproductive tract sequelae is supported by numerous studies, the magnitude of this risk is poorly defined and adequately powered, prospective studies have not yet been conducted. Current recommendations against screening are designed to limit antibiotic exposure to symptomatic people where there is a clear benefit to treatment.

DISCUSSION AND SUMMARY

MG infections induce genital tract inflammation in most infected individuals and can be chronic. MG is an established and common cause of male urethritis. A strong body of evidence links MG to female reproductive tract syndromes but the magnitude of risk is uncertain because of the lack of prospective studies defining the natural history of infection. The risk of asymptomatic infection is controversial and additional clinical trial evidence is needed to determine whether screening and treatment can prevent sequelae. Treatment of symptomatic infection is challenging because MG is susceptible to only a few classes of antibiotics. Macrolide resistance is widespread and although moxifloxacin remains effective in most cases in the United States, fluoroquinolone resistance is rising. Treatment in pregnancy is particularly difficult; only azithromycin and pristinamycin are not contraindicated in pregnant people, and pristinamycin is not available in the United States. Clinicians should carefully consider appropriate antimicrobials in the context of antimicrobial resistance detection to optimize treatment success in symptomatic individuals.

CLINICS CARE POINTS

- MG should be suspected in cases of NGU, cervicitis, and PID. NAAT testing is required to diagnose MG infection because clinical signs and symptoms are similar to *C trachomatis*.
- Few antibiotics are effective against MG given its unique biology and high rates of antimicrobial resistance. Macrolides are not effective in many geographic areas and where macrolide resistance detection assays are unavailable, sequential therapy with doxycycline followed by moxifloxacin is currently the treatment of choice.
- Screening asymptomatic people is not recommended given the uncertainty around sequelae associated with asymptomatic infection and the need to limit antibiotic pressure on this organism. Tests of cure in asymptomatic people are not recommended for similar reasons.

DISCLOSURE

G.E. Wood has received research funds from SpeeDx, Pty, Australia, Hologic, Inc., and Abbott. C.S. Bradshaw has received research funds from SpeeDx and diagnostics kits from Cepheid and Hologic; and is supported by a National Health and Medical Research Council Investigator Leadership Grant. L.E. Manhart has received research funds from Hologic, United States and Nabriva Therapeutics, Ireland; and honoraria from Hologic, Inc., Nabriva Therapeutics, and Health Advances, LLC, United States.

REFERENCES

1. Iverson-Cabral SL, Manhart LE, Totten PA. Detection of *Mycoplasma genitalium*-reactive cervicovaginal antibodies among infected women. Clin Vaccine Immunol 2011;18(10):1783–6.
2. Clausen HF, Fedder J, Drasbek M, et al. Serological investigation of *Mycoplasma genitalium* in infertile women. Hum Reprod 2001;16(9):1866–74.
3. Svenstrup HF, Jensen JS, Gevaert K, et al. Identification and characterization of immunogenic proteins of *Mycoplasma genitalium*. Clin Vaccine Immunol 2006; 13(8):913–22.
4. Iverson-Cabral SL, Astete SG, Cohen CR, et al. Intrastrain heterogeneity of the *mgpB* gene in *Mycoplasma genitalium* is extensive in vitro and in vivo and suggests that variation is generated via recombination with repetitive chromosomal sequences. Infect Immun 2006;74(7):3715–26.
5. Burgos R, Wood GE, Iverson-Cabral SL, et al. *Mycoplasma genitalium* nonadherent phase variants arise by multiple mechanisms and escape antibody-dependent growth inhibition. Infect Immun 2018;86(4). 008666-e917.

6. Wood GE, Iverson-Cabral SL, Patton DL, et al. Persistence, immune response, and antigenic variation of *Mycoplasma genitalium* in an experimentally infected pig-tailed macaque (*Macaca nemestrina*). Infect Immun 2013;81(8):2938–51.

7. Iverson-Cabral SL, Astete SG, Cohen CR, et al. *mgpB* and *mgpC* sequence diversity in *Mycoplasma genitalium* is generated by segmental reciprocal recombination with repetitive chromosomal sequences. Mol Microbiol 2007;66(1):55–73.

8. Wood GE, Iverson-Cabral SL, Gillespie CW, et al. Sequence variation and immunogenicity of the *Mycoplasma genitalium* MgpB and MgpC adherence proteins during persistent infection of men with non-gonococcal urethritis. PLoS One 2020;15(10):e0240626.

9. Iverson-Cabral SL, Wood GE, Totten PA. Analysis of the *Mycoplasma genitalium* MgpB adhesin to predict membrane topology, investigate antibody accessibility, characterize amino acid diversity, and identify functional and immunogenic epitopes. PLoS One 2015;10(9):e0138244.

10. Arfi Y, Lartigue C, Sirand-Pugnet P, et al. Beware of Mycoplasma anti-immunoglobulin strategies. mBio 2021;12(6):e0197421.

11. Dehon PM, McGowin CL. The immunopathogenesis of *Mycoplasma genitalium* infections in women: a narrative review. Sex Transm Dis 2017;44(7):428–32.

12. McGowin CL, Radtke AL, Abraham K, et al. *Mycoplasma genitalium* infection activates cellular host defense and inflammation pathways in a 3-dimensional human endocervical epithelial cell model. J Infect Dis 2013;207(12):1857–68.

13. McGowin CL, Annan RS, Quayle AJ, et al. Persistent *Mycoplasma genitalium* infection of human endocervical epithelial cells elicits chronic inflammatory cytokine secretion. Infect Immun 2012;80(11):3842–9.

14. You X, Wu Y, Zeng Y, et al. *Mycoplasma genitalium*-derived lipid-associated membrane proteins induce activation of MAPKs, NF-kappaB and AP-1 in THP-1 cells. FEMS Immunol Med Microbiol 2008;52(2):228–36.

15. Wu Y, Qiu H, Zeng Y, et al. *Mycoplasma genitalium* lipoproteins induce human monocytic cell expression of proinflammatory cytokines and apoptosis by activating nuclear factor kappaB. Mediators Inflamm 2008;2008:195427.

16. McGowin CL, Ma L, Martin DH, et al. *Mycoplasma genitalium*-encoded MG309 activates NF-kappaB via Toll-like receptors 2 and 6 to elicit proinflammatory cytokine secretion from human genital epithelial cells. Infect Immun 2009;77(3):1175–81.

17. Martinez MA, Das K, Saikolappan S, et al. A serine/threonine phosphatase encoded by MG_207 of *Mycoplasma genitalium* is critical for its virulence. BMC Microbiol 2013;13:44.

18. Baczynska A, Funch P, Fedder J, et al. Morphology of human Fallopian tubes after infection with *Mycoplasma genitalium* and *Mycoplasma hominis*: in vitro organ culture study. Hum Reprod 2007;22(4):968–79.

19. Daubenspeck JM, Totten AH, Needham J, et al. *Mycoplasma genitalium* biofilms contain poly-GlcNAc and contribute to antibiotic resistance. Front Microbiol 2020;11:585524.

20. Jensen JS, Blom J, Lind K. Intracellular location of *Mycoplasma genitalium* in cultured Vero cells as demonstrated by electron microscopy. Int J Exp Pathol 1994;75(2):91–8.

21. Ueno PM, Timenetsky J, Centonze VE, et al. Interaction of *Mycoplasma genitalium* with host cells: evidence for nuclear localization. Microbiology 2008;154(Pt 10):3033–41.

22. McGowin CL, Popov VL, Pyles RB. Intracellular *Mycoplasma genitalium* infection of human vaginal and cervical epithelial cells elicits distinct patterns of inflammatory cytokine secretion and provides a possible survival niche against macrophage-mediated killing. BMC Microbiol 2009;9:139.

23. McGowin CL, Spagnuolo RA, Pyles RB. *Mycoplasma genitalium* rapidly disseminates to the upper reproductive tracts and knees of female mice following vaginal inoculation. Infect Immun 2010;78(2):726–36.

24. Taylor-Robinson D, Furr PM, Hetherington CM. The pathogenicity of a newly discovered human mycoplasma (strain G37) for the genital tract of marmosets. J Hyg 1982;89(3):449–55.

25. Tully JG, Taylor-Robinson D, Rose DL, et al. Urogenital challenge of primate species with *Mycoplasma genitalium* and characteristics of infection induced in chimpanzees. J Infect Dis 1986;153(6):1046–54.

26. Taylor-Robinson D, Tully JG, Barile MF. Urethral infection in male chimpanzees produced experimentally by *Mycoplasma genitalium*. Br J Exp Pathol 1985; 66(1):95–101.

27. Moller BR, Taylor-Robinson D, Furr PM, et al. Acute upper genital-tract disease in female monkeys provoked experimentally by *Mycoplasma genitalium*. Br J Exp Pathol 1985;66(4):417–26.

28. Wood GE, Patton DL, Cummings PK, et al. Experimental infection of pig-tailed macaques (*Macaca nemestrina*) with *Mycoplasma genitalium*. Infect Immun 2017;85(2).

29. Aguila LKT, Patton DL, Gornalusse GG, et al. Ascending reproductive tract infection in pig-tailed macaques inoculated with *Mycoplasma genitalium*. Infect Immun 2022;e0013122. https://doi.org/10.1128/iai.00131-22.

30. Baumann L, Cina M, Egli-Gany D, et al. Prevalence of *Mycoplasma genitalium* in different population groups: systematic review and meta-analysis. Sex Transm Infect 2018;94(4):255–62.

31. Stafford IA, Hummel K, Dunn JJ, et al. Retrospective analysis of infection and antimicrobial resistance patterns of *Mycoplasma genitalium* among pregnant women in the southwestern USA. BMJ Open 2021;11(6):e050475.

32. Hu M, Souder JP, Subramaniam A, et al. Prevalence of *Mycoplasma genitalium* infection and macrolide resistance in pregnant women receiving prenatal care. Int J Gynaecol Obstet 2022. https://doi.org/10.1002/ijgo.14443.

33. Nyemba DC, Haddison EC, Wang C, et al. Prevalence of curable STIs and bacterial vaginosis during pregnancy in sub-Saharan Africa: a systematic review and meta-analysis. Sex Transm Infect 2022;98(7):484–91.

34. Manhart LE, Gaydos CA, Taylor SN, et al. Characteristics of *Mycoplasma genitalium* urogenital infections in a diverse patient sample from the United States: results from the Aptima *Mycoplasma genitalium* Evaluation Study (AMES). J Clin Microbiol 2020;58(7).

35. Gaydos CA, Manhart LE, Taylor SN, et al. Molecular testing for *Mycoplasma genitalium* in the United States: results from the AMES prospective multicenter clinical study. J Clin Microbiol 2019;57(11). https://doi.org/10.1128/JCM.01125-19.

36. Sonnenberg P, Ison CA, Clifton S, et al. Epidemiology of *Mycoplasma genitalium* in British men and women aged 16-44 years: evidence from the third National Survey of Sexual Attitudes and Lifestyles (Natsal-3). Int J Epidemiol 2015; 44(6):1982–94.

37. Torrone EA, Kruszon-Moran D, Philips C, et al. Prevalence of urogenital *Mycoplasma genitalium* infection, United States, 2017 to 2018. Sex Transm Dis 2021;48(11):e160–2.
38. Hamill MM, Onzia A, Wang T-H, et al. High burden of untreated syphilis, drug resistant *Neisseria gonorrhoeae*, and other sexually transmitted infections in men with urethral discharge syndrome in Kampala, Uganda. BMC Infect Dis 2022;22(1):440.
39. Manhart LE, Holmes KK, Hughes JP, et al. *Mycoplasma genitalium* among young adults in the United States: an emerging sexually transmitted infection. Am J Public Health 2007;97(6):1118–25.
40. Ronda J, Gaydos CA, Perin J, et al. Does the sex risk quiz predict *Mycoplasma genitalium* infection in urban adolescents and young adult women? Sex Transm Dis 2018;45(11):728–34.
41. Hjorth SV, Bjornelius E, Lidbrink P, et al. Sequence-based typing of *Mycoplasma genitalium* reveals sexual transmission. J Clin Microbiol 2006;44(6):2078–83.
42. Guiraud J, Lounnas M, Boissière A, et al. Lower *mgpB* diversity in macrolide-resistant *Mycoplasma genitalium* infecting men visiting two sexually transmitted infection clinics in Montpellier, France. J Antimicrob Chemother 2021; 76(1):43–7.
43. Fernandez-Huerta M, Bodiyabadu K, Esperalba J, et al. Multicenter clinical evaluation of a novel multiplex real-time PCR (qPCR) assay for detection of fluoroquinolone resistance in *Mycoplasma genitalium*. J Clin Microbiol 2019. https://doi. org/10.1093/jac/dkaa410. pii: JCM.0.
44. Dumke R, Rust M, Glaunsinger T. MgpB types among *Mycoplasma genitalium* strains from men who have sex with men in Berlin, Germany, 2016-2018. Pathog (Basel, Switzerland) 2019;9(1). https://doi.org/10.3390/pathogens9010012.
45. Dumke R. Molecular tools for typing *Mycoplasma pneumoniae* and *Mycoplasma genitalium*. Front Microbiol 2022;13:904494.
46. Chua T-P, Bodiyabadu K, Machalek DA, et al. Prevalence of *Mycoplasma genitalium* fluoroquinolone-resistance markers, and dual-class-resistance markers, in asymptomatic men who have sex with men. J Med Microbiol 2021;70(9). https://doi.org/10.1099/jmm.0.001429.
47. Fookes MC, Hadfield J, Harris S, et al. *Mycoplasma genitalium*: whole genome sequence analysis, recombination and population structure. BMC Genom 2017; 18(1):993.
48. Horner PJ, Martin DH. *Mycoplasma genitalium* infection in men. J Infect Dis 2017;216(suppl_2):S396–405.
49. Cina M, Baumann L, Egli-Gany D, et al. *Mycoplasma genitalium* incidence, persistence, concordance between partners and progression: systematic review and meta-analysis. Sex Transm Infect 2019;95(5):328–35.
50. Xiao L, Waites KB, Van Der Pol B, et al. *Mycoplasma genitalium* infections with macrolide and fluoroquinolone resistance-associated mutations in heterosexual African American couples in Alabama. Sex Transm Dis 2019;46(1):18–24.
51. Slifirski JB, Vodstrcil LA, Fairley CK, et al. *Mycoplasma genitalium* infection in adults reporting sexual contact with infected partners, Australia, 2008-2016. Emerg Infect Dis 2017;23(11):1826–33.
52. Romano SS, Jensen JS, Lowens MS, et al. Long duration of asymptomatic *Mycoplasma genitalium* infection after syndromic treatment for nongonococcal urethritis. Clin Infect Dis 2018. https://doi.org/10.1093/cid/ciy843.
53. Ring A, Balakrishna S, Imkamp F, et al. High rates of asymptomatic *Mycoplasma genitalium* infections with high proportion of genotypic resistance to first-line

macrolide treatment among men who have sex with men enrolled in the Zurich Primary HIV Infection Study. Open Forum Infect Dis 2022;9(6):ofac217.

54. Cohen CR, Nosek M, Meier A, et al. *Mycoplasma genitalium* infection and persistence in a cohort of female sex workers in Nairobi, Kenya. Sex Transm Dis 2007;34(5):274–9.

55. Balkus JE, Manhart LE, Jensen JS, et al. *Mycoplasma genitalium* infection in Kenyan and US women. Sex Transm Dis 2018;45(8):514–21.

56. Vandepitte J, Weiss HA, Kyakuwa N, et al. Natural history of *Mycoplasma genitalium* infection in a cohort of female sex workers in Kampala, Uganda. Sex Transm Dis 2013;40(5):422–7.

57. Oakeshott P, Aghaizu A, Hay P, et al. Is *Mycoplasma genitalium* in women the "new chlamydia?" A community-based prospective cohort study. Clin Infect Dis 2010;51(10):1160–6.

58. Sena AC, Lee JY, Schwebke J, et al. A silent epidemic: the prevalence, incidence and persistence of *Mycoplasma genitalium* among young, asymptomatic high-risk women in the United States. Clin Infect Dis 2018;67(1):73–9.

59. Smieszek T, White PJ. Apparently-different clearance rates from cohort studies of *Mycoplasma genitalium* are consistent after accounting for incidence of infection, recurrent infection, and study design. PLoS One 2016;11(2):e0149087.

60. Taylor-Robinson D, Jensen JS. *Mycoplasma genitalium*: from Chrysalis to multicolored butterfly. Clin Microbiol Rev 2011;24(3):498–514.

61. Workowski KA, Bachmann LH, Chan PA, et al. Sexually transmitted infections treatment guidelines. MMWR Recomm reports Morb Mortal Wkly report Recomm reports 2021;70(4):1–187.

62. Bachmann LH, Kirkcaldy RD, Geisler WM, et al. Prevalence of *Mycoplasma genitalium* infection, antimicrobial resistance mutations and symptom resolution following treatment of urethritis. Clin Infect Dis 2020;71(10):e624–32.

63. Wetmore CM, Manhart LE, Lowens MS, et al. Demographic, behavioral, and clinical characteristics of men with nongonococcal urethritis differ by etiology: a case-comparison study. Sex Transm Dis 2011;38(3):180–6.

64. Peel J, Aung E, Bond S, et al. Recent advances in understanding and combatting *Mycoplasma genitalium*. Fac Rev 2020;9:3.

65. Read TRH, Murray GL, Danielewski JA, et al. Symptoms, sites, and significance of *Mycoplasma genitalium* in men who have sex with men. Emerg Infect Dis 2019;25(4):719–27.

66. Mahlangu MP, Muller EE, Venter JME, et al. The prevalence of *Mycoplasma genitalium* and association with human immunodeficiency virus infection in symptomatic patients, Johannesburg, South Africa, 2007-2014. Sex Transm Dis 2019;46(6):395–9.

67. Chow EPF, Lee D, Bond S, et al. Nonclassical pathogens as causative agents of proctitis in men who have sex with men. Open Forum Infect Dis 2021;8(7):ofab137.

68. Bissessor M, Tabrizi SN, Bradshaw CS, et al. The contribution of *Mycoplasma genitalium* to the aetiology of sexually acquired infectious proctitis in men who have sex with men. Clin Microbiol Infect 2016;22(3):260–5.

69. Ong JJ, Aung E, Read TRH, et al. Clinical characteristics of anorectal *Mycoplasma genitalium* infection and microbial cure in men who have sex with men. Sex Transm Dis 2018;45(8):522–6.

70. Latimer RL, Shilling HS, Vodstrcil LA, et al. Prevalence of *Mycoplasma genitalium* by anatomical site in men who have sex with men: a systematic review and meta-analysis. Sex Transm Infect 2020;96(8):563–70.

71. Jensen JS, Cusini M, Gomberg M, et al. 2021 European guideline on the management of *Mycoplasma genitalium* infections. J Eur Acad Dermatol Venereol 2022;36(5):641–50.
72. de Vries HJC, Nori AV, Kiellberg Larsen H, et al. 2021 European guideline on the management of proctitis, proctocolitis and enteritis caused by sexually transmissible pathogens. J Eur Acad Dermatology Venereol 2021;35(7):1434–43.
73. Moi H, Reinton N, Moghaddam A. *Mycoplasma genitalium* in women with lower genital tract inflammation. Sex Transm Infect 2009;85(1):10–4.
74. Högdahl M, Kihlström E. Leucocyte esterase testing of first-voided urine and urethral and cervical smears to identify *Mycoplasma genitalium*-infected men and women. Int J STD AIDS 2007;18(12):835–8.
75. Anagrius C, Loré B, Jensen JS. *Mycoplasma genitalium*: prevalence, clinical significance, and transmission. Sex Transm Infect 2005;81(6):458–62.
76. Olson E, Gupta K, Van Der Pol B, et al. *Mycoplasma genitalium* infection in women reporting dysuria: a pilot study and review of the literature. Int J STD AIDS 2021;32(13):1196–203.
77. Latimer RL, Vodstrcil LA, Plummer EL, et al. The clinical indications for testing women for *Mycoplasma genitalium*. Sex Transm Infect 2022;98(4):277–85.
78. Wiesenfeld HC, Manhart LE. *Mycoplasma genitalium* in women: current knowledge and research priorities for this recently emerged pathogen. J Infect Dis 2017;216(suppl_2):S389–95.
79. Lis R, Rowhani-Rahbar A, Manhart LE. *Mycoplasma genitalium* infection and female reproductive tract disease: a meta-analysis. Clin Infect Dis 2015;61(3):418–26.
80. Dehon PM, Hagensee ME, Sutton KJ, et al. Histological evidence of chronic *Mycoplasma genitalium*-induced cervicitis in HIV-infected women: a retrospective cohort study. J Infect Dis 2016;213(11):1828–35.
81. Moller BR, Taylor-Robinson D, Furr PM. Serological evidence implicating *Mycoplasma genitalium* in pelvic inflammatory disease. Lancet (London, England) 1984;1(8386):1102–3.
82. Mitchell CM, Anyalechi GE, Cohen CR, et al. Etiology and diagnosis of pelvic inflammatory disease: looking beyond gonorrhea and *Chlamydia*. J Infect Dis 2021;224(12 Suppl 2):S29–35.
83. Lewis J, Horner PJ, White PJ. Incidence of pelvic inflammatory disease associated with *Mycoplasma genitalium* infection: evidence synthesis of cohort study data. Clin Infect Dis 2020;71(10):2719–22.
84. Bjartling C, Osser S, Persson K. *Mycoplasma genitalium* in cervicitis and pelvic inflammatory disease among women at a gynecologic outpatient service. Am J Obstet Gynecol 2012;206(6):476.e1–8.
85. Dean G, Soni S, Pitt R, et al. Treatment of mild-to-moderate pelvic inflammatory disease with a short-course azithromycin-based regimen versus ofloxacin plus metronidazole: results of a multicentre, randomised controlled trial. Sex Transm Infect 2021;97(3):177–82.
86. Latimer RL, Read TRH, Vodstrcil LA, et al. Clinical features and therapeutic response in women meeting criteria for presumptive treatment for pelvic inflammatory disease associated with *Mycoplasma genitalium*. Sex Transm Dis 2019;46(2):73–9.
87. Towns JM, Williamson DA, Bradshaw CS. Case of *Mycoplasma genitalium* pelvic inflammatory disease with perihepatitis. Sex Transm Infect 2021;97(8):628.
88. Han T, Nolan SM, Regard M. *Mycoplasma genitalium* as a cause of pelvic inflammatory disease. J Pediatr Adolesc Gynecol 2020;33(6):739–41.

89. Haggerty CL, Totten PA, Astete SG, et al. Failure of cefoxitin and doxycycline to eradicate endometrial *Mycoplasma genitalium* and the consequence for clinical cure of pelvic inflammatory disease. Sex Transm Infect 2008;84(5):338–42.

90. Trent M, Yusuf HE, Perin J, et al. Clearance of *Mycoplasma genitalium* and *Trichomonas vaginalis* among adolescents and young adults with pelvic inflammatory disease: results from the Tech-N study. Sex Transm Dis 2020;47(11): e47–50.

91. Bjartling C, Osser S, Persson K. The association between *Mycoplasma genitalium* and pelvic inflammatory disease after termination of pregnancy. BJOG 2010;117(3):361–4.

92. Taylor BD, Zheng X, O'Connell CM, et al. Risk factors for *Mycoplasma genitalium* endometritis and incident infection: a secondary data analysis of the T cell Response Against Chlamydia (TRAC) Study. Sex Transm Infect 2018;94(6): 414–20.

93. Svenstrup HF, Fedder J, Kristoffersen SE, et al. *Mycoplasma genitalium*, *Chlamydia trachomatis*, and tubal factor infertility: a prospective study. Fertil Steril 2008;90(3):513–20.

94. Ma C, Du J, Dou Y, et al. The associations of genital mycoplasmas with female infertility and adverse pregnancy outcomes: a systematic review and meta-analysis. Reprod Sci 2021;28(11):3013–31.

95. Idahl A, Le Cornet C, González Maldonado S, et al. Serologic markers of *Chlamydia trachomatis* and other sexually transmitted infections and subsequent ovarian cancer risk: results from the EPIC cohort. Int J Cancer 2020;147(8): 2042–52.

96. Peipert JF, Zhao Q, Schreiber CA, et al. Intrauterine device use, sexually transmitted infections, and fertility: a prospective cohort study. Am J Obstet Gynecol 2021;225(2):157.e1–9.

97. Ashshi AM, Batwa SA, Kutbi SY, et al. Prevalence of 7 sexually transmitted organisms by multiplex real-time PCR in Fallopian tube specimens collected from Saudi women with and without ectopic pregnancy. BMC Infect Dis 2015; 15:569.

98. Refaat B, Ashshi AM, Batwa SA, et al. The prevalence of *Chlamydia trachomatis* and *Mycoplasma genitalium* tubal infections and their effects on the expression of IL-6 and leukaemia inhibitory factor in Fallopian tubes with and without an ectopic pregnancy. Innate Immun 2016;22(7):534–45.

99. Jurstrand M, Jensen JS, Magnuson A, et al. A serological study of the role of *Mycoplasma genitalium* in pelvic inflammatory disease and ectopic pregnancy. Sex Transm Infect 2007;83(4):319–23.

100. Frenzer C, Egli-Gany D, Vallely LM, et al. Adverse pregnancy and perinatal outcomes associated with *Mycoplasma genitalium*: systematic review and meta-analysis. Sex Transm Infect 2022;98(3):222–7.

101. Khosropour CM, Jensen JS, Soge OO, et al. High prevalence of vaginal and rectal *Mycoplasma genitalium* macrolide resistance among female sexually transmitted disease clinic patients in Seattle, Washington. Sex Transm Dis 2020;47(5):321–5.

102. Lillis RA, Nsuami MJ, Myers L, et al. Utility of urine, vaginal, cervical, and rectal specimens for detection of *Mycoplasma genitalium* in women. J Clin Microbiol 2011;49(5):1990–2.

103. Cosentino LA, Campbell T, Jett A, et al. Use of nucleic acid amplification testing for diagnosis of anorectal sexually transmitted infections. J Clin Microbiol 2012; 50(6):2005–8.

104. Hay B, Dubbink JH, Ouburg S, et al. Prevalence and macrolide resistance of *Mycoplasma genitalium* in South African women. Sex Transm Dis 2015;42(3): 140–2.
105. Dicker LW, Mosure DJ, Berman SM, et al. Gonorrhea prevalence and coinfection with chlamydia in women in the United States, 2000. Sex Transm Dis 2003;30(5): 472–6.
106. Srinivasan S, Chambers LC, Tapia KA, et al. Urethral microbiota in men: association of *Haemophilus influenzae* and *Mycoplasma penetrans* with nongonococcal urethritis. Clin Infect Dis 2021;73(7):e1684–93.
107. Latimer RL, Vodstrcil L, De Petra V, et al. Extragenital *Mycoplasma genitalium* infections among men who have sex with men. Sex Transm Infect 2020; 96(1):10–8.
108. Balkus JE, Manhart LE, Lee J, et al. Periodic presumptive treatment for vaginal infections may reduce the incidence of sexually transmitted bacterial infections. J Infect Dis 2016;213(12):1932–7.
109. Hillier SL, Bernstein KT, Aral S. A review of the challenges and complexities in the diagnosis, etiology, epidemiology, and pathogenesis of pelvic inflammatory disease. J Infect Dis 2021;224(12 Suppl 2):S23–8.
110. Lokken EM, Balkus JE, Kiarie J, et al. Association of recent bacterial vaginosis with acquisition of *Mycoplasma genitalium*. Am J Epidemiol 2017;186(2): 194–201.
111. Shipitsyna E, Khusnutdinova T, Budilovskaya O, et al. Bacterial vaginosis-associated vaginal microbiota is an age-independent risk factor for *Chlamydia trachomatis*, *Mycoplasma genitalium* and *Trichomonas vaginalis* infections in low-risk women, St. Petersburg, Russia. Eur J Clin Microbiol Infect Dis 2020; 39(7):1221–30.
112. Wiesenfeld HC, Meyn LA, Darville T, et al. A randomized controlled trial of ceftriaxone and doxycycline, with or without metronidazole, for the treatment of acute pelvic inflammatory disease. Clin Infect Dis 2021;72(7):1181–9.
113. Napierala Mavedzenge S, Weiss HA. Association of *Mycoplasma genitalium* and HIV infection: a systematic review and meta-analysis. AIDS 2009;23(5): 611–20.
114. Zhao N, Li KT, Gao Y-Y, et al. *Mycoplasma genitalium* and *Mycoplasma hominis* are prevalent and correlated with HIV risk in MSM: a cross-sectional study in Shenyang, China. BMC Infect Dis 2019;19(1):494.
115. Barker EK, Malekinejad M, Merai R, et al. Risk of human immunodeficiency virus acquisition among high-risk heterosexuals with nonviral sexually transmitted infections: a systematic review and meta-analysis. Sex Transm Dis 2022;49(6): 383–97.
116. Manhart LE, Mostad SB, Baeten JM, et al. High *Mycoplasma genitalium* organism burden is associated with shedding of HIV-1 DNA from the cervix. J Infect Dis 2008;197(5):733–6.
117. Gatski M, Martin DH, Theall K, et al. *Mycoplasma genitalium* infection among HIV-positive women: prevalence, risk factors and association with vaginal shedding. Int J STD AIDS 2011;22(3):155–9.
118. Mavedzenge SN, Van Der Pol B, Weiss HA, et al. The association between *Mycoplasma genitalium* and HIV-1 acquisition in African women. AIDS 2012;26(5): 617–24.
119. Deguchi T, Yasuda M, Horie K, et al. Drug resistance-associated mutations in *Mycoplasma genitalium* in female sex workers, Japan. Emerg Infect Dis 2015; 21(6):1062–4.

120. Deguchi T, Yasuda M, Yokoi S, et al. Failure to detect *Mycoplasma genitalium* in the pharynges of female sex workers in Japan. J Infect Chemother 2009;15(6): 410–3.

121. Chrisment D, Machelart I, Wirth G, et al. Reactive arthritis associated with *Mycoplasma genitalium* urethritis. Diagn Microbiol Infect Dis 2013;77(3):278–9.

122. Taylor-Robinson D, Gilroy CB, Horowitz S, et al. *Mycoplasma genitalium* in the joints of two patients with arthritis. Eur J Clin Microbiol Infect Dis 1994;13(12): 1066–9.

123. Tully JG, Rose DL, Baseman JB, et al. *Mycoplasma pneumoniae* and *Mycoplasma genitalium* mixture in synovial fluid isolate. J Clin Microbiol 1995;33(7): 1851–5.

124. Chu K-A, Chen W, Hsu CY, et al. Increased risk of rheumatoid arthritis among patients with *Mycoplasma pneumonia*: a nationwide population-based cohort study in Taiwan. PLoS One 2019;14(1):e0210750.

125. Asif AA, Roy M, Ahmad S. Rare case of *Ureaplasma parvum* septic arthritis in an immunocompetent patient. BMJ Case Rep 2020;13(9). https://doi.org/10.1136/bcr-2020-236396.

126. Horner PJ, Taylor-Robinson D. Association of *Mycoplasma genitalium* with balanoposthitis in men with non-gonococcal urethritis. Sex Transm Infect 2011; 87(1):38–40.

127. Björnelius E, Jensen JS, Lidbrink P. Conjunctivitis associated with *Mycoplasma genitalium* infection. Clin Infect Dis 2004;39(7):e67–9.

128. Jensen JS, Cusini M, Gomberg M, et al. European guideline on *Mycoplasma genitalium* infections. J Eur Acad Dermatol Venereol 2016;30(10):1650–6.

129. Salado-Rasmussen K, Tolstrup J, Sedeh FB, et al. Clinical importance of superior sensitivity of the Aptima TMA-based assays for *Mycoplasma genitalium* detection. J Clin Microbiol 2022;60(4):e0236921.

130. Vodstrcil LA, Plummer EL, Doyle M, et al. Combination therapy for *Mycoplasma genitalium*, and new insights into the utility of *parC* mutant detection to improve cure. Clin Infect Dis 2022;75(5):813–23.

131. Murray GL, Bradshaw CS, Bissessor M, et al. Increasing macrolide and fluoroquinolone resistance in *Mycoplasma genitalium*. Emerg Infect Dis 2017;23(5): 809–12.

132. Murray GL, Bodiyabadu K, Danielewski J, et al. Moxifloxacin and sitafloxacin treatment failure in *Mycoplasma genitalium* infection: association with parC mutation G248T (S83I) and concurrent gyrA mutations. J Infect Dis 2020;221(6): 1017–24.

133. Murray GL, Bodiyabadu K, Vodstrcil LA, et al. *parC* variants in *Mycoplasma genitalium*: trends over time and association with moxifloxacin failure. Antimicrob Agents Chemother 2022;66(5):e0027822.

134. Hamasuna R, Le PT, Kutsuna S, et al. Mutations in ParC and GyrA of moxifloxacin-resistant and susceptible *Mycoplasma genitalium* strains. PLoS One 2018;13(6):e0198355.

135. Wood GE, Jensen NL, Astete S, et al. Azithromycin and doxycycline resistance profiles of US *Mycoplasma genitalium* strains and their association with treatment outcomes. J Clin Microbiol 2021;JCM0081921. https://doi.org/10.1128/JCM.00819-2.

136. Waites KB, Crabb DM, Atkinson TP, et al. Omadacycline is highly active in vitro against *Mycoplasma genitalium*. Microbiol Spectr 2022;e0365422. https://doi.org/10.1128/spectrum.03654-22.

137. Pitt R, Boampong D, Day M, et al. Challenges of in vitro propagation and anti-microbial susceptibility testing of *Mycoplasma genitalium*. J Antimicrob Chemother 2022;77(11):2901–7.
138. Jensen JS, Bradshaw C. Management of *Mycoplasma genitalium* infections: can we hit a moving target? BMC Infect Dis 2015;15:343.
139. Machalek DA, Tao Y, Shilling H, et al. Prevalence of mutations associated with resistance to macrolides and fluoroquinolones in *Mycoplasma genitalium*: a systematic review and meta-analysis. Lancet Infect Dis 2020;20(11):1302–14.
140. Parmar NR, Mushanski L, Wanlin T, et al. High prevalence of macrolide and fluoroquinolone resistance-mediating mutations in *Mycoplasma genitalium*-positive urine specimens from Saskatchewan. Sex Transm Dis 2021;48(9):680–4.
141. McIver R, Jalocon D, McNulty A, et al. Men who have sex with men with *Mycoplasma genitalium*-positive nongonococcal urethritis are more likely to have macrolide-resistant strains than men with only female partners: a prospective study. Sex Transm Dis 2019;46(8):513–7.
142. Li Y, Su X, Le W, et al. *Mycoplasma genitalium* in symptomatic male urethritis: macrolide use is associated with increased resistance. Clin Infect Dis 2020; 70(5):805–10.
143. Dionne-Odom J, Geisler WM, Aaron KJ, et al. High prevalence of multidrug-resistant *Mycoplasma genitalium* in human immunodeficiency virus-infected men who have sex with men in Alabama. Clin Infect Dis 2018;66(5):796–8.
144. Durukan D, Doyle M, Murray G, et al. Doxycycline and sitafloxacin combination therapy for treating highly resistant *Mycoplasma genitalium*. Emerg Infect Dis 2020;26(8):1870–4.
145. Read TRH, Fairley CK, Murray GL, et al. Outcomes of resistance-guided sequential treatment of *Mycoplasma genitalium* infections: a prospective evaluation. Clin Infect Dis 2019;68(4):554–60.
146. Peyriere H, Makinson A, Marchandin H, et al. Doxycycline in the management of sexually transmitted infections. J Antimicrob Chemother 2018;73(3):553–63.
147. Gossé M, Nordbø SA, Pukstad B. Evaluation of treatment with two weeks of doxycycline on macrolide-resistant strains of *Mycoplasma genitalium*: a retrospective observational study. BMC Infect Dis 2021;21(1):1225.
148. Molina J-M, Charreau I, Chidiac C, et al. Post-exposure prophylaxis with doxycycline to prevent sexually transmitted infections in men who have sex with men: an open-label randomised substudy of the ANRS IPERGAY trial. Lancet Infect Dis 2018;18(3):308–17.
149. Luetkemeyer A, Dombrowski J, Cohen S, et al. Doxycycline post-exposure prophylaxis for STI prevention among MSM and transgender women on HIV PrEP or living with HIV: high efficacy to reduce incident STI's in a randomized trial. In: The 24th international AIDS Conference. Montreal, Canada; 2022:Abstr 13231.
150. Berçot B, Charreau I, Rousseau C, et al. High prevalence and high rate of antibiotic resistance of *Mycoplasma genitalium* infections in men who have sex with men: a substudy of the ANRS IPERGAY pre-exposure prophylaxis trial. Clin Infect Dis 2021;73(7):e2127–33.
151. Chua T-P, Danielewski J, Bodiyabadu K, et al. Impact of 16S rRNA single nucleotide polymorphisms on *Mycoplasma genitalium* organism load with doxycycline treatment. Antimicrob Agents Chemother 2022;66(5):e0024322.
152. Le Roy C, Touati A, Balcon C, et al. Identification of 16S rRNA mutations in *Mycoplasma genitalium* potentially associated with tetracycline resistance in vivo but not selected in vitro in *M. genitalium* and *Chlamydia trachomatis*. J Antimicrob Chemother 2021. https://doi.org/10.1093/jac/dkab016.

153. Getman D, Cohen S, Jiang A. Distribution of macrolide resistant *Mycoplasma genitalium* in urogenital tract specimens from women enrolled in a US clinical study cohort. Clin Infect Dis 2022. https://doi.org/10.1093/cid/ciac602.
154. Gadeau AP, Mouches C, Bove JM. Probable insensitivity of mollicutes to rifampin and characterization of spiroplasmal DNA-dependent RNA polymerase. J Bacteriol 1986;166(3):824–8. https://doi.org/10.1093/cid/ciac602.
155. Renaudin H, Tully JG, Bebear C. In vitro susceptibilities of *Mycoplasma genitalium* to antibiotics. Antimicrob Agents Chemother 1992;36(4):870–2.
156. Falk L, Jensen JS. Successful outcome of macrolide-resistant *Mycoplasma genitalium* urethritis after spectinomycin treatment: a case report. J Antimicrob Chemother 2017;72(2):624–5.
157. Doyle M, Vodstrcil LA, Plummer EL, et al. Nonquinolone options for the treatment of *Mycoplasma genitalium* in the era of increased resistance. Open Forum Infect Dis 2020;7(8):ofaa291.
158. Damião Gouveia AC, Unemo M, Jensen JS. In vitro activity of zoliflodacin (ETX0914) against macrolide-resistant, fluoroquinolone-resistant and antimicrobial-susceptible *Mycoplasma genitalium* strains. J Antimicrob Chemother 2018;73(5):1291–4.
159. Paukner S, Gruss A, Jensen JS. In vitro activity of lefamulin against sexually transmitted bacterial pathogens. Antimicrob Agents Chemother 2018;62(5). https://doi.org/10.1128/AAC.02380-17.
160. Read TRH, Jensen JS, Fairley CK, et al. Use of pristinamycin for macrolide-resistant *Mycoplasma genitalium* infection. Emerg Infect Dis 2018;24(2):328–35.
161. Takahashi S, Hamasuna R, Yasuda M, et al. Clinical efficacy of sitafloxacin 100 mg twice daily for 7 days for patients with non-gonococcal urethritis. J Infect Chemother Off J Japan Soc Chemother 2013;19(5):941–5.
162. Hook EW 3rd, Golden M, Jamieson BD, et al. A phase 2 trial of oral solithromycin 1200 mg or 1000 mg as single-dose oral therapy for uncomplicated gonorrhea. Clin Infect Dis 2015;61(7):1043–8.
163. Jensen JS, Nørgaard C, Scangarella-Oman N, et al. In vitro activity of the first-in-class triazaacenaphthylene gepotidacin alone and in combination with doxycycline against drug-resistant and -susceptible *Mycoplasma genitalium*. Emerg Microbes Infect 2020;9(1):1388–92.

Sexual Transmission of Viral Hepatitis

Audrey R. Lloyd, MD[a], Ricardo A. Franco, MD[b],*

KEYWORDS

- Hepatitis A • Hepatitis B • Hepatitis C • Hepatitis D • Sexual transmission
- Prevention • Viral hepatitis elimination

KEY POINTS

- Major breakthroughs mark the historic scientific advances in viral hepatitis.
- Sexual transmission of viral hepatitis has been recognized since the modern era of viral hepatitis scientific discoveries.
- While widely recognized in hepatitis B, sexual transmision of hepatitis A and C is endemic in at risk groups and pose challenges to disease control.
- Expanded vaccinations and use of curative therapies in vulnerable populations are key to viral hepatitis control and elimination.

INTRODUCTION

Hepatitis, from the Greek root "hepar" (liver) and suffix "itis" (inflammation), has been a major plague to mankind.[1] In descriptions of jaundice on clay tablets 5,000 years ago—and seemingly tied to stigma then—Sumerians believed that patients with the skin-yellowing condition had their livers—the home of the soul—victimized by the devil Ahhazu.[2] When reporting on epidemic jaundice and fulminant cases, Hippocrates (460–375 BC) shared visionary elaboration that "jaundice appears when the bile enters into motion and is worn under the skin," suddenly sweeping away divine origin beliefs.[1] Although Greeks and Romans observed epidemic jaundice, divine malediction remained to blame during the middle age, believed to affect people who were "impure" who needed to be "isolated."

Ensuing wars in early modern times sparked many outbreaks of epidemic jaundice, confirming the notion of contagion and transmissibility. Indeed, during the American Civil War more than 70,000 Union troops were disabled by the disease, and countless

---

[a] Division of Infectious Diseases, Department of Medicine and Pediatrics, University of Alabama at Birmingham Heersink School of Medicine, Children's Harbor Building, 1600 7th Avenue South, Room 308, Birmingham, AL 35223, USA; [b] Division of Infectious Diseases, Department of Medicine, University of Alabama at Birmingham Heersink School of Medicine, 1917 Clinic Dewberry, 3220 5th Avenue South, Room 1044A, Birmingham, AL 35222, USA
* Corresponding author.
E-mail address: rfranco@uabmc.edu

Infect Dis Clin N Am 37 (2023) 335–349
https://doi.org/10.1016/j.idc.2023.02.010
0891-5520/23/© 2023 Elsevier Inc. All rights reserved.

soldiers were afflicted by the 2 World Wars.[1] In addition to epidemic jaundice, several reports from the late nineteenth and early twentieth centuries also linked hepatitis clusters to vaccination, blood drawing, and parenteral treatment of syphilitic and diabetic patients with contaminated needles.[3] By midcentury, there was a clear differentiation of 2 forms of hepatitis. The epidemic form, or hepatitis A (HA, the long-known epidemic jaundice), transmitted by contaminated water and food usually lasted 1 to 2 months and had a very low mortality. The sporadic form, or hepatitis B (HB, also called serum hepatitis), is disseminated by transfusions with infected blood, contaminated syringes, and intimate sexual contact, especially among men who have sex with men (MSM). The latter had a more protracted course and, in many cases, ended after many years in cirrhosis and hepatic insufficiency,[4] and this strongly suggested that the 2 conditions were likely to result from different etiologic agents, as shown by the modern era of hepatitis research.[5]

In the 2000 years since Hippocrates coined the term *ikterus*, no single event has been more pivotal to the understanding and prevention of viral hepatitis than the discovery of the "Australia antigen" by Blumberg in 1967.[6] From the outset, reports of cases in which Australia antigen–positive hepatitis was transmitted from male patients to their intimate female contacts by a nonparenteral route implied that the disease may be sexually transmitted.[7] Similarly, several other of epidemiological studies linked acute Australia antigen-positive hepatitis to sexual contacts, history of other sexually transmitted infections (STIs), same gender sex among men, and non-European immigrants.[8] The hypothesis that the virus could be transmitted by menstrual blood[9] and the demonstration of Australia antigen in the semen of 10 of 19 antigenemic men tested further indicated that hepatitis could, in some cases, be a disease truly transmitted through sex.[10] It had also become clear at the time that both Australia antigen–negative and Australia antigen–positive hepatitis could transmit both parenterally and by nonparenteral person-to-person contact—the latter occurring primarily by the fecal-oral route with hepatitis A and sexual transmission being one of the possible acquisition routes of transmission of hepatitis B.[11]

In the ensuing decades, evidence established sex as being one of the routes of transmission for hepatitis types A, C, and D as well. Although hepatitis G, GB, and TT may also transmit sexually, these organisms are not known to cause human disease. Similarly, there has been no evidence that hepatitis E is sexually transmitted.[12] In this article, the authors further elaborate their understanding and recent developments of sexually transmitted forms of viral hepatitis of clinical importance.

HEPATITIS A

Hepatitis A virus (HAV) is a member of the Picornaviridae family and is a small single-stranded nonenveloped, RNA virus transmitted mainly through the fecal oral route, as well as by close personal contact. The highest concentration of infectious particles is present in stool 2 weeks before clinical illness or jaundice appears, supporting asymptomatic transmission.[13] Coinfection with human immunodeficiency virus (HIV) may prolong HAV viremia, possibly prolonging viral shedding.[14] Worldwide, especially in areas of poor access to sanitation and clean drinking water, infection is almost universal among young children, with estimated 46.9 million cases in 2010.[15] In countries with high endemicity, greater than 90% of adults and greater than 80% of older children may show evidence of past infection in seroprevalence studies.[16] In the 90s, improving levels of sanitation in many countries have led to a decrease in childhood HAV infection with a concomitant increase in adults susceptible to symptomatic disease and outbreaks.[17] In the United States, outbreaks occur through ingestion of contaminated food as the one linked to contaminated strawberries in 2022[18] and through contact in group living homes.[19] HAV can also survive in the environment outside of the body for months allowing for transmission via contaminated fomites.[20] Parenteral spread can also occur in injecting drug users (IDUs), hemophiliacs using contaminated factor VIII, and other recipients of blood products.[21] In most cases, HAV infection leads to mild illness in children and self-limited gastrointestinal illness in adults. However, HAV can precipitate fulminant liver failure, especially in older adults or those with preexisting liver injury. In outbreaks by the opioid epidemic in the United States, acute hepatitis A accounted for 179 deaths in 2020.[22] The presence of serum immunoglobulin G antibodies against HAV (anti-HAV) indicates immunity from infection or vaccination.

Sexual Transmission

Most of the MSM do not seem to be at increased risk of sexual transmission, nor is there evidence for heterosexual spread of HAV.[23] Nevertheless, detailed diaries of sexual behavior in a prospective cohort of MSM in the early 80s linked incident HAV infection with frequent oral-anal contact.[24] Reports of HAV outbreaks started to emerge in the 90s among MSM in large cities including Melbourne, New York, London, Amsterdam, and Tokyo. Infection was linked with visits to saunas and darkrooms, sex with anonymous partners, group sex, oroanal and digital-rectal intercourse, and number of partners.[25,26] Subsequent molecular epidemiological studies documented the circulation of specific HAV strains within populations of MSM. Genotype clustering occurred within MSM networks, whereas distinct genotypes occurred among simultaneous cases linked to children returning from HAV-endemic countries and their contacts.[27] Transmission among travelers was sporadic, with a seasonal pattern associated with the summer holidays. The MSM clusters were larger and persisted over longer periods, suggesting ongoing endemic spread within the local MSM community.[28] A collaborative study in Denmark, Germany, the Netherlands, Norway, Spain, and the United Kingdom detected closely related and longitudinally stable HAV strain clustering among MSM in isolates collected from 1997 to 2005.[29] It seemed that specific strains circulated exclusively among MSM over long periods and across a wide geographic region, suggesting endemic HAV transmission as well.

Recent Epidemiological Trends

In 2016, a large uptick in HAV cases emerged in the United States, with 294% more infections reported from 2016 to 2018 compared with 2013 to 2015, especially among unhoused and incarcerated persons and people who inject drugs (PWID),[30] including 260 reported cases among MSM from 8 states in the period 2017 to 2018.[31] In 133 cases with molecular typing available, genotype IA identified in 95% of cases and IB in 5%. Among 126 genotype IA sequences, 43% were genetically identical to 1 of 3 strains associated with the 2016–2018 HAV outbreaks among MSM in the European Union (RIVM-HAV16–090; VRD_521_2016; and V16–25801).[31,32] The other 44% were identified as strains that were known to be circulating among MSM in the United States during this time period. In response to the large increase in HAV cases in the United States, the Centers for Disease Contol and Prevention (CDC) has instituted the Global Hepatitis Outbreak and Surveillance Technology (GHOST) system in 2017. It has been noted since a shifting emergence of genotype IB as the majority strain during another large person-to-person multistate outbreak.[33] This ongoing outbreak have accrued 11,920 total reported cases, 7,254 hospitalizations (61%), and 82 deaths in 37 states.[34]

Likewise CDC, the European Centre for Disease Prevention and Control tracked a large HAV outbreak from 2016 to 2018, affecting a disproportionate number of MSM, with 4475 confirmed cases across 22 European countries. Circulating strains were found to be specific to MSM and had 99.3% sequence homology to one of the known 3 HAV genotype IA outbreak strains (VRD_521_2016; RIVM-HAV16–090; and V16–25801).[32] Investigators also noted a drastically different male to female ratio (M:F) in cases involving the outbreak strains. In May 2017, the M:F ratio was noted to be as high as 11.8 as compared with an M:F of 4.8 among all HAV cases reported between March and May, 2017. Comparatively, outbreaks in 16 European countries before the 2016 outbreak (2012–2016) had an average M:F of 1.0:1.7.[35] When evaluated in 2018, 92% of outbreak confirmed cases were among unvaccinated men.[35] As an illustrative example, in an outbreak in Milan, Italy during the same time, 48.7% of affected people self-identified as MSM.[36] Most of them (93.7%) shared high nucleotide identity with 1 of the 3 viral epidemic strains linked to the European HAV outbreak.[32] Notably, only 3.4% of people involved in the Milan outbreak were vaccinated against HAV.[36] HAV outbreaks associated with European strains were also described in Asia and South America specifically among MSM, further underscoring the potential reach of sexual transmission in hepatitis A.[37–39]

Prevention

The hepatitis A (Hep A) vaccine is safe and highly efficacious, providing long-lasting protection.[40] Hep A vaccination has been recommended for PWID and MSM by the Advisory Committee on Immunization Practices (ACIP) since 1996.[41] With the introduction of routine childhood Hep A vaccination in 2006, the overall rates of susceptibility to HAV infection (no anti-HAV) have continued to decrease for most of the population.[42] During outbreaks, administering a single dose of Hep A vaccine to high-risk groups is highly effective in controlling outbreaks.[43] Despite high effectiveness, vaccination rates among high-risk groups remains low. The National Health and Nutrition Examination Survey (years 2007–2016) found high rates of HAV susceptibility and low rates of Hep A vaccination among PWID (72.9% and only 18.9%, respectively). Rates of vaccination were better among MSM but still at 34.8%, far less than the estimated threshold for preventing sustained epidemics (70% anti-HAV positivity in the population).[44] Predictors of susceptibility to HAV and no history of Hep A vaccination included being aged 30 to 49 years, being non-Hispanic white or black, having low income, and having no health insurance.[42] US insurance claims analysis shows that, even when Hep A vaccination is initiated, only 27% of patients complete vaccination series.[45] Although a single dose of Hep A vaccine has been shown to offer protective anti-HAV levels persisting up to 11 years in most people, HIV coinfection, especially in men and those with low CD4 lymphocyte counts, may decrease Hep A vaccination efficacy, lending importance to completing a full vaccine schedule in this population.[46] Increased vaccination and outreach to at-risk groups is needed to further prevent HAV outbreaks and morbidity. Potential areas for improvement include administration of Hep A vaccine during routine visits for HIV preexposure prophylaxis (PrEP),[47] at Emergency Department encounters,[48] or during visits to harm reduction settings such as syringe service programs.

HEPATITIS B

The hepatitis B virus (HBV) is a small partially double-stranded DNA virus with a circular genome.[49] Acute HBV infection is a subclinical illness in around two-thirds of healthy adults and leads to chronic HBV infection in 1% to 5% of cases.[50] Although the HBV is not directly cytotoxic to hepatocytes, the ensuing immune response can lead to the development of hepatocellular carcinoma, fibrosis, cirrhosis, and eventual liver failure in people with chronic hepatitis B (CHB).[51] CHB is defined as the persistence of hepatitis B surface antigen (HBsAg) and is the cause of extensive disease burden worldwide, with an estimated 290 million people living with chronic infection.[52] In the United States, HBV infections remained responsible for 1752 deaths at a rate of 0.45 per 100,000 cases in 2020.[53] Although rates of chronic HBV infection have decreased significantly, the incidence of acute HBV infections has remained stubbornly stable from 2013 to 2019.[54] Of note, a 32% decrease in reported acute HBV infections was seen in 2020; however, it remains to be seen if this was a true sustainable decline or an artifact of decreased screening, decreased health care contact, and increased isolation seen during the COVID-19 epidemic.[54]

Sexual Transmission

HBV is efficiently transmitted via sexual contact. HBsAg or HBV DNA has been detected in body fluids and mucosal surfaces including semen, menstrual blood/vaginal discharge, saliva, feces, anal canal, rectal mucosa, and rectal mucosal lesions.[25] In endemic regions, most of the HBV transmission is through mother to child at birth (vertical transmission) or from infected to uninfected children before the age of 5 years. Widespread pediatric vaccination and the use of hepatitis B immunoglobulin have made vertical transmission a rare occurrence in the United States (only 10 reported cases from 2005 to 2020).[54] Multiple studies have reported high levels of past or present HBV infection among groups believed to be at higher risk via sexual exposure, including persons attending STI clinics, commercial sex workers, and MSM.[25] Sexual transmission continues to play a major role in incidental HBV in the United States, accounting for 32% of acute HBV infections from 2013 to 2018.[55] The CDC has estimated 103,000 prevalent sexually transmitted HBV infections in those aged 15 years and older in 2018.[56]

People living with HIV (PLHIV) are approximately 1.4 times more likely than people without HIV to be HBsAg-positive. Globally, the prevalence of coinfection is around 7.6% among PLHIV but may range as high as 69% (in sub-Saharan Africa), depending on the region and population.[57] As HIV is around 100 times less infectious compared with HBV sexually, and is transmitted through many of the same pathways, diagnosis of either infection should prompt evaluation for the other and preventative measures— HIV pre-exposure prophylaxis (PrEP) and/or Hep B vaccination.[58] In pregnant women living with HIV, timely identification of HBV and selection of tenofovir-based antiretroviral regimen may reduce vertical transmission of HBV as well as HIV.

Prevention

In 1982 the CDC recommended vaccination of at-risk individuals based on results of a surface Ag recombinant vaccine trial (**Box 1**).[59] Current recombinant HBV vaccines offer safe and effective protection against HBV infection. A hepatitis B surface antibody response of 10 mIU/mL or greater is considered protective and is achieved in greater than 90% of healthy recipients after a 3-dose series.[60] Protection from hepatitis B vaccines is long-lasting. Vaccination with the Heptavax plasma–derived HBV vaccine on a 0-, 1-, and 6-month schedule showed protective immunity 35 years after the initial series without need for a booster.[61] Multiple studies have demonstrated childhood vaccination at birth, age 1 month, and age 6 months with recombinant Hep B vaccine delivers reliable protection to 98% of children that lasts well into adolescence.[62] Previous vaccination recommendations contemplated adults who met certain risk-based criteria such as MSM, injection drug use, and health care workers. However, uptake was sub-par and per the 2018 National Health Interview Survey, only 40.3% for adults aged 19 to 49 years had Hep B vaccination coverage

---

Box 1
1982 centers for disease control and prevention definition of high-risk individuals

- Health care providers, clients, and staff at institutions for the developmentally disabled
- Hemodialysis patients
- MSM
- PWID
- Recipients of clotting factors for bleeding disorders
- Household and sexual contacts of a person with CHB infection
- Populations with high rates of HBV infection (Alaska Natives, Pacific Islanders, and immigrants and refugees from countries in which HBV is endemic)
- Inmates of long-term correctional facilities

Data from Centers for Disease Control and Prevention. Achievements in Public Health: Hepatitis B Vaccination–United States, 1982–2002. MMWR Morbidity and mortality weekly report. 2002;51(25):549-552, 563.

(>3 doses).[63] Assessing for risk factors has proved a strain on providers, with 68% reporting that patients would not disclose high-risk behaviors and nearly 45% endorsing they did not have time to routinely assess patients for risk factors.[64] Such evidence prompted the ACIP to change their recommendations from risk-based to universal vaccination for all people aged 19 to 51 years in March 2022.[65] The goal is to incentivize vaccination and screening for HBV infection by removing often stigmatizing and uncomfortable risk-based screening questions and promote the still-evolving physician awareness and vaccination uptake in target populations. An August 2022 survey found that only 50% of family physicians were aware of the new guidelines and only 8% had implemented these guidelines in their office.[66] Low rates of hepatitis B vaccination completion is enhanced by provider awareness gaps.[45] Such findings hold public health importance given the disproportionate burden of acute HBV infection among non-Hispanic Black people and Appalachia communities and high rates of chronic HBV infection among Asian/Pacific Islander persons (17.6 cases per 100,000 people), almost 12 times the rates among non-Hispanic Whites.[54]

HEPATITIS C

Hepatitis C virus (HCV) is a common blood-borne infection worldwide, with a prevalence estimated as 2.3 million adults living with the disease in the United States.[67] HCV is an RNA virus capable of causing chronic hepatitis, cirrhosis, hepatocellular carcinoma, and end-stage liver disease. Mortality attributed to HCV reached all-time highs in 2014 (nearly 20,000 deaths per year) and surpassed the total combined number of deaths from 60 other infectious diseases reported to CDC, including HIV, pneumococcal disease, and tuberculosis.[68] Since then, declines in death rates are on track of CDC viral hepatitis elimination goals by 2030, a result of expanded use of curative direct-acting antivirals (DAAs).[69] However, prevalent infections are highest in the Western and Southern regions and Washington, DC and among American Indians/Alaska Natives, Blacks, and baby boomers. Furthermore, incidence is increasing among younger adults (380% in those aged 20–39 years) and intensified by the opioid crisis, posing challenges for effective disease control.[70] HCV transmits primarily through asymptomatic percutaneous exposure (injection drug use, receipt of blood or blood products, occupational exposures) as well as nosocomial transmission in health care settings with inadequate infection control.[71] Other less efficient routes of transmission include mother-to-child transmission and sexual transmission between partners.

Sexual Transmission

Investigators have detected low levels of HCV RNA in saliva, cervical, and seminal plasma, but it remains unclear whether those represent transmissible virus.[72] Regarding condomless penile vaginal intercourse, the weight of evidence is that there is no increased risk among heterosexual couples in regular relationships (or events are exceedingly rare at the very least). In a meta-analysis (Tohme and Holmberg), the risk increases among persons with multiple sexual partners, but this association may be confounded by increased likelihood of injection drug use with increased number of partners[73]; this was especially the case in cross-sectional studies lacking phylogenetic testing of transmission events. In the HCV Partners Study, a prospective follow-up of 500 heterosexual, monogamous couples for 10 years, detailed phylogenetic analysis of 20 incident partner infections showed that 6 of them had concordant sero/genotype. Of those, 3 were closely related phylogenetically, giving an estimated risk of 1 transmission per 190,000 sexual contacts.[74] Other large prospective studies corroborate the notion that transmission events in this setting are exceedingly rare.[75,76] In these studies combined, there was no increased risk of sexual transmission of HCV, even after an estimated 750,000 vaginal and anal contacts between couples. The probability of such transmission would be less than 1 in 10 million sex contacts.[73] The HCV Partners Study assessed median contacts per month for vaginal intercourse during menses (0, range 0–10), anal intercourse (0, range 0–20), and oral sex (3, range 0–100), with these practices reported by 65%, 30%, and greater than 90% of couples, respectively. The proportion of HCV-concordant couples compared with those with one uninfected partner engaging in riskier sexual activities was numerically, but not statistically, higher: vaginal intercourse during menses (100% and 66%, p = 0.55), anal intercourse (67% and 30%, p = 0.22), and lack of condom use (100% and 70%, p = 0.56). The number of transmission events in the HCV Partners Study may have been too low to conclusively exclude an association with specific sex practices, especially because of the very low estimated overall transmission risk among *monogamous* couples, even if engaging in the specific sexual practices discussed earlier. Oral sex was highly common in both groups (with and without HCV transmission), and no differences were therefore noted.[74]

In the other hand, there seems to be a real increased risk of HCV sexual transmission for women coinfected with HIV or other STIs.[73] Among HIV-infected women with no history of injection drug use participating in the Women's Interagency HIV Study, sex with a male IDU was associated with prevalent HCV, and among all participants, being HIV infected was associated with a nearly 2-fold increased risk of being HCV coinfected.[77] In this population, risks factors for sexually acquired HCV include multiple sex partners, high-risk sexual practices (ie, anonymous partners, sex in the setting of drug use, exchanging sex for money/drugs, sex with IDU), presence or history of other STIs, and exposure to blood via partner violence.[73]

Multiple reports emerged in the late 90s and early 2000s of clusters of acute HCV infection among MSM, primarily among MSM who are coinfected with HIV.[25] Risk factors include unprotected anal intercourse, especially as the receptive partner; inconsistent condom use; drug use during sex; current or previous STIs, especially ulcerative STIs including lymphogranuloma venereum proctitis, syphilis, and herpes simplex; multiple or anonymous and casual sex partners; group sex; sexual practices that result in bleeding or damage to mucosa; fisting; and use of shared sex toys.[25,78,79] The risk of sexual acquisition of HCV is especially higher for HIV-infected compared with HIV-uninfected MSM.[73] Molecular epidemiology has defined HCV transmission clusters within MSM networks further. Clusters of HCV variants among MSM have shown lineage divergences over time (implying increased transmission),[80] distinct sequences from those in IDU or other unrelated patients, circulation of otherwise unusual genotypes (such as subtype 4d in Germany) and distinct from circulating IDU and non-MSM clusters,[81] or forming large international transmission networks encompassing individuals from United Kingdom, France, Germany, Australia, and the Netherlands.[82] An Australian study, however, showed that clusters were made of individuals with both injection drug use–related and sex-related acquisition risks and MSM, suggesting as well that both injection and sexual route of transmission can be active within the same social networks.[83]

Recent Epidemiological Trends

In the last decade, the body of evidence examining the sexual routes of mucosal HCV transmission in MSM has grown further, yet underscoring the role of activities where blood-to-blood contact may occur (ie, fisting, sharing sex toys) and settings whereby at-risk activities are more likely to take place (ie, group sex, "chemsex" including "slamming") and highlighting a crescendo epidemic of sexually transmitted HCV among HIV-positive MSM.[84] In 2017, Foster and colleagues[72] provided direct evidence that HCV is shed into the rectum in HIV-infected men in sufficient quantity to directly transmit to an inserted penis or be passed indirectly through fomite-like transmission to the rectum of a sex partner. In this timeframe, 2 major breakthroughs have deeply affected the landscape of sexual transmission in HCV. First, DAAs with high levels of tolerability and cure rates of greater than 95% became increasingly available, playing large role in HCV control.[85] Second, landmark studies demonstrated that universal test and treatment approach as well as the demonstration that HIV cannot be sexually transmitted from PLHIV with an undetectable viremia (undetectable = untransmittable [U = U] campaign) and PrEP are very effective HIV biomedical prevention strategies for MSM.[84] The scale-up of these interventions has reduced HIV incidence in MSM and also changed patterns of sexual networks and behavior towards lower fears of HIV acquisition and greater risk taking.[86] This has contributed to increased HCV incidence among HIV-negative MSM who were eligible for or on PrEP, especially in settings where unrestricted access to DAAs had halved the incidence of acute hepatitis C, all potentially refueling the HCV epidemic in HIV-positive MSM. In this regard, a meta-analysis by Hosseini-Hooshyar and colleagues compiling 41 studies predominantly conducted in Europe concluded that the incidence of reinfection following successful therapy among PLHIV was 3.76 cases per 100 person-years overall, 6.01 among MSM, and 3.29 among people who inject drugs. Such findings highlights the need of continued DAA scale-up, ongoing HCV screening, and treatment in order to reduce viremic burden and risk of reinfection.[87]

Prevention

Given HCV genetic variability and envelope complexity, there is no vaccine for the prevention of hepatitis C. Encouragingly, efforts toward a vaccine continue into a range of novel approaches that aided understanding of how neutralizing antibodies work and potential advantages of adopting envelope protein sequences for vaccine candidates, both informing rational vaccine design.[88] Although the risk for sexually transmitting hepatitis C is probably low if blood is not involved, the consistent use of condoms for sexual activity can reduce the risk of STI in general, including HIV and hepatitis

B. People with chronic hepatitis C should discuss the risk of hepatitis C transmission, which is low but not absent, with their sex partners. An open conversation regarding sexual and drug-use practices (limiting the number of sex partners, use of barrier methods, avoiding or limiting conducive sexual practices) should be beneficial.

As DAAs costs reduce and access become less restrictive, hepatitis C treatment as prevention is taking hold in European countries and is a promising prospect in the United States, especially in states with wider access to DAAs and harm reduction.[89] Primarily geared toward PWIDs, such programs also affect populations at greatest risk of sexual transmission of HCV, as seen in the experience with universal access to DAAs in Netherlands since 2015. Nationwide DAA scale-up among HIV-positive MSM led to decreases in acute hepatitis C by half in ensuing years and significant declines in high baseline rates of reinfection posttreatment.[90] Further effectiveness studies are forthcoming in elucidating the long-term impact of DAAs in prevention and elimination efforts.

HEPATITIS D

Hepatitis delta virus (HDV) is a defective RNA virus that does not encode its own envelope proteins and depends on the expression of HBsAg in the same cell to complete its life cycle. Being a result of either coinfection by HBV and HDV or HDV superinfection of patients chronically infected with HBV, chronic hepatitis D is arguably the most aggressive type of viral hepatitis associated with an increased risk of cirrhosis, liver decompensation, and hepatocellular carcinoma.[91]

Because of heterogeneous and nonstandardized screening practices and the inaccessibility to testing in many endemic areas, the exact global prevalence of infection remains unknown, and estimates vary widely between 15 and 72 million people affected by HDV. The highest prevalence is in Mongolia, where HDV infects 60% of HBsAg-positive individuals. Other endemic areas include the Amazon basin, West Africa, the Mediterranean basin, and Eastern Europe.[92] In the United States, HDV infection is rare. Screening recommendations are limited to high-risk populations, and suboptimal testing rates underestimate true prevalence.[93]

As HBV, HDV transmit by blood and blood-derived products and sexual contact. Vertical transmission is however rare. In high endemic populations, transmission occurs mainly through intrafamilial and iatrogenic spread in association with poor hygiene conditions. In low endemic regions in the northern hemisphere, IDU is the main transmission route. Sexual transmission, although less frequent than for HBV or HIV, seems to be important in regions where HBV infection is endemic, such as Taiwan.[94] HBV vaccination protects effectively against both HBV and HDV infection, and HBV vaccine introduction has shown clear correlation with decreases in HDV incidence.[91]

IMPLICATIONS FOR PUBLIC HEALTH

Sexual transmission of viral hepatitis disproportionately affects minorities and the vulnerable. Access to treatment, treatment as prevention, and vaccinations halt transmission of viral hepatitis and improves the quality of life of people living with HBV and HCV. Worldwide and in the United States, public health efforts continue to fall short of disease control targets.[52,95] Worldwide, only 5% of the estimated 94 million people who qualify for hepatitis B antiviral therapy are actually on treatment,[52] and 7% of the estimated 71 million people infected with hepatitis C have been successfully treated.[96] The 2021 National Academy of Medicine (NAM) report "Sexually Transmitted Infections: Adopting a Sexual Health Paradigm" calls for integrating sexual health, intersectionality, and social determinants in addressing STI epidemics tailored to priority populations, including those at risk of viral hepatitis.[97] NAM perspective is in line with the US Viral Hepatitis Action Plan 2020–2025 goals: reduce new viral hepatitis infections through vaccination promotion and harm reduction expansion and integrated care with perinatal programs.[95] Sexual transmission of viral hepatitis holds significance due to the shared burden, latest unfavorable trends, persisting health inequities, and surveillance limitations shared by STIs and viral hepatitis.[97] Both remain underfunded and neglected fields of practice yet incurring staggering direct medical costs, long-term sequelae, and mortality.

CLINICS CARE POINTS

- Hepatitis A virus vaccination of at-risk adults (PWID, homeless, inmates, MSM) is key to prevent and halt outbreaks, and mitigate endemic transmission in sexual networks.

- Adults between 19 and 51 years of age are now universally eligible to receive hepatitis B vaccination, expanding prevention beyond traditional at-risk groups and routine vaccination of children.

- Expanded vaccination of adults with hepatitis B vaccine is a helpful tool against challenges with routine risk assessment in clinic and invaluable at control of increases in cases fueled by opioid epidemic.

- Hepatitis C screening is recommended for all adults between 18 and 79 years of age (including in prenatal care), once in lifetime and regularly for PWID. Expanded screening, allied with simplified evaluation algorithms and well tolerated treatments with DAAs, are meant to prevent transmission by means of prompt diagnosis and cure, very important to halt disease burden in MSM sexual networks.

FUNDING

This work has been supported by NIH/NIAID P30 Grant 2P30AI027767-31.

REFERENCES

1. Trepo C. A brief history of hepatitis milestones. Liver Int 2014;1(34 Suppl):29–37.
2. Payen JL. De la jaunisse à l'hépatite C, 5000 ans d'histoire. Paris: Editions EDK; 2002.
3. MacCallum FO. Early studies of viral hepatitis. Br Med Bull 1972;28:105–8.
4. Murray R. Viral hepatitis. Bull NY Acad Med 1955;31:341–58.
5. Pérez V. Viral hepatitis: historical perspectives from the 20th to the 21st century. Arch Med Res 2007;38(6):593–605.
6. Alter H. Baruch Blumberg (1925–2011). Nature 2011;473:155.
7. Hersh T, Melnick J, Goyal RK, et al. Nonparenteral transmission of viral hepatitis type B (Australia antigen-associated serum hepatitis). N Engl J Med 1971;285:1363–4.
8. Heathcote J, Sherlock S. Spread of acute type-B hepatitis in London. Lancet 1973;1:1468–70.
9. Mazzur S. Menstrual blood as a vehicle of Australia-antigen transmission. Lancet 1973;1:749.
10. Heathcote J, Cameron CH, Dane DS. Hepatitis-B antigen in saliva and semen. Lancet 1974;1:71–3.
11. Fass RJ. Sexual Transmission of Viral Hepatitis? JAMA 1974;230(6):861–2.

12. Brook MG. Sexually acquired hepatitis. Sex Transm Infect 2002;78(4):235–40.
13. Tassopoulos NC, Papaevangelou GJ, Ticehurst JR, et al. Fecal excretion of Greek strains of hepatitis A virus in patients with hepatitis A and in experimentally infected chimpanzees. J Infect Dis 1986;154(2):231–7.
14. Ida S., Tachikawa N., Nakajima A., et al., Influence of human immunodeficiency virus type 1 infection on acute hepatitis A virus infection, *Clin Infect Dis*, 34 (3), 2002, 379–385.
15. Kirk MD, Pires SM, Black RE, et al. World Health Organization estimates of the global and regional disease burden of 22 foodborne bacterial, protozoal, and viral diseases, 2010: a data synthesis. PLoS Med 2015;12(12):e1001921.
16. Fathalla SE, Al-Jama AA, Al-Sheikh IH, et al. Seroprevalence of hepatitis A virus markers in eastern Saudi Arabia. Saudi Med J 2000;21:945–9.
17. Lee SD. Asian perspectives on viral hepatitis A. J Gastroenterol Hepatol 2000; 15(suppl):G94–9.
18. Centers for Disease Control and Prevention, Multistate outbreak of hepatitis A virus infections linked to fresh organic strawberries. Available at: https://www.cdc.gov/hepatitis/outbreaks/2022/hav-contaminated-food/index.htm. Accessed March 26, 2023.
19. Coulepis AG, Locarnini SA, Westaway EG, et al. Biophysical and biochemical characterization of hepatitis A virus. Intervirology 1982;18(3):107–27.
20. Abad FX, Pintó RM, Bosch A. Survival of enteric viruses on environmental fomites. Appl Environ Microbiol 1994;60(10):3704–10.
21. Grinde B, Stene-Johansen K, Sharma B, et al. Characterisation of an epidemic of hepatitis A virus involving intravenous drug abusers—infection by needle sharing? J Med Virol 1997;53:69–75.
22. Centers for Disease Control and Prevention. Numbers and rates of deaths with hepatitis A virus infection listed as a cause of death among residents, by demographic characteristics — United States, 2016-2020. Available at: https://www.cdc.gov/hepatitis/statistics/2020surveillance/hepatitis-a/table-1.4.htm. Accessed March 26, 2023.
23. Corona R, Stroffolini T, Giglio A, et al. Lack of evidence for increased risk of hepatitis A infection in homosexual men. Epidemiol Infect 1999;123:89–93.
24. Corey L, Holmes KK. Sexual transmission of hepatitis A in homosexual men: incidence and mechanism. N Engl J Med 1980;302:435–8.
25. Gorgos L. Sexual transmission of viral hepatitis. Infect Dis Clin North Am 2013; 27(4):811–36.
26. Leentvaar-Kuijpers A, Kool JL, Veugelers PJ, et al. An outbreak of hepatitis A among homosexual men in Amsterdam 1991–1993. Int J Epidemiol 1995;24: 218–22.
27. van Steenbergen JE, Tjon G, van den Hoek A, et al. Two years' prospective collection of molecular and epidemiological data shows limited spread of hepatitis A virus outside risk groups in Amsterdam, 2000-2002. J Infect Dis 2004;189: 471–82.
28. Tjon G, Xiridou M, Coutinho R, et al. Different transmission patterns of hepatitis A virus for two main risk groups as evidenced by molecular cluster analysis. J Med Virol 2007;79:488–94.
29. Stene-Johansen K, Tjon G, Schreier E, et al. Molecular epidemiological studies show that hepatitis A virus is endemic among active homosexual men in Europe. J Med Virol 2007;79:356–65.
30. Centers for Disease Control and Prevention, Number of reported cases* of hepatitis A virus infection and estimated infections† — United States, 2013-2020, Viral

Hepatitis 2020 8/17/2022 10/10/2022]; Available at: https://www.cdc.gov/hepatitis/statistics/2020surveillance/hepatitis-a/figure-1.1.htm. Accessed December 19, 2022.

31. Foster M.A., Hofmeister M.G., Albertson J.P., et al., Hepatitis A virus infections among men who have sex with men - eight U.S. States, 2017-2018, *MMWR Morb Mortal Wkly Rep*, 70 (24), 2021, 875–878.

32. European Centre for Disease Prevention and Control, Epidemiological update: Hepatitis A outbreak in the EU/EEA mostly affecting men who have sex with men, Available at: https://www.ecdc.europa.eu/en/news-events/epidemiological-update-hepatitis-outbreak-eueea-mostly-affecting-men-who-have-sex-men-2, 2018. Accessed December 19, 2022.

33. Ramachandran S, Xia GL, Dimitrova Z, et al. Changing Molecular Epidemiology of Hepatitis A Virus Infection, United States, 1996-2019. Emerg Infect Dis 2021; 27(6):1742–5.

34. Centers for Disease Control and Prevention, Widespread person-to-person out-breaks of hepatitis A across the United States, *Viral Hepatitis*, 2022, Available at: https://www.cdc.gov/hepatitis/outbreaks/2017March-HepatitisA.htm. Accessed December 19, 2022.

35. Ndumbi P., Freidl G.S., Williams C.J., et al., Hepatitis A outbreak disproportion-ately affecting men who have sex with men (MSM) in the European Union and European Economic Area, June 2016 to May 2017, *Euro Surveill*, 2018 23 (33):1700641.

36. Aulicino G, Faccini M, Lamberti A, et al. Hepatitis A epidemic in men who have sex with men (MSM) in Milan, Italy. Acta Biomed 2020;91(3–s):106–10.

37. Chen W.C., Chiang P.H., Liao Y.H., et al., Outbreak of hepatitis A virus infection in Taiwan, June 2015 to September 2017, *Euro Surveill*, 2019, 24(14):1800133.

38. Tanaka S, Kishi T, Ishihara A, et al. Outbreak of hepatitis A linked to European out-breaks among men who have sex with men in Osaka, Japan, from March to July 2018. Hepatol Res 2019;49(6):705–10.

39. Chuffi S, Gomes-Gouvea MS, Casadio LVB, et al. The molecular characterization of hepatitis A virus strains circulating during hepatitis A outbreaks in São Paulo, Brazil, from September 2017 to May 2019. Viruses 2021;14(1):73.

40. Nelson NP, Weng MK, Hofmeister MG, et al. Prevention of Hepatitis A Virus Infec-tion in the United States: recommendations of the advisory committee on immu-nization practices, 2020. MMWR Recomm Rep (Morb Mortal Wkly Rep) 2020; 69(5):1–38.

41. Prevention of hepatitis A through active or passive immunization: recommenda-tions of the advisory committee on immunization practices (ACIP), MMWR Re-comm Rep (Morb Mortal Wkly Rep), 45 (Rr-15), 1996, 1–30.

42. Yin S, Barker L, Ly KN, et al. Susceptibility to Hepatitis A Virus Infection in the United States, 2007–2016. Clin Infect Dis 2020;71(10):e571–9.

43. Ott JJ, Wiersma ST. Single-dose administration of inactivated hepatitis A vaccina-tion in the context of hepatitis A vaccine recommendations. Int J Infect Dis 2013; 17(11):e939–44.

44. Regan DG, Wood JG, Benevent C, et al. Estimating the critical immunity threshold for preventing hepatitis A outbreaks in men who have sex with men. *Epidemiol Infect* 2016;144(7):1528–37.

45. LaMori J, Feng X, Pericone CD, et al. Hepatitis vaccination adherence and completion rates and factors associated with low compliance: A claims-based analysis of U.S. adults. PLoS One 2022;17(2):e0264062.

46. Fritzsche C., Bergmann L., Loebermann M., et al., Immune response to hepatitis A vaccine in patients with HIV, *Vaccine*, 37 (16), 2019, 2278–2283.

47. Cohall A, Zucker J, Krieger R, et al. Missed Opportunities for Hepatitis A Vaccination Among MSM Initiating PrEP. J Community Health 2020;45(3):506–9.

48. Bukhsh M.A., Thyagarajan R., Todd B., et al., An electronic medical record-based intervention to improve hepatitis A vaccination rates in the emergency department during a regional outbreak, *BMJ Open Qual*, 11 (4), 2022, e001876.

49. Landers TA, Greenberg HB, Robinson WS. Structure of hepatitis B Dane particle DNA and nature of the endogenous DNA polymerase reaction. J Virol 1977;23(2): 368–76.

50. Hyams KC. Risks of chronicity following acute hepatitis B virus infection: a review. Clin Infect Dis 1995;20(4):992–1000.

51. Khanam A, Chua JV, Kottilil S. Immunopathology of Chronic Hepatitis B Infection: Role of Innate and Adaptive Immune Response in Disease Progression. Int J Mol Sci 2021;22(11).

52. Global prevalence, treatment, and prevention of hepatitis B virus infection in 2016: a modelling study. Lancet Gastroenterol Hepatol 2018;3(6):383–403.

53. Centers for Disease Control and Prevention, Numbers and rates* of deaths with hepatitis B virus infection listed as a cause of death† among residents, by state or jurisdiction — United States, 2016-2020, *Viral Hepatitis*, 2022, Available at: https://www.cdc.gov/hepatitis/statistics/2020surveillance/hepatitis-b/table-2.7.htm. Accessed December 19, 2022.

54. Centers for Disease Control and Prevention. Viral Hepatitis Surveillance Report – United States, 2020. https://www.cdc.gov/hepatitis/statistics/2020surveillance/index.htm. Published September 2022. Accessed March 26, 2023.

55. Roberts H, Jiles R, Harris AM, et al. Incidence and Prevalence of Sexually Transmitted Hepatitis B, United States, 2013-2018. Sex Transm Dis 2021;48(4):305–9.

56. Kreisel K.M., Spicknall I.H., Gargano J.W., et al., "Sexually transmitted infections among US women and men: prevalence and incidence estimates, 2018.", *Sex Transm Dis*, 48 (4), 2021, 208–214.

57. Platt L., French C.E., McGowan C.R., et al., Prevalence and burden of HBV co-infection among people living with HIV: A global systematic review and meta-analysis, *J Viral Hepat*, 27 (3), 2020, 294–315.

58. Mena G, García-Basteiro AL, Bayas JM. Hepatitis B and A vaccination in HIV-infected adults: a review. Hum Vaccin Immunother 2015;11(11): 2582–98.

59. Szmuness W., Stevens C.E., Zang E.A., et al., A controlled clinical trial of the efficacy of the hepatitis B vaccine (Heptavax B): a final report, Hepatology, 1 (5), 1981, 377–385.

60. Bruce MG, Bruden D, Hurlburt D, et al. Protection and antibody levels 35 years after primary series with hepatitis B vaccine and response to a booster dose. Hepatology 2022;76(4):1180–9.

61. Bruce MG, Bruden D, Hurlburt D, et al. Antibody Levels and Protection After Hepatitis B Vaccine: Results of a 30-Year Follow-up Study and Response to a Booster Dose. J Infect Dis 2016;214(1):16–22.

62. Middleman AB, Baker CJ, Kozinetz CA, et al. Duration of protection after infant hepatitis B vaccination series. Pediatrics 2014;133(6):e1500–7.

63. Centers for Disease Control and Prevention, ACIP evidence to recommendations for a universal hepatitis B (HepB) vaccination strategy in adults, Available at: https://www.cdc.gov/vaccines/acip/recs/grade/hepb-adults-etr.html. Accessed December 19, 2022.

64. Daley MF, Hennessey KA, Weinbaum CM, et al. Physician practices regarding adult hepatitis B vaccination: a national survey. Am J Prev Med 2009;36(6):491–6.

65. Weng M.K., Doshani M., Khan M.A., et al., Universal Hepatitis B Vaccination in Adults Aged 19-59 Years: Updated Recommendations of the Advisory Committee on Immunization Practices - United States, 2022, *MMWR Morb Mortal Wkly Rep*, 71 (13), 2022, 477–483.

66. Kuwahara RK, Jabbarpour Y, Westfall JM. Increased physician awareness is needed to implement universal hepatitis B vaccination. Am Fam Physician 2022;106(2):132–3.

67. Hofmeister MG, Rosenthal EM, Barker LK, et al. Estimating prevalence of hepatitis C virus infection in the United States, 2013-2016. Hepatology 2019;69:1020–31.

68. Ly KN, Hughes EM, Jiles RB, et al. Rising Mortality Associated With Hepatitis C Virus in the United States, 2003-2013. Clin Infect Dis 2016;62(10):1287–8.

69. Centers for Disease Control and Prevention, National Center for Health Statistics. Multiple Cause of Death 1999-2018 on CDC WONDER Online Database, released in 2020, Available at: http://wonder.cdc.gov/mcd-icd10.html. Accessed December 19, 2022.

70. Holtzman D, Asher AK, Schillie S. The Changing Epidemiology of Hepatitis C Virus Infection in the United States During the Years 2010 to 2018. Am J Public Health 2021;111(5):949–55.

71. Health care-Associated Hepatitis B and C Outbreaks (≥ 2 cases) Reported to the Centers for Disease Control and Prevention (CDC) 2008-2019. CDC, Division of Viral Hepatitis, National Center for HIV, Viral Hepatitis, STD, and TB Prevention. May 11th 2020. Available at: https://www.cdc.gov/hepatitis/statistics/healthcareoutbreak table.htm. Accessed November 6, 2022.

72. Foster AL, Gaisa MM, Hijdra RM, et al. Shedding of Hepatitis C Virus Into the Rectum of HIV-infected Men Who Have Sex With Men. Clin Infect Dis 2017; 64(3):284–8.

73. Tohme RA, Holmberg SD. Is sexual contact a major mode of hepatitis C virus transmission? Hepatology 2010;52(4):1497–505.

74. Terrault NA, Dodge JL, Murphy EL, et al. Sexual transmission of hepatitis C virus among monogamous heterosexual couples: the HCV partners study. Hepatology 2013;57(3):881–9.

75. Vandelli C, Renzo F, Romanò L, et al. Lack of evidence of sexual transmission of hepatitis C among monogamous couples: results of a 10-year prospective follow-up study. Am J Gastroenterol 2004;99:855–9.

76. Marincovich B, Castilla J, del Romero J, et al. Absence of hepatitis C virus transmission in a prospective cohort of heterosexual serodiscordant couples. Sex Transm Infect 2003;79:160–2.

77. Frederick T, Burian P, Terrault N, et al. Factors associated with prevalent hepatitis C infection among HIV-infected women with no reported history of injection drug use: the Women's Interagency HIV Study (WIHS). AIDS Patient Care STDS 2009; 23:915–23.

78. Centers for Disease Control (CDC). Sexual transmission of hepatitis C virus among HIV-infected men who have sex with men–New York City, 2005-2010. MMWR Morb Mortal Wkly Rep 2011;60:945–50.

79. Gambotti L, Batisse D, Colin-de-Verdiere N, et al. Acute hepatitis C infection in HIV positive men who have sex with men in Paris, France, 2001-2004. Euro Surveill 2005;10:115–7.

80. Danta M, Brown D, Bhagani S, et al. Recent epidemic of acute hepatitis C virus in HIV-positive men who have sex with men linked to high-risk sexual behaviours. AIDS 2007;21:983–91.
81. Vogel M, van de Laar T, Kupfer B, et al. Phylogenetic analysis of acute hepatitis C virus genotype 4 infections among human immunodeficiency virus-positive men who have sex with men in Germany. Liver Int 2010;30:1169–72.
82. van de Laar T, Pybus O, Bruisten S, et al. Evidence of a large, international network of HCV transmission in HIV-positive men who have sex with men. Gastroenterology 2009;136:1609–17.
83. Matthews GV, Pham ST, Hellard M, et al. Patterns and characteristics of hepatitis C transmission clusters among HIV-positive and HIV-negative individuals in the Australian trial in acute hepatitis C. Clin Infect Dis 2011;52:803–11.
84. European Treatment Network for HIV. Hepatitis and Global Infectious Diseases (NEAT-ID) Consensus Panel*. Recently acquired and early chronic hepatitis C in MSM: Recommendations from the European treatment network for HIV, hepatitis and global infectious diseases consensus panel. AIDS 2020;34(12):1699–711.
85. World health OrganizationCombating hepatitis B and C to reach elimination by 2030. Geneva: World Health Organization; 2016.
86. Traeger MW, Schroeder SE, Wright EJ, et al. Effects of preexposure prophylaxis for the prevention of human immunodeficiency virus infection on sexual risk behavior in men who have sex with men: a systematic review and meta-analysis. Clin Infect Dis 2018;67:676686.
87. Hosseini-Hooshyar S, Hajarizadeh B, Bajis S, et al. Risk of hepatitis C reinfection following successful therapy among people living with HIV: a global systematic review, meta-analysis, and meta-regression. Lancet HIV 2022;9(6):e414–27.
88. Duncan JD, Urbanowicz RA, Tarr AW, et al. (Basel) 2020;8(1):90.
89. Ward JW, Hinman AR, Alter HJ. Time for the Elimination of Hepatitis C Virus as a Global Health Threat. The Liver: Biology and Pathobiology. Sixth Edition. John Wiley & Sons Ltd; 2020.
90. Smit C, Boyd A, Rijnders BJA, et al. Op de Coul ELM, van der Valk M, Reiss P; ATHENA observational cohort. HCV micro-elimination in individuals with HIV in the Netherlands 4 years after universal access to direct-acting antivirals: a retrospective cohort study. Lancet HIV 2021;8(2):e96–105.
91. Mentha N, Clément S, Negro F, et al. A review on hepatitis D: from virology to new therapies. J Adv Res 2019;17:3–15.
92. Stockdale A.J., Kreuels B., Henrion M.R.Y., et al., Hepatitis D prevalence: problems with extrapolation to global population estimates, Gut, 69 (2), 2020, 396–397.
93. Patel EU, Thio CL, Boon D, et al. Prevalence of Hepatitis B and Hepatitis D virus infections in the United States, 2011–2016. Clin Infect Dis 2019;69(4):709–12.
94. Liaw YF, Chiu KW, Chu CM, et al. Heterosexual transmission of hepatitis delta virus in the general population of an area endemic for hepatitis B virus infection: a prospective study. J Infect Dis 1990;162:1170–2.
95. U.S. Department of Health and Human Services. National Strategic Plan A Roadmap to Elimination for the United States. Available at: https://www.hhs.gov/sites/default/files/Viral-Hepatitis-National-Strategic-Plan-2021-2025.pdf.   Accessed March 26, 2023.
96. Thomas DL. State of the Hepatitis C Virus Care Cascade. Clin Liver Dis 2020; 16(1):8–11.
97. National Academies of Sciences, Engineering, and Medicine. Sexually transmitted infections: adopting a sexual health paradigm. Washington, DC: The National Academies Press; 2021. https://doi.org/10.17226/25955.

Genital Herpes Infection
Progress and Problems

Nicholas Van Wagoner, MD, PhD[a],*, Fuad Qushair, BS[b],
Christine Johnston, MD, MPH[c]

KEYWORDS

- Genital herpes • Herpes simplex virus • HSV-1 • HSV-2 • Genital ulcer disease

KEY POINTS

- Genital herpes is a prevalent sexually transmitted infection caused by herpes simplex virus type 1 (HSV-1) or type 2 (HSV-2).
- Genital herpes, the leading cause of genital ulcer disease, causes significant global morbidity. Transmission to neonates causes neonatal disease and HSV-2 infection substantially increases the risk of HIV acquisition.
- Diagnosis of genital herpes requires a high index of suspicion due to recurrent, self-limited symptoms which may be unrecognized and is made with virologic testing from genital lesions or with serologic assays to detect antibodies in blood.
- Treatment of genital herpes relies on acyclic guanosine analogs used as suppressive therapy to prevent recurrences and decrease the risk of transmission or as episodic therapy to treat recurrences. Suppressive therapy doses are higher for people with HIV and pregnant people.
- Novel approaches to diagnose, treat, and prevent genital herpes are needed. Specific gaps are accurate, widely available serologic tests, novel antiviral medications, and prophylactic or therapeutic vaccines.

EPIDEMIOLOGY OF HSV-1 AND HSV-2: SEROPREVALENCE AND BURDEN OF DISEASE

Genital herpes (GH) is caused by 2 related yet distinct viruses: herpes simplex viruses (HSV) type-1 (HSV-1) and type-2 (HSV-2).[1] In 2016, there were an estimated 491.5 million people worldwide aged 15 to 49 years infected with HSV-2 (13.2% seroprevalence) and 3.75 billion people aged 0 to 49 years infected with HSV-1 (66.6% seroprevalence).[2] Seroprevalence is highest in the African region (**Fig. 1**). In the 2015 to 2016

[a] Division of Infectious Diseases, Department of Medicine, University of Alabama Heersink School of Medicine, VH 102A, 1720 2nd Avenue South, Birmingham, AL 35294, USA;
[b] University of Alabama Heersink School of Medicine, 1720 2nd Avenue South, Birmingham, AL 35294, USA; [c] Division of Allergy and Infectious Diseases, Department of Medicine, University of Washington, 325 9th Avenue Box 359928, Seattle, WA 98104, USA
* Corresponding author.
E-mail address: nvanwagoner@uabmc.edu

Infect Dis Clin N Am 37 (2023) 351–367
https://doi.org/10.1016/j.idc.2023.02.011
0891-5520/23/© 2023 Elsevier Inc. All rights reserved.
id.theclinics.com

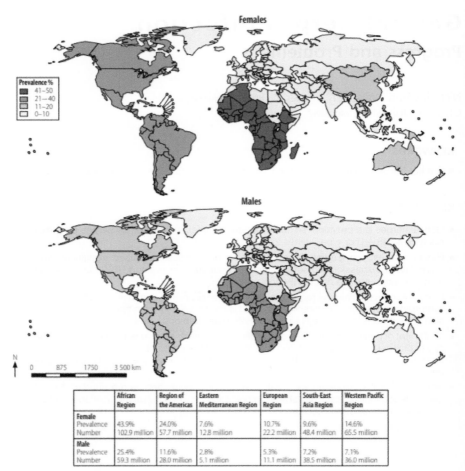

	African Region	Region of the Americas	Eastern Mediterranean Region	European Region	South-East Asia Region	Western Pacific Region
Female						
Prevalence	43.9%	24.0%	7.6%	10.7%	9.6%	14.6%
Number	102.9 million	57.7 million	12.8 million	22.2 million	48.4 million	65.5 million
Male						
Prevalence	25.4%	11.6%	2.8%	5.3%	7.2%	7.1%
Number	59.3 million	28.0 million	5.1 million	11.1 million	38.5 million	36.0 million

Fig. 1. Map of regional estimates of the number and prevalence of herpes simplex virus type 2 infections in females and males, 15 to 49 years of age in 2016. (*From* James, C., et al., Herpes simplex virus: global infection prevalence and incidence estimates, 2016. Bull World Health Organ, 2020. 98(5): p. 315–329.)

report from the United States (U.S.) National Health and Nutrition Examination Survey (NHANES), 11.9% of the population aged 14 to 49 years had HSV-2 infection.[3] In 2018, there were an estimated 18.6 million prevalent cases and 572,000 incident cases among 18 to 49-year-olds in the U.S.[4] In Canada, mean pooled seroprevalence was estimated at 10.0% in the general population with higher seroprevalence among persons attending sexual health clinics and in persons living with HIV.[5] Similarly, in Mexico seroprevalence varies by population and ranges from 5.9% to 86%.[6,7]

HSV-1 seroprevalence in NHANES 2015 to 2016 was 47.8% in 14 to 49 year-olds and is declining over time,[3] particularly among children and adolescents.[3,8] HSV-1 seroprevalence in Canada approximates 50%.[9] A systematic analysis of HSV-1 in Latin America and the Caribbean, including Mexico, reported an overall pooled mean HSV-1 seroprevalence of 83.1%.[10] While most cases of GH are due to HSV-2, HSV-1 is responsible for an increasing number of first-episode GH, particularly in high-income settings.[1] It is hypothesized that the decline in acquisition during childhood contributes to the increasing number of genital HSV-1 infections, as people enter their sexual lives without pre-existing HSV-1 immunity. In 2016, modeling studies estimated the global burden of genital HSV-1 infection at 192.0 million (5.2% prevalence in ages 15–49).[2]

Disparities in the burden of HSV-2 infection exist. Women account for 65% of infections, likely due to biologic factors. Seroprevalence increases with increasing age and number of sexual partners.[3] Prevalence is higher among non-Hispanic black populations, reflecting structural racism[3,4] that contributes to racial disparities in STIs including inequalities in social determinants of health and lack of equity in and access to quality health care.

GH varies greatly in symptom severity. Many people have subclinical infection or infrequent genital recurrences while others have a more frequent or severe symptomatic infection. HSV is the most common cause of GUD worldwide.[11] In 2016, 187 million people had HSV-related GUD: 178 million and 9 million cases were attributed to HSV-2 and HSV-1, respectively.[12] This translated to 8 billion days of HSV-2-related GUD and substantial economic burden[12] including the direct cost for treatment and indirect costs from loss of productivity.[13] In the U.S., the lifetime cost of incident GH infections is estimated at $90.7 million. This does not include the costs of treating neonatal herpes or associated with the increased risk of acquiring HIV in persons with HSV-2.[14]

In 2016, there were an estimated 14,000 cases of neonatal herpes (10 cases/ 100,000 live births).[15] While neonatal herpes data in the U.S. are limited due to the lack of reporting requirements, in settings where reporting of neonatal HSV is required, rates are as high as 31.5 cases/100,000 live births.[16]

HSV-2 infection increases inflammation in the genital tract, which is hypothesized to contribute to increased susceptibility to HIV infection.[17] In 2016, 420,000 cases of HIV were attributable to HSV-2, giving a population attributable fraction (PAF) of 29.6%.[18] Among heterosexual populations, the PAF is even higher, at 37.5%,[19] underscoring the importance of developing strategies to prevent and treat HSV-2 infection.

TRANSMISSION AND NATURAL HISTORY OF HERPES SIMPLEX VIRUSES INFECTION

While HSV-2 was long assumed to evolve directly from HSV-1, genomic sequencing demonstrates that HSV-2 evolved from Great Ape herpesviruses and was likely transmitted to humans around 1 million years ago as a zoonotic infection.[20] Both HSV-1 and HSV-2 have sophisticated mechanisms to evade aspects of the host immune system which contribute to their asymptomatic transmission and acquisition.[21] HSV-1 and HSV-2 enter skin and mucosa through breaks in the epidermis and replicate in the dermal layers locally while also invading sensory nerve endings. Virus is transported retrogradely to the sacral dorsal root ganglia, where it establishes a latent, chronic infection that cannot be cleared.[22] Periodic reactivations of the virus result in its anterograde transport down the sensory neurons to the skin/mucosa, which causes recurrent GH or subclinical shedding, which may lead to transmission. HSV-2 is more trophic to the sacral dorsal root ganglia than HSV-1. HSV-2 infection is associated with more frequent genital recurrences and more frequent shedding compared to HSV-1.[23] HSV-1 oral exposures also cause infection in the trigeminal ganglion, causing oral or ocular disease.

Both HSV-1 and HSV-2 are transmitted through intimate contact of skin and mucosal surfaces. HSV-1 can be transmitted through either oral or genital sex to either the oral or genital compartment of the partner (**Fig. 2**). HSV-2 is typically transmitted

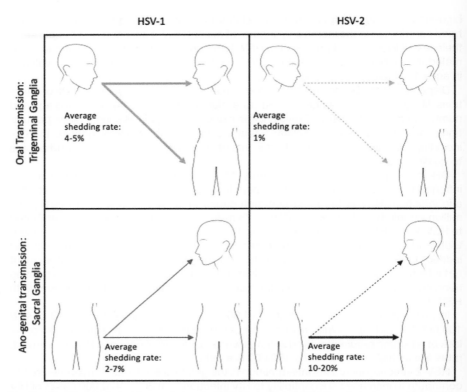

Fig. 2. Likelihood of viral transmission by HSV type, site of infection in index partner. HSV-1 and HSV-2 are transmitted through intimate contact of skin and mucosal surfaces. Dashed arrows designate possible but rare transmission. Shedding rates are higher in the first year of infection and vary between people. Shedding rates are higher in people with a history of symptomatic GH and in people who are immunocompromised.

from genital tract to genital tract through genital sex. While HSV-1 oral infection decreases the risk of symptomatic primary genital HSV-2 infection, it does not protect against HSV-2 acquisition.[24] In contrast, genital HSV-2 infection protects against the acquisition of genital HSV-1 infection. Antibody responses are critical to protect against infection, particularly in the setting of neonatal herpes, which may explain why neonatal herpes is most often associated with maternal HSV acquisition during pregnancy.[25]

Reactivation of HSV-2 in the genital tract is associated with chronic inflammation, production of pro-inflammatory cytokines, and recruitment of CD4+ and CD8+ T cells to contain viral replication.[25] The chronic inflammation seen in GH is independent of symptoms. Increased numbers of mucosal CCR5+ CD4+ T-cells in people with HSV-2 infection is the likely mechanism by which HSV-2 increases the risk of HIV acquisition.[26] In addition, CD8+ tissue-resident memory T cells patrol the genital mucosa after reactivation.[27] CD4+ and CD8+ T cell responses are likely required for effective prevention of recurrences.

Clinical manifestations

HSV primary infection occurs when the virus is acquired in the absence of HSV-1/HSV-2 antibodies. HSV nonprimary infection is defined as HSV-1 or HSV-2 acquisition in a person with pre-existing HSV antibodies. Clinical manifestations typically occur within 1 week of acquisition and can include both genital symptoms, such as painful lesions, dysuria, urinary retention, pruritus, vaginal/urethral discharge, tender inguinal adenopathy, and systemic symptoms (ie, fevers, headaches, malaise).[28] Herpetic lesions in primary infection may be extensive occurring bilaterally on the genitals and extending to adjacent skin. Herpes lesions may also occur in the peri-anal region, the buttocks or upper thighs.[28] Lesions classically progress through stages of erythema, papules, vesicles, ulcers, and crusts with full resolution within 2 to 3 weeks without antiviral therapy.[28] Systemic symptoms are reported more often in women than men.[28]

Innate and adaptive immune responses play important roles in controlling the severity of disease and frequency of recurrence in GH.[29] Interference with either arm of the immune response can result in atypical, prolonged, and severe manifestations, disseminated disease, and the development of resistance to antivirals. Persons living with HIV (PLWH) and with CD4+ T cell count less than 100 cells/mm^3, are susceptible to frequent HSV recurrence[30] and hypertrophic lesions mimicking malignancies have been described.[31] Similarly, other immunosuppressed populations (ie, solid organ transplant and stem cell transplant recipients, persons with malignancy), and in particular, those with reduced cell-mediated immune responses report frequent HSV recurrence.[32] The prevalence of acyclovir-resistant HSV is higher in immunocompromised populations and is hypothesized to result from prolonged replication and survival of less pathogenic virus when the immune response is impaired.[33] Acyclovir resistance if often seen in atypical presentations of GH.

GH recurrences are typically self-limited and mild to moderate in severity. Prodromal symptoms described as tingling, burning, or shooting pain often precede the recurrence by 12 to 24 hours, followed by the development of lesions predominantly on epithelialized skin. Lesions are typically unilateral and fewer in number compared to lesions associated with primary infection.[28] Atypical skin manifestations (ie, fissures, excoriations) can result from HSV reactivation. Without antiviral therapy, lesions typically heal within 1 to 2 weeks. The frequency of recurrence varies widely and occurs more often in the year following infection and declines over time.[34] Recurrences are less frequent in GH caused by HSV-1 compared to HSV-2.[35]

HSV-associated urethritis, cervicitis, and proctitis are seen most often in primary infection. Studies suggest that HSV-associated urethritis is more often caused by HSV-1 and associated with a history of oral-penile exposure,[36] with symptoms of dysuria, meatitis, lymphadenopathy, and urethral discharge. Genital ulcers are absent in approximately 30% of persons with HSV urethritis.[36,37] HSV cervicitis is characterized by diffuse erosive and hemorrhagic lesions of the ectocervical epithelium, and ulceration.[38,39] HSV proctitis can occur in people who have receptive anal sex and may present with rectal burning, pain, and tenesmus[40]. HSV is the most common cause of gram stain-negative proctitis and is a frequent cause of proctitis among PLWH.[41] Anal ulceration is seen in the minority of persons with HSV proctitis.[41]

When acquired during pregnancy, HSV causes typical symptoms of GH. Rarely, disseminated infection can occur in the absence of genital or skin lesions, and there are several case reports of fulminant hepatitis occurring during pregnancy.[42]

Transmission of HSV to the neonate occurs with exposure to HSV-1 or HSV-2 *in utero*, peripartum or postpartum. *In utero* transmission accounts for 5% of neonatal HSV.[43] Postpartum infection occurs when the infant comes into direct contact with orolabial or cutaneous lesions. Peripartum acquisition of neonatal herpes is the most common route of neonatal HSV.[43] The greatest risk for transmission to the neonate occurs when HSV is acquired during pregnancy; additional risk factors include use of fetal-scalp electrodes and prolonged rupture of membranes.[44] Clinical manifestations of neonatal HSV are classified as: skin, eye, and mucous membrane (SEM) disease, central nervous system (CNS) disease, and disseminated disease. Neonatal herpes typically presents in the first 1 to 3 weeks after birth. SEM disease is characterized by vesicular and ulcerative skin lesions. Nonspecific symptoms of poor oral intake, irritability, or temperature instability may also be present.[43] CNS disease may present with lethargy, bulging fontanelle, or seizure in addition to the above nonspecific symptoms. Cutaneous lesions are present in approximately two-thirds of cases.[43] Disseminated disease presents with sepsis, respiratory failure, liver failure, and disseminated intravascular coagulopathy.[45] SEM disease has low morbidity and mortality. Even with the use of antiviral therapy, neurologic sequalae are common in CNS disease and mortality is 30% for disseminated disease.[46,47] Clinicians should maintain a high index of suspicion for neonatal herpes among neonates presenting with failure to thrive, fevers, temperature instability, or neurologic symptoms. Prompt initiation of antiviral therapy reduces morbidity and mortality.

DIAGNOSIS OF GENITAL HERPES

Diagnosis of GH is complicated by the self-limited nature of outbreaks which are often absent at the time of clinical evaluation. History and physical examination offer valuable information, but diagnosis of GH should always be confirmed using type-specific assays that differentiate between HSV-1 and HSV-2. Nucleic acid amplification tests (NAAT) and viral culture can be performed on samples collected from lesions; NAAT is preferred due to high sensitivity and specificity compared to culture[48] and several FDA-approved assays are available.[49]

Serologic assays test for antibodies to HSV. IgM-antibody tests do not distinguish primary infection from recurrences and are not recommended.[50,51] Type-specific immunoglobulin (Ig) G-based antibody tests are the test of choice.

Several IgG-based enzyme immunoassays (EIA) and chemiluminescent immunoassays (CLIA) for glycoprotein G2 (HSV-2) or glycoprotein G1 (HSV-1) are commercially available and provide a quantitative "Index-value" based on colorimetric change. Their sensitivity ranges from 80% to 98%.[52] False-negatives can occur early in infection prior to the development of HSV type-specific IgG. In cases where HSV is suspected and EIA is negative, repeat testing 12 weeks after suspected acquisition is recommended.[52] HSV-2 assays have high rates of false positivity at low Index-values, particularly, in low-prevalence populations.[53] Cross-reactivity with HSV-1 antibodies may contribute. Confirmation of low positive Index-values (<3.0) with a second HSV type-specific assay is recommended[52] to avoid giving patients an inaccurate diagnosis.

Utilization and interpretation of diagnostic tests for GH depend on clinical scenario. Evaluation of patients presenting with GUD should include history and physical examination followed by virologic and serologic tests for HSV-1 and HSV-2. Interpretation of the potential assay result combinations is described in **Fig. 3**A. The diagnosis of GH using type-specific antibody tests alone is more challenging. Although most HSV-2 infections are localized to the sacral ganglia, HSV-1 antibody may represent oral or anogenital infection and detection of HSV-1 type-specific antibody alone should not be used to diagnose HSV-1 GH.[52] Type-specific HSV-2 serologic assays may be used in the absence of GUD to diagnose GH in certain scenarios (**Fig. 3**B). HSV-2 serologic screening in the general population is not recommended.[52]

MANAGEMENT AND TREATMENT

The acyclic nucleoside analogs acyclovir, and its prodrug valacyclovir, and famciclovir are approved to treat GH. These guanosine nucleoside analogs require initial

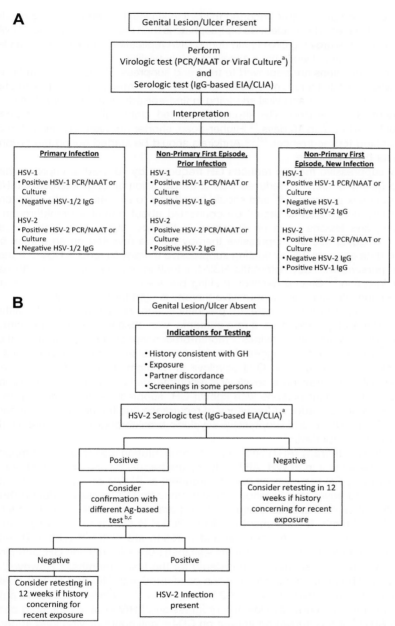

Fig. 3. Testing algorithm and test interpretation for GH in the presence (*A*) and absence (*B*) of genital lesions. [a]PCR preferred over viral culture. NAAT, nucleic acid amplification test; PCR, polymerase chain reaction. EIA/CLIA, enzyme immunoassay/chemiluminescence immunoassay. [a]HSV-1 IgG does not distinguish orolabial from genital infection. [b]Biokit or Western Blot recommended. If confirmatory tests are unavailable, patients should be counseled about the limitations of available testing before obtaining serologic tests, and health care providers should be aware that false-positive results occur. [c]Required for all persons with low index value (optimal values not established for all tests). (*Data from* Corey L,

phosphorylation by the HSV-encoded thymidine kinase, followed by phosphorylation by cellular kinases. This nucleotide triphosphate is then incorporated by HSV DNA polymerase into the growing DNA chain during DNA replication and leads to chain termination.[32,54] These antivirals have excellent safety profiles.[55]

These medications are approved to treat and suppress GH outbreaks and prevent transmission. While there is no cure for GH, antiviral treatment shortens the duration of clinical manifestations and viral shedding in first-episode and recurrent disease.[56,57] Treatment of first-episode GH should be started empirically as soon as possible and continued for 7 to 10 days.[52] Higher-dose, shorter duration regimens (1–5 days) are indicated for recurrences.[52,58] Antivirals should be started during the prodromal phase for best response.

Daily suppressive therapy reduces GH frequency by 70%-80%, improves health-related quality of life,[59–61] reduces HSV-2 transmission among heterosexual HSV-2 discordant sex partners,[62,63] and should be offered to all patients with symptomatic HSV-2 infection. Patients should be counseled about potential breakthrough viral shedding and lesions while on suppressive therapy, even when high doses are used.[64] Ongoing use of suppressive therapy can be revisited on an annual basis. Limited data are available evaluating suppressive therapy to reduce HSV-2 transmission in persons with asymptomatic HSV-2 infection and among those with genital HSV-1 infection.[52] Shared decision making between patient and provider is useful to determine whether daily suppressive therapy is right for the patient.

Acyclovir is considered safe in pregnancy and breast feeding[65,66] although increased risk of gastroschisis, a rare outcome, was observed among pregnant people receiving antiherpetic antivirals 1 month-preconception through month 3 of pregnancy.[67] Animal models suggest low risk for adverse pregnancy outcomes with valacyclovir and famciclovir. Oral acyclovir is recommended for first-episode and recurrent GH and intravenous acyclovir is recommended in severe disease in pregnant people.[52] In pregnant persons with known GH, suppressive acyclovir beginning at 36 weeks gestation reduced frequency of recurrence and the need for Cesarean delivery.[68] Despite the use of suppressive acyclovir, breakthrough cases of neonatal herpes have been reported.[69]

Antiretroviral therapy (ART) and immune reconstitution are important components of GH management in PLWH. ART reduces the frequency and severity of reactivation; however, GH recurrences are still frequent in PLWH co-infected with HSV-2 on ART[70]. Moreover, the likelihood of symptomatic GH increases during the first 6 months after ART initiation, especially in persons with CD4+ T-cell count less than 200 cell/mm3. Management of GH in PLWH is similar to its management in other populations but antiviral dose and duration are higher[52] (**Table 1**). Among PLWH initiating ART with CD4+ counts less than 200 cell/mm3 and GH, antiherpetic suppressive therapy should be considered for the first 6 months.[52] However, suppressive antiherpetic therapy in persons coinfected with HIV and HSV-2 does not reduce the risk for either HIV or HSV-2 transmission.[71,72] While suppressive antiherpetic therapy may modestly slow the progression of HIV in dually infected persons not on ART[73], it has shown no impact on CD4+ cell count or viral load in persons dually infected on ART.[74]

◄————————————————————————————————————

Benedetti J, Critchlow C, et al. Treatment of primary first-episode genital herpes simplex virus infections with acyclovir: results of topical, intravenous and oral therapy. J Antimicrob Chemother. 1983;12 Suppl B:79–88.)

Table 1
Preferred genital herpes treatment and suppressive regimens

	General Population	HIV	Pregnant
Primary initial infection			
Acyclovir	400 mg orally 3 times/d for 7–10 d	400 mg orally 3 times/d for 7–10 d	400 mg orally 3 times/d for 7–10 d
Famciclovir	250 mg orally 3 times/d for 7–10 d	250 mg orally 3 times/d for 7–10 d	
Valacyclovir	1 gm orally 2 times/d for 7–10 d	1 gm orally 2 times/d for 7–10 d	1 gm orally 2 times/d for 7–10 d
Episodic/recurrent infection[a]			
Acyclovir	800 mg orally 2 times/d for 5 d OR 800 mg orally 3 times/d for 2 d	400 mg orally 3 times/d for 5–10 d	400 mg orally 3 times/d for 5 d OR 800 mg orally 2 times/d for 5 d
Famciclovir	1 gm orally 2 times/d for 1 d OR 500 mg once, followed by 250 mg 2 times/d for 2 d OR 125 mg 2 times/d for 5 d	500 mg orally 2 times/d for 5–10 d	
Valacyclovir	500 mg orally 2 times/d for 3 d OR 1 gm orally once daily for 5 d	1 gm orally 2 times/d for 5–10 d	500 mg orally 2 times/d for 3 d OR 1 gm orally daily for 5 d
Suppression	General Population	HIV	Pregnant at 36 wk Gestation
Acyclovir	400 mg orally 2 times/d	400–800 mg orally 2–3 times/d	400 mg orally 3 times/d
Famciclovir	250 mg orally 2 times/d	500 mg orally 2 times/d	N/A
Valacyclovir	500 mg orally once a day[a] OR 1 gm orally once a day[b]	500 mg orally 2 times/d	500 mg orally 2 times/d

N/A, no specific guidance for pregnant persons.

[a] Doses have been studied for genital HSV-2. Similar doses can be used for genital HSV-1, although the risk of recurrences and transmission is lower than with genital HSV-2 infection.

[b] For those with ≥9 recurrences/y.

The lack of clinical response to guanosine nucleoside analogs suggests acyclovir resistance. Risk factors for the development of acyclovir resistance include prolonged exposure to antivirals, suboptimal dosing, immunosuppression, and ongoing viral replication.[75,76] Resistance most often results from mutations in the gene encoding the viral thymidine kinase (UL23) but may also result from mutation of the viral DNA polymerase (UL30).[32] Foscarnet, a pyrophosphate analogue that inhibits HSV DNA replication, is the treatment of choice for resistant HSV.[52] However, foscarnet use is limited, with only intravenous formulations and significant side effects including nephrotoxicity and electrolyte abnormalities. HSV strains with mutations in UL30 are resistance to both guanosine nucleoside analogs and foscarnet.[77] Case reports describe the use of topical imiquimod, which stimulates localized immune activation, or intralesional or topical cidofovir, a cytosine analogue that inhibits HSV DNA polymerase to treat acyclovir-resistant HSV.[31,78] Helicase-primase inhibitors have potent activity against HSV and are under investigation in human trials and may offer alternative treatment in resistant HSV.[32]

Prevention

Limited tools in addition to suppressive therapy are available to prevent GH transmission. Consistent and correct condom use is associated with a 30% decreased risk of HSV-2 acquisition compared to no condoms use.[79] Studies suggest that condom use is differentially protective in penile-vaginal sex reducing per sex act risk of HSV-2 transmission among HIV-1, HSV-2 serodiscordant couples from cis-men to cis-women by 96% and from cis-women to cis-men by only 65%.[80] The impact of condoms for prevention of transmission during anal sex is not known. HIV prevention studies suggest that penile circumcision may reduce acquisition in cis-men who exclusively have sex with cis-women and reduces cis-male to cis-female HSV-2 transmission.[79,81] Reduction in HSV-2 acquisition is observed in persons taking the acyclic nucleoside phosphonate tenofovir for HIV Pre-Exposure Prophylaxis (PrEP).[81] In one study intravaginal tenofovir gel reduced acquisition of HSV-2.[82] However, this result was not replicated in a second trial, potentially impacted by low adherence to the study drug.[69] Tenofovir as a part of PrEP was shown to protect against incident symptomatic HSV-2 infection in MSM and transgender women.[69] At this time tenofovir use for the sole purpose of preventing GH is not recommended.

COUNSELING

GH is highly stigmatized, and patients often experience distress when learning the diagnosis.[83,84] Accurate, timely information that is patient-centered and fact-based is critical for patient health and wellbeing. **Table 2** provides approaches to frequently asked questions and to patient counseling. GH counseling tools and talking points are also available through the Centers for Disease Control and Prevention and the Canadian Government.[52,85]

THE FUTURE OF GENITAL HERPES PREVENTION AND MANAGEMENT

The high prevalence of genital HSV-1 and HSV-2 infection and the significant impact of recurrent GUD make improvements in diagnostics, prevention, and treatment a high priority. Improvements in the accuracy of serologic diagnostics and wider availability of NAAT testing would allow for more people to know their GH status. Antiviral therapies with new mechanisms of action and delivery mechanisms may allow for greater access to suppressive therapies. Ongoing research into the

Table 2
Counseling messages for persons diagnosed with genital herpes

	Key Points
Transmission	• Transmission occurs through direct skin to skin or mucous membrane contact • Condoms reduce but do not eliminate the possibility of transmission. Use condoms to cover the entire area of exposure • HSV can be transmitted when symptoms are absent • Suppressive antiviral therapy can reduce the risk of transmission
Feelings of shame or guilt	• Sex is a normal and important part of life • Persons living with genital herpes achieve healthy and sexually fulfilling relationships • Having someone to talk to can help. Support groups are available • Genital Herpes is very common • Suppressive therapy helps prevent outbreaks
Pregnancy or Fertility Concerns	• Fertility is not affected • Transmission to the fetus is uncommon and suppression during the last weeks of pregnancy decreases the risk of viral shedding during childbirth
Effect on current partner	• Sex partners should be informed of diagnosis and tested • Most people don't know that they have genital herpes • Available tests are not able to determine when someone became infected.
Finding future sex partners	• Counsel on how to reduce transmission • Risk of transmission is higher during outbreaks • Suppressive therapy and condoms can reduce the risk of transmission • Many people with genital herpes go on to have healthy sex lives
Who they should inform	• The last sexual partner they had, and any current or future ones
Afraid of partner reaction to news	• Support groups are available to discuss with people who are in the same situation • Couple's or individual counseling could help with this anxiety • Reassure that you are there to support the patient
Health Concerns	• Most people with genital herpes have occasional genital outbreaks which can be treated or prevented with antiviral therapy • The virus persists in the body but is mostly in a latent state • Genital herpes does not cause cancer • Genital herpes can increase your risk of acquiring HIV infection if exposed, consider PrEP

development of prophylactic and therapeutic vaccines may provide optimized prevention strategies, and monoclonal antibodies are being developed to prevent neonatal herpes and recurrences.[86] In addition, HSV cure strategies, which include gene editing, are being developed.[87] Work addressing health equity must be pursued to rectify the disparities in GH prevalence among racial and sexual minority populations.

CLINICS CARE POINTS

- Clinical manifestations in primary infection may include genital and systemic symptoms and are more severe than those observed in recurrences.GH can cause atypical and severe clinical manifestations in immunocompromised and pregnant persons.
- Confirm GH using type-specific assays that differentiate between HSV-1 and HSV-2.
- Nucleic acid amplification tests are more sensitive than viral culture and are the preferred test to diagnose GH from genital lesions.
- Type-specific IgG-based antibody tests are the test of choice for HSV serologic testing. However, these assays have high rates of false positivity at low Index-values. Confirm low positive Index-values (<3.0) with a second HSV type-specific assay to avoid inaccurate diagnosis.
- HSV-2 serologic screening is not recommended in the general population.
- Antiviral treatment shortens the duration of clinical manifestations and viral shedding. Start antiviral therapy as soon as possible.
- Suppressive therapy reduces recurrences and transmission in some populations.
- In pregnancy, treat first-episode and recurrent GH with acyclovir or valacyclovir. In severe disease, treat with intravenous acyclovir.
- In pregnant persons, start suppressive acyclovir beginning at 36 weeks gestation to reduce frequency of recurrence and the need for Cesarean delivery.
- In PLWH, a CD4 count less than 200 cells/mm3, and GH, consider suppressive therapy for GH for the first 6 months of ART.
- GH is highly stigmatized, and patients often experience distress when learning the diagnosis. Accurate, timely information is critical for patient health and wellbeing.

DISCLOSURE

N. Van Wagoner and F. Qushair have no disclosures. C. Johnston receives grant funding from Gilead, United States and has served as a consultant to GlaxoSmithKline and Assembly Biosciences. She receives royalties from UpToDate.

REFERENCES

1. Chemaitelly H, Nagelkerke N, Omori R, et al., Characterizing herpes simplex virus type 1 and type 2 seroprevalence declines and epidemiological association in the United States, *PLoS One*, 2019;14(6):e0214151.
2. James C, Harfouche M, Welton NJ, et al. Herpes simplex virus: global infection prevalence and incidence estimates, 2016, *Bull World Health Organ*, 2020;98(5):315–329.
3. McQuillan G, Kruszon-Moran D, Flagg EW, et al. Prevalence of Herpes Simplex Virus Type 1 and Type 2 in Persons Aged 14-49: United States, 2015-2016. NCHS Data Brief 2018;304:1–8.
4. Spicknall IH, Flagg EW, Torrone EA. Estimates of the Prevalence and Incidence of Genital Herpes, United States, 2018. Sex Transm Dis 2021;48(4):260–5.

5. AlMukdad S, Farooqui US, Harfouche M, et al. Epidemiology of herpes simplex virus type 2 in canada, australia, and new zealand: Systematic review, meta-analyses, and meta-regressions. Sex Transm Dis 2022;49(6):403–13.
6. García-Cisneros S, Sánchez-Alemán M, Conde-Glez CJ, et al. Performance of elisa and western blot to detect antibodies against hsv-2 using dried blood spots. J Infect Public Health 2019;12(2):224–8.
7. Uribe-Salas F, Conde-Glez CJ, Juarez-Figueroa L, et al. Socio-demographic characteristics and sex practices related to herpes simplex virus type 2 infection in mexican and central american female sex workers. Epidemiol Infect 2003; 131(2):859–65.
8. Bradley H, Markowitz LE, Gibson T, et al. Seroprevalence of herpes simplex virus types 1 and 2–united states, 1999-2010. J Infect Dis 2014;209(3):325–33.
9. Gorfinkel IS, Aoki F, McNeil S, et al. Seroprevalence of hsv-1 and hsv-2 antibodies in canadian women screened for enrolment in a herpes simplex virus vaccine trial. Int J STD AIDS 2013;24(5):345–9.
10. Sukik L, Alyafei M, Harfouche M, et al. Herpes simplex virus type 1 epidemiology in latin america and the caribbean: Systematic review and meta-analytics. PLoS One 2019;14(4):e0215487.
11. Paz-Bailey G, Ramaswamy M, Hawkes SJ, et al. Herpes simplex virus type 2: Epidemiology and management options in developing countries. Sex Transm Infect 2007;83(1):16–22.
12. Looker KJ, Johnston C, Welton NJ, et al. The global and regional burden of genital ulcer disease due to herpes simplex virus: A natural history modelling study. BMJ Glob Health 2020;5(3):e001875.
13. Silva S, Ayoub HH, Johnston C, et al. Estimated economic burden of genital herpes and hiv attributable to herpes simplex virus type 2 infections in 90 low- and middle-income countries: A modeling study. PLoS Med 2022;19(12):e1003938.
14. Chesson HW, Spicknall IH, Bingham A, et al. The estimated direct lifetime medical costs of sexually transmitted infections acquired in the united states in 2018. Sex Transm Dis 2021;48(4):215–21.
15. Looker KJ, Magaret AS, May MT, et al. First estimates of the global and regional incidence of neonatal herpes infection. Lancet Glob Health 2017;5(3):e300–9.
16. Matthias J, du Bernard S, Schillinger JA, et al. Estimating neonatal herpes simplex virus incidence and mortality using capture-recapture, florida. Clin Infect Dis 2021;73(3):506–12.
17. Shannon B, Yi TJ, Thomas-Pavanel J, et al. Impact of asymptomatic herpes simplex virus type 2 infection on mucosal homing and immune cell subsets in the blood and female genital tract. J Immunol 2014;192(11):5074–82.
18. Looker KJ. Welton NJ. Sabin KM. et al. Global and regional estimates of the contribution of herpes simplex virus type 2 infection to hiv incidence: A population attributable fraction analysis using published epidemiological data, *Lancet Infect Dis*, 2020;20(2):240–249.
19. Silhol R, Coupland H, Baggaley RF, et al. What is the burden of heterosexually acquired hiv due to hsv-2? Global and regional model-based estimates of the proportion and number of hiv infections attributable to hsv-2 infection. J Acquir Immune Defic Syndr 2021;88(1):19–30.
20. Wertheim JO, Hostager R, Ryu D, et al. Discovery of novel herpes simplexviruses in wild gorillas, bonobos, and chimpanzees supports zoonotic origin of hsv-2. Mol Biol Evol 2021;38(7):2818–30.
21. Kurt-Jones EA, Orzalli MH, Knipe DM. Innate immune mechanisms and herpes simplex virus infection and disease. Adv Anat Embryol Cell Biol 2017;223:49–75.

22. Diefenbach RJ, Miranda-Saksena M, Douglas MW, et al. Transport and egress of herpes simplex virus in neurons. Rev Med Virol 2008;18(1):35–51.
23. Langenberg AG, Corey L, Ashley RL, et al. A prospective study of new infections with herpes simplex virus type 1 and type 2. Chiron hsv vaccine study group. N Engl J Med 1999;341(19):1432–8.
24. Corey L, Holmes KK. Genital herpes simplex virus infection: Current concepts in diagnosis, therapy and prevention. Ann Int Med 1983;98:973–83.
25. Patel CD, Backes IM, Taylor SA, et al. Maternal immunization confers protection against neonatal herpes simplex mortality and behavioral morbidity. Sci Transl Med 2019;11(487).
26. Zhu J, Hladik F, Woodward A, et al. Persistence of hiv-1 receptor-positive cells after hsv-2 reactivation is a potential mechanism for increased hiv-1 acquisition. Nat Med 2009;15(8):886–92.
27. Zhu J, Peng T, Johnston C, et al. Immune surveillance by cd8aa+ skin-resident t cells in human herpes virus infection. Nature 2013;497(7450):494–7.
28. Corey L, Adams HG, Brown ZA, et al. Genital herpes simplex virus infections: Clinical manifestations, course, and complications. Ann Intern Med 1983;98(6): 958–72.
29. Chew T, Taylor KE, Mossman KL. Innate and adaptive immune responses to herpes simplex virus. Viruses 2009;1(3):979–1002.
30. Bagdades EK, Pillay D, Squire SB, et al. Relationship between herpes simplex virus ulceration and cd4+ cell counts in patients with hiv infection. Aids 1992;6(11): 1317–20.
31. Leeyaphan C, Surawan TM, Chirachanakul P, et al. Clinical characteristics of hypertrophic herpes simplex genitalis and treatment outcomes of imiquimod: A retrospective observational study. Int J Infect Dis 2015;33:165–70.
32. Schalkwijk HH, Snoeck R, Andrei G. Acyclovir resistance in herpes simplex viruses: Prevalence and therapeutic alternatives. Biochem Pharmacol 2022;206: 115322.
33. Piret J, Boivin G. Resistance of herpes simplex viruses to nucleoside analogues: mechanisms, prevalence, and management. Antimicrob Agents Chemother 2011;55(2):459–72.
34. Benedetti JK, Zeh J, Corey L. Clinical reactivation of genital herpes simplex virus infection decreases in frequency over time. Ann Intern Med 1999;131(1):14–20.
35. Engelberg R, Carrell D, Krantz E, et al. Natural history of genital herpes simplex virus type 1 infection. Sex Transm Dis 2003;30(2):174–7.
36. Ong JJ, Morton AN, Henzell HR, et al. Clinical characteristics of herpes simplex virus urethritis compared with chlamydial urethritis among men. Sex Transm Dis 2017;44(2):121–5.
37. Bradshaw CS, Tabrizi SN, Read TR, et al. Etiologies of nongonococcal urethritis: Bacteria, viruses, and the association with orogenital exposure. J Infect Dis 2006; 193(3):336–45.
38. Marrazzo JM, Martin DH. Management of women with cervicitis. Clin Infect Dis 2007;44(Suppl 3):S102–10.
39. Holmes KK, Sparling PF, Stamm WE, et al. *Sexually transmitted diseases*. New York: The McGraw-Hill Companies; 2007.
40. Pinto-Sander N, Parkes L, Fitzpatrick C, et al. Symptomatic sexually transmitted proctitis in men who have sex with men. Sex Transm Infect 2019;95(6):471.
41. Bissessor M, Fairley CK, Read T, et al. The etiology of infectious proctitis in men who have sex with men differs according to hiv status. Sex Transm Dis 2013; 40(10):768–70.

42. McCormack AL, Rabie N, Whittemore B, et al. Hsv hepatitis in pregnancy: A review of the literature. Obstet Gynecol Surv 2019;74(2):93–8.
43. James SH, Kimberlin DW. Neonatal herpes simplex virus infection. Infect Dis Clin North Am 2015;29(3):391–400.
44. Brown ZA, Benedetti J, Ashley R, et al. Neonatal herpes simplex virus infection in relation to asymptomatic maternal infection at the time of labor. N Engl J Med 1991;324(18):1247–52.
45. Mahant S, Hall M, Schondelmeyer AC, et al. Neonatal herpes simplex virus infection among medicaid-enrolled children: 2009-2015. Pediatrics 2019;143(4).
46. Kimberlin DW, Whitley RJ, Wan W, et al. Oral acyclovir suppression and neurodevelopment after neonatal herpes. N Engl J Med 2011;365(14):1284–92.
47. Kimberlin DW, Lin CY, Jacobs RF, et al. Natural history of neonatal herpes simplex virus infections in the acyclovir era. Pediatrics 2001;108(2):223–9.
48. Strick LB, Wald A. Diagnostics for herpes simplex virus: is PCR the new gold standard? Mol Diagn Ther 2006;10(1):17–28.
49. U.S Food and Drug Administration. Nucleic Acid Based Tests. In Vitro Diagnostics. Available at: https://www.fda.gov/medical-devices/in-vitro-diagnostics/nucleic-acid-based-tests. Accessed January 28, 2023.
50. Page J, Taylor J, Tideman RL, et al. Is hsv serology useful for the management of first episode genital herpes? Sex Transm Infect 2003;79(4):276–9.
51. Morrow R, Friedrich D. Performance of a novel test for IgM and IgG antibodies in subjects with culture-documented genital herpes simplex virus-1 or -2 infection. Clin Microbiol Infect 2006;12(5):463–9.
52. Workowski KA, Bachmann LH, Chan PA, et al. Sexually transmitted infections treatment guidelines, 2021. MMWR Recomm Rep 2021;70(4):1–187.
53. Agyemang E, Le QA, Warren T, et al. Performance of commercial enzyme-linked immunoassays for diagnosis of herpes simplex virus-1 and herpes simplex virus-2 infection in a clinical setting. Sex Transm Dis 2017;44(12):763–7.
54. Elion GB, Furman PA, Fyfe JA, et al. Selectivity of action of an antiherpetic agent, 9-(2-hydroxyethoxymethyl) guanine. Proc Natl Acad Sci U S A 1977;74(12):5716–20.
55. Johnson RE, Mullooly JP, Valanis BG, et al. Utilization and safety of oral acyclovir over an 8-year period. Pharmacoepidemiol Drug Saf 1997;6(2):101–13.
56. Corey L, Benedetti J, Critchlow C, et al. Treatment of primary first-episode genital herpes simplex virus infections with acyclovir: Results of topical, intravenous and oral therapy. J Antimicrob Chemother, 1983;12 (Suppl B):79-88.
57. Sacks SL, Aoki FY, Diaz-Mitoma F, et al. Patient-initiated, twice-daily oral famciclovir for early recurrent genital herpes. A randomized, double-blind multicenter trial. Canadian famciclovir study group. Jama 1996;276(1):44–9.
58. Spruance S, Aoki FY, Tyring S, et al. Short-course therapy for recurrent genital herpes and herpes labialis. J Fam Pract 2007;56(1):30–6.
59. Reitano M, Tyring S, Lang W, et al. Valaciclovir for the suppression of recurrent genital herpes simplex virus infection: A large-scale dose range-finding study. International valaciclovir hsv study group. J Infect Dis 1998;178(3):603–10.
60. Diaz-Mitoma F, Sibbald RG, Shafran SD, et al. Oral famciclovir for the suppression of recurrent genital herpes: A randomized controlled trial. Collaborative famciclovir genital herpes research group. Jama 1998;280(10):887–92.
61. Mertz GJ, Loveless MO, Levin MJ, et al. Oral famciclovir for suppression of recurrent genital herpes simplex virus infection in women. A multicenter, double-blind, placebo-controlled trial. Collaborative famciclovir genital herpes research group. Arch Intern Med 1997;157(3):343–9.

62. Corey L, Wald A, Patel R, et al. Once-daily valacyclovir to reduce the risk of transmission of genital herpes. N Engl J Med 2004;350(1):11–20.
63. Patel R, Tyring S, Strand A, et al. Impact of suppressive antiviral therapy on the health related quality of life of patients with recurrent genital herpes infection. Sex Transm Infect 1999;75(6):398–402.
64. Johnston C, Saracino M, Kuntz S, et al. Standard-dose and high-dose daily antiviral therapy for short episodes of genital hsv-2 reactivation: Three randomised, open-label, cross-over trials. Lancet 2012;379(9816):641–7.
65. Pasternak B, Hviid A. Use of acyclovir, valacyclovir, and famciclovir in the first trimester of pregnancy and the risk of birth defects. JAMA 2010;304(8):859–66.
66. Stone KM, Reiff-Eldridge R, White AD, et al. Pregnancy outcomes following systemic prenatal acyclovir exposure: Conclusions from the international acyclovir pregnancy registry, 1984-1999. Birth Defects Res A Clin Mol Teratol 2004; 70(4):201–7.
67. Ahrens KA, Anderka MT, Feldkamp ML, et al. Antiherpetic medication use and the risk of gastroschisis: Findings from the national birth defects prevention study, 1997-2007. Paediatr Perinat Epidemiol 2013;27(4):340–5.
68. Watts DH, Brown ZA, Money D, et al. A double-blind, randomized, placebo-controlled trial of acyclovir in late pregnancy for the reduction of herpes simplex virus shedding and cesarean delivery. Am J Obstet Gynecol 2003;188(3):836–43.
69. Marrazzo JM, Rabe L, Kelly C, et al. Tenofovir gel for prevention of herpes simplex virus type 2 acquisition: Findings from the voice trial. J Infect Dis 2019; 219(12):1940–7.
70. Posavad CM, Wald A, Kuntz S, et al. Frequent reactivation of herpes simplex virus among hiv-1-infected patients treated with highly active antiretroviral therapy. J Infect Dis 2004;190(4):693–6.
71. Mujugira A, Magaret AS, Celum C, et al. Daily acyclovir to decrease herpes simplex virus type 2 (hsv-2) transmission from hsv-2/hiv-1 coinfected persons: A randomized controlled trial. J Infect Dis 2013;208(9):1366–74.
72. Celum C, Wald A, Lingappa JR, et al. Acyclovir and transmission of hiv-1 from persons infected with hiv-1 and hsv-2. N Engl J Med 2010;362(5):427–39.
73. Lingappa JR, Baeten JM, Wald A, et al. Daily acyclovir for hiv-1 disease progression in people dually infected with hiv-1 and herpes simplex virus type 2: A randomised placebo-controlled trial. Lancet 2010;375(9717):824–33.
74. Van Wagoner N, Geisler WM, Bachmann LH, et al. The effect of valacyclovir on hiv and hsv-2 in hiv-infected persons on antiretroviral therapy with previously unrecognised hsv-2. Int J STD AIDS 2015;26(8):574–81.
75. Englund JA, Zimmerman ME, Swierkosz EM, et al. Herpes simplex virus resistant to acyclovir. A study in a tertiary care center. Ann Intern Med 1990;112(6):416–22.
76. Sellar RS, Peggs KS. Management of multidrug-resistant viruses in the immunocompromised host. Br J Haematol 2012;156(5):559–72.
77. Schmit I, Boivin G. Characterization of the DNA polymerase and thymidine kinase genesof herpes simplex virus isolates from AIDS patients in whom acyclovirand foscarnet therapy sequentially failed. J Infect Dis 1999;180(2):487–90.
78. Jumpertz M, Blaizot R, Couppié P, et al. Intravenous cidofovir for pseudotumoral genital herpes simplex virus infection in two persons living with human immunodeficiency virus (hiv). Int J Dermatol 2023;62(4):e212-e213.
79. Martin ET, Krantz E, Gottlieb SL, et al. A pooled analysis of the effect of condoms in preventing hsv-2 acquisition. Arch Intern Med 2009;169(13):1233–40.

80. Magaret AS, Mujugira A, Hughes JP, et al. Effect of condom use on per-act hsv-2 transmission risk in hiv-1, hsv-2-discordant couples. Clin Infect Dis 2016;62(4): 456–61.
81. Grund JM, Bryant TS, Jackson I, et al. Association between male circumcision and women's biomedical health outcomes: A systematic review. Lancet Glob Health 2017;5(11):e1113–22.
82. Abdool Karim SS, Abdool Karim Q, Kharsany AB, et al. Tenofovir gel for the prevention of herpes simplex virus type 2 infection. N Engl J Med 2015;373(6):530–9.
83. Melville J, Sniffen S, Crosby R, et al. Psychosocial impact of serological diagnosis of herpes simplex virus type 2: A qualitative assessment. Sex Transm Infect 2003; 79(4):280–5.
84. Romanowski B, Zdanowicz YM, Owens ST. In search of optimal genital herpes management and standard of care (INSIGHTS): doctors' and patients' perceptions of genital herpes. Sex Transm Infect 2008;84(1):51–6.
85. Steben M., and Fisher W.A., Genital Herpes Counselling Tool. Government of Canada 2019 [cited 2023 January 22, 2023].
86. Backes IM, Byrd BK, Slein MD, et al. Maternally transferred mabs protect neonatal mice from hsv-induced mortality and morbidity. J Exp Med 2022; 219(12).
87. Aubert M, Strongin DE, Roychoudhury P, et al. Gene editing and elimination of latent herpes simplex virus in vivo. Nat Commun 2020;11(1):4148.

An Ulcer by Any Other Name
Non-herpes and Non-syphilis Ulcerative Sexually Transmitted Infections

Ronnie M. Gravett, MD*, Jeanne Marrazzo, MD, MPH

KEYWORDS

- Genital ulcer disease • Ulcer • Lymphogranuloma venereum • Chancroid
- Donovanosis • Mpox virus

KEY POINTS

- Ulcerative sexually transmitted infection (STI) syndromes overlap, so travel and exposure history lay the foundation for diagnosis.
- Ulcerative STIs co-occur with HIV often and increase the risk of HIV acquisition.
- Laboratory resources to confirm the diagnosis may not be available, so syndromic management may be reasonable.

INTRODUCTION

Ulcerative sexually transmitted infections (STIs), often termed genital ulcer disease (GUD), encompass a variety of pathogens beyond herpes simplex virus (HSV) or syphilis. Owing to this variety, these ulcerative diseases may mystify even the most seasoned and experienced sexual health clinicians. Ulcerative infections are not solely relegated to the genitals; indeed, oral, anal, and genital ulcers may be caused by sexually transmitted pathogens. History and physical examination can inform the diagnosis but ultimately dedicated laboratory testing (as available) is necessary for confirmation.[1,2] Even still, more than a quarter of GUD may never have a confirmed diagnosis.[3] Ulcerative STIs and GUD have been consistently associated with increased chances of HIV acquisition as well as a higher incidence among people living with HIV.[4] This narrative review will focus on the history, epidemiology, clinical features, diagnosis, and management of ulcerative STIs, aside from HSV and syphilis, with emphasis on new and emerging literature.

Division of Infectious Diseases, Department of Medicine, Heersink School of Medicine, University of Alabama at Birmingham, THT 215, 1900 University Boulevard, Birmingham, AL 35294, USA
* Corresponding author.
E-mail address: rgravett@uabmc.edu

Infect Dis Clin N Am 37 (2023) 369–380
https://doi.org/10.1016/j.idc.2023.02.005
0891-5520/23/© 2023 Elsevier Inc. All rights reserved.

id.theclinics.com

LYMPHOGRANULOMA VENEREUM

Lymphogranuloma venereum (LGV), caused by the intracellular pathogen *Chlamydia trachomatis*, causes a particularly morbid clinical syndrome, contrasting with other chlamydial syndromes.[2,5–7] *C trachomatis* serovars L1, L2, and L3 cause LGV, whereas serovars D-K cause the common sexually transmitted urethral, cervical, and anorectal mucosal infections. The LGV syndrome stems from the lymphoinvasive nature of the L1-3 serovars and its progression from a mucosal inoculation into deeper tissues and subsequent potentially serious complications.

History and Epidemiology

Historically, LGV was characterized as a rare tropical disease primarily affecting cisgender, heterosexual persons with the classic presentation as a genital ulcer on the penis, vagina, or vulva and associated inguinal lymphadenopathy.[8] During the last 2 decades, this epidemiology shifted tremendously. Now, the significant majority of new LGV cases occur among gay, bisexual, and other men who have sex with men (MSM). This shift, initially reported in Europe, has now led to changes in LGV trends globally.[9–17] LGV currently overwhelmingly affects MSM and primarily causes a proctocolitis syndrome.[7,18] Among MSM, early reports in LGV trends revealed a significant burden among those living with HIV but more recent reports indicate a significant increase among HIV-negative MSM also.[9,12,15–17,19–24] This is likely a reflection of mixing of sexual networks among MSM with less regard to serostatus or sexual serosorting, which could be attributed to increased use of preexposure prophylaxis and treatment as prevention.

Clinical Features

The invasive nature of LGV distinguishes it from other ulcerative STIs. Classically, LGV starts with a relatively painless genital papule that would then ulcerate, which may go unnoticed. Simultaneously, the pathogen would invade the lymphatic system, leading to profound inguinal lymphadenopathy. These buboes would show the characteristic "groove sign" as the inguinal ligament traverses over enlarged lymph nodes but this inguinal lymphadenopathy is not present in anorectal infection due to drainage to different regional lymph nodes. The current LGV outbreak consistently features a severe anorectal proctitis, characterized by a papule that transforms into a perianal or perirectal ulcer, anal discharge, or drainage that may be bloody or mucopurulent, severe pain, and tenesmus. LGV may be misdiagnosed as inflammatory bowel disease or even malignancy.[25,26] Urethral LGV is much less common comparatively.[27] Interestingly, asymptomatic LGV-specific *C trachomatis* infection has been noted in retrospective specimen analysis, which makes it difficult to detect at a population level because LGV testing is generally directed by clinical syndrome.[28,29] If LGV remains untreated, then it may progress to a severe fibrosing stage with possible strictures and even elephantiasis.[20,30]

Diagnosis

Specific nucleic acid amplification testing (NAAT) is the primary methodology for confirming LGV but this is challenging given it is not widely available. LGV, by case definition, will test positive for *C trachomatis* using widely available NAAT testing aimed at serovar D-K infection.[31] Further typing to detect an LGV-specific genovar is available via certain laboratories using laboratory-derived assays but these are not United States Food and Drug Administration (FDA)-approved.[32] Culture is possible for *C trachomatis* but this is technically challenging and does not delineate LGV biovar versus mucosal biovar. Serology is available and has been used for diagnosing LGV but this is neither widely available nor especially sensitive nor specific and may be less useful in anorectal disease.[33]

Treatment

Doxycycline 100 mg PO bid for 21 days is the long-established treatment of LGV.[2,5] This is based on expert opinion, retrospective observation, and some clinical trials. If doxycycline cannot be used due to allergy or other factor, such as pregnancy, then azithromycin 1 g weekly for 3 weeks is a reasonable alternative. Beyond that, salvage therapies may include erythromycin or moxifloxacin.[5] Adjunctive therapy such as bubo aspiration or abscess drainage can help with symptomatic management as well.

CHANCROID

Caused by the gram-negative pathogen, *Haemophilus ducreyi*, chancroid is a declining cause of ulcerative STIs, yet it is a now recognized as cause of chronic skin ulceration.[34] *H ducreyi* has been divided into 2 classes, Class I and Class II, based on genomic and proteomic analyses, yet both classes may be isolated from chancroid genital disease as well as chronic skin ulcers.[35–37]

Epidemiology and Transmission

Epidemiologic trends for chancroid, and *H ducreyi* infections in general, are challenging to monitor due to the difficulty in confirming diagnoses. Direct skin contact transmits the pathogen rather effectively at even a very low organism burden with only 30 colony forming units causing clinically apparent papules.[38] The largest proportion of chancroid occurs in Africa, although with considerable variation across the continent, India, and the South Pacific.[39] In the United States, since 2000, less than 100 cases have been diagnosed each year, and fewer than 5 cases have been diagnosed per year since 2016.[40] Although chancroid remains a cause of GUD, more recent reports from Zimbabwe and South Africa have reported far fewer cases.[41,42]

Clinical Features

The hallmark feature of chancroid is one or multiple painful ulcers that may be accompanied by inguinal lymphadenopathy. Often after an average incubation of 3 to 7 days after exposure, the lesion begins as a papule and progresses to a pustule that then ulcerates, and these ulcers may even coalesce.[2,34,43] The edges of the ulcer are not typically indurated or heaped, and they may be ragged without significant surrounding inflammation. Ulcer bases may feature granulating exudate. Inguinal lymphadenitis may be large and painful. Systemic symptoms are not typically present.

Diagnosis

Chancroid diagnosis can be confirmed with NAAT or culture but these are technically challenging and not widely available. In fact, there is no FDA-approved NAAT test available for *H ducreyi*, so NAATs must be laboratory-derived. The fastidious organism requires hemin supplementation with microaerophilic incubation at 33°C to 35°C to culture, so in vitro isolation can be challenging.[34,44] Because confirmed diagnosis is so challenging, the case definition of chancroid includes typical clinical features of a one or more painful ulcers, the presentation of the ulcers and syndrome are consistent with chancroid, and negative results for comprehensive testing for syphilis (lesion-directed or serologic testing at least 1 week after onset) and HSV (culture or NAAT).[2]

Management

Chancroid treatment has largely remained unchanged as cases dwindle globally. Many options are available for treating chancroid: azithromycin 1 g orally once in a single dose, ceftriaxone 250 mg as a single intramuscular injection dose, ciprofloxacin 500 mg BID orally for 3 days, or erythromycin 500 mg orally tid for 7 days.[2] Notably, a Cochrane review did not show that macrolides were better than other treatment options.[45]

GRANULOMA INGUINALE

Granuloma inguinale (GI), also termed donovanosis, is caused by an infection with *Klebsiella granulomatis*, and similar to chancroid, incident cases of this pathogen seem to be declining globally. *K granulomatis* is an intracellular pathogen with the pathognomonic Donovan bodies, bipolar densities that stain with Giemsa or silver.[44]

Epidemiology

New cases of GI are declining considerably even in areas with the highest rates, such as equatorial Africa, India, and Papua New Guinea.[46,47] South African prevalence during the last several years is only roughly 2% as diagnosed by molecular assay because stain-confirmed cases were not identified.[48] Interestingly, by medical billing codes, 50 cases were identified among US armed services members serving in endemic areas from 2011 to 2020.[49]

Clinical Features

Similar to other ulcerative STIs, the initial lesion begins as an indurated papule that then later ulcerates. However, the incubation period may be very long, up to 50 days, and the lesion progresses more slowly when compared with other ulcerative STIs.[50] The most common, or even classic, presentation is a beefy-red, nontender ulcer that bleeds easily. Three other less common manifestations may be seen: hypertrophic, verrucous with elevated ragged edge; necrotic with extensive tissue damage, drainage, and often foul odor; and sclerotic with fibrosing scar tissue.[50–52] Contrasting to LGV and chancroid, true lymphadenitis is not common, although there may be subcutaneous swelling which could be mistaken for the bubo associated with LGV, a phenomenon sometimes termed a pseudobubo. Lesions more often occur on the coronal sulcus, prepuce, and glans penis in persons with a penis and the labia minora and fourchette in persons with a vagina.[44,51] Cervical lesions have also been described. Extragenital lesions affecting the oropharynx have uncommonly been described also.

Diagnosis

Diagnostic microscopy with Giema or silver stain on tissue biopsy, crush prep, or smear showing pathognomonic Donovan bodies can more readily establish the diagnosis. Staining reveals intracytoplasmic or intravacuolar organisms. NAAT tests are not commercially available, and laboratory-derived NAATs are uncommon. Culture for this pathogen has been very difficult and rarely accomplished. Thus, diagnosis often relies on consistent clinical examination and history in an endemic area after syndromic treatment of syphilis, genital herpes, and chancroid has not demonstrated improvement.

Treatment

Treatment should be continued until lesions are healed and no less than 3 weeks. Azithromycin is the first line regimen, as either 1 g weekly or 500 mg daily.[2,50,51]

Doxycycline 100 mg orally twice daily, trimethoprim sulfamethoxazole 160 mg/800 mg orally twice daily, and erythromycin 500 mg 4 times daily are alternatives. Resolution is often slow, and healing progresses from ulcer margins inward.

MPOX VIRUS

Emerging unexpectedly, the 2022 outbreak of mpox virus (MPV) should not be considered a resurgence; rather, the MPV outbreak beginning in 2022 is seemingly quite different than earlier MPV outbreaks. MPV is an orthopoxvirus that has historically been described as 2 clades, Clade 1 (previously Congo Basin Clade) and Clade 2 (West African Clade) but more recent phylogenetic studies demonstrate that the new 2022 outbreak may be due to a novel clade, Clade 3, that arose from Clade 2.[53] MPV has been long established as an endemic and zoonotic disease causing infrequent, clustered outbreaks until 2022, when a large, multinational outbreak occurred. Akin to LGV, MPV evolved significantly in both epidemiology and clinical features.

Epidemiology and Transmission

In years past, MPV was largely limited to endemic areas in central and western Africa, where an animal reservoir remains active with small mammals (not monkeys as suggested by the name), or as imported cases from endemic areas.[54,55] More recent outbreaks beginning in Nigeria in 2017 to 2018 demonstrated person-to-person spread, making public health control measures even more imperative.[56–58] Many of these outbreaks remained clustered and were managed with classic infection control practices: isolation, contact tracing, and, in some cases, vaccination for preexposure and postexposure prophylaxis.[54] Despite this, cases still occur outside of endemic areas and often without report of known exposure.[59,60] The 2022 MPV outbreak is considerably different. First, this outbreak overwhelmingly affects gay, bisexual, and other men who have sex with men (GBM).[61,62] Second, MPV is well established to transmit through direct skin-to-skin contact, which remains true, yet mounting evidence shows that MPV is efficiently transmitted sexually, supported by genital, anal, and oropharyngeal lesions, presence of viable MPV in semen samples, and also transmission among sexual contacts and within sociosexual networks.[63–65] Additionally, STIs and HIV accompany MPV infection frequently, and persons living with HIV are significantly affected by MPV.[66–68]

Clinical Features

The hallmark clinical feature of MPV is the classic rash, characterized by a progression of lesions that may affect any body part as well as systemic syndrome with fever, chills, myalgias.[61,62,69] The skin lesions, which are often quite painful or itchy, may progress from a papule to vesicle to umbilicated pustule to ulcer before finally crusting and healing in resolution. As we have learned from other STIs manifesting as dermatoses, not all clinical syndromes strictly follow this progression. In fact, MPV may present as scattered, pustular lesions, fooling the clinician into thinking these lesions may be acne or folliculitis if no adequate sexual or exposure history is discussed. Importantly, MPV has been heralded by the emergence of exquisitely painful lesions on the genitals, anus, and within the oropharynx, sites not previously frequently affected by MPV. These lesions can lead to scarring and permanent disfigurement, especially if the condition remains untreated. MPV affecting the eye and eye structures has also been described.[70] Although the 2022 outbreak may belong to a novel clade with expected lower mortality, severe cases resulting in hospitalization and deaths due to

MPV have now been reported in persons with weakened immune systems, such as advanced, uncontrolled HIV.[71]

Diagnosis

Unless the classic rash and syndrome is present, this diagnosis may be challenging given potential variation in skin lesions. A case may be suspected based on characteristic rash with a consistent sexual or exposure history within 21 days of symptom onset but MPV is confirmed using NAAT tests detecting MPV DNA or by MPV recovered in viral culture.[72]

Prevention and Management

In contrast to the coronavirus disease 2019 pandemic, tools for managing the MPV were established, although not widely available. Similar to the early HIV epidemic, behavioral changes among those with the highest risk for MPV acquisition, that is, GBM, can temper the trajectory of the outbreak but these behavioral changes must be adjunctive to equitable implementation of proven effective biomedical strategies, such as vaccination.[73] Currently, there are 2 products available for vaccination: modified vaccinia Ankara (MVA) vaccine, a live replication-deficient virus, and ACAM2000, a live attenuated virus. MVA seems most promising for preventing MPV infection. It produces robust neutralizing antibody titers and is safe among HIV-negative persons as well as persons living with HIV, yet real-world clinical efficacy data are lacking, although growing.[74,75] Early, noncontrolled prospective data support MVA as an effective vaccination for preventing MPV infection, and infections after MVA vaccination are few and have generally occurred before peak antibody titers.[76,77] Although MVA may be effective at prevention, its availability limits its effectiveness to protect priority populations; in effort to mitigate the shortage, intradermal administration using 20% of the standard reaches similar levels of neutralizing antibodies and may be viable strategy to reach greater number of persons at risk.[78,79] MVA vaccination may also be used as postexposure prophylaxis strategy if administered within 4 days of an exposure. It is imperative that MPV vaccination be implemented equitably to the persons disproportionately affected; using LGBTQ + events, particularly events highlighting LGBTQ + communities of color, vaccination can be centralized to reach the communities with greatest need.[80,81] Furthermore, MPV vaccination can serve as an opportunity to reach this priority population with wrap-around HIV services, such as testing and linkage to treatment or preexposure prophylaxis.[73,82]

Treatment of MPV is largely considered supportive for symptomatic management, but for persons with severe disease with systemic involvement, lesions in vulnerable areas, for example, genitals, anus, eyes, or oropharynx, or in persons with significant immunocompromise, tecovirimat can be used as a directed antiviral treatment. Tecovirimat has been FDA-approved via the "animal rule" but it is under Investigational New Drug authorization.[83–86] Additionally, cidofovir and brincidofovir are active against MPV but clinical efficacy data are lacking and higher chance for adverse effects reduce their utility.[87,88]

SUMMARY

Ulcerative STIs persist globally and domestically, although chancroid and GI are clearly significantly declining.[39,89] Yet, although some diseases are declining, new outbreaks of MPV and LGV are gaining traction after an epidemiologic evolution. Ulcerative syndromes overlap considerably: papules progressing to pustules and finally to ulcers is not necessarily specific to any one condition. Thus, particular attention to the nature of lesion, exposure history, and regional endemicity are vital to making the diagnosis. Syndromic approach to managing GUD may have contributed to a decline in some cases.[39,41,90,91] Critically, syndromic management, although initially directed at syphilis and HSV, is a key component in regions where resources for a confirmed diagnosis are limited.[1] Beyond treatment of these syndromes, treatment of LGV, chancroid, and GI may overlap enough (ie, doxycycline or azithromycin as primary or alternative treatment) such that there is may be some efficacy without confirmed diagnosis, although duration of treatment will be different pending on likely disease.

These infections cause substantial morbidity and increase the chances of acquiring HIV.[4] Ulcerative STIs not only cause a mucosal defect that becomes the open door for HIV but they also lead to inflammation and lymphocyte recruitment to be the targets of invading HIV virions.[4,92] Indeed, HIV and ulcerative STIs co-occur at high rates, which is more likely a consequence of sociosexual networks. Understanding this, ulcerative STI management should serve as an opportunity to screen for HIV and link to either treatment or prevention services.[2]

As clinicians encounter ulcerative diseases affecting the genitals, anus, and even oropharynx, a thorough history exploring sexual and travel exposures and careful physical examination are crucial to diagnosing and managing these syndromes.[1,2] A comprehensive approach managing these syndromes, including attention to HIV risk, can reduce the morbidity burden and continue to reduce the impact of these diseases as they decline.

CLINICS CARE POINTS

- Ulcerative STI syndromes can be challenging to diagnosis with confirmatory testing.
- Syndromic management may be reasonable while awaiting confirmatory results.
- It is imperative to treat ulcerative STIs to slow transmission, reduce morbidity, and prevent acquisition.

DISCLOSURE

The authors have nothing to disclose.

REFERENCES

1. World Health Organization. Guidelines for the management of symptomatic sexually transmitted infections. Geneva: World Health Organization © World Health Organization; 2021. p. 2021.
2. Workowski KA, Bachmann Laura H, Chan Philip A, et al. Sexually Transmitted Infections Treatment Guidelines, 2021. MMWR Recomm Rep (Morb Mortal Wkly Rep) 2021;70(No RR-4):1–187.
3. DiCarlo RP, David HDH. The Clinical Diagnosis of Genital Ulcer Disease in Men. Clin Infect Dis 1997;25(2):292–8.
4. Mayer KH, Venkatesh KK. Interactions of HIV, Other Sexually Transmitted Diseases, and Genital Tract Inflammation Facilitating Local Pathogen Transmission and Acquisition. Am J Reprod Immunol 2011;65(3):308–16.
5. de Vries HJC, de Barbeyrac B, de Vrieze NHN, et al. European guideline on the management of lymphogranuloma venereum. J Eur Acad Dermatol Venereol 2019;33(10):1821–8.

6. de Vrieze NH, van Rooijen M, Schim van der Loeff MF, et al. Anorectal and inguinal lymphogranuloma venereum among men who have sex with men in Amsterdam, The Netherlands: trends over time, symptomatology and concurrent infections. Sex Transm Infect 2013;89(7):548–52.

7. Gravett RM, Marrazzo J. What's Old Is New: the Evolution of Lymphogranuloma Venereum Proctitis in Persons Living with HIV. Curr Infect Dis Rep 2022;24(8): 97–104.

8. Mabey D, Peeling RW. Lymphogranuloma venereum. Sexually Transmitted Infections 2002;78(2):90–2.

9. Cabello Úbeda A, Fernández Roblas R, García Delgado R, et al. Anorectal Lymphogranuloma Venereum in Madrid: A Persistent Emerging Problem in Men Who Have Sex With Men. Sex Transm Dis 2016;43(7):414–9.

10. Centers for Disease Control and Prevention. Lymphogranuloma venereum among men who have sex with men–Netherlands, 2003-2004. MMWR Morbidity and mortality weekly report 2004;53(42):985–8.

11. Childs T, Simms I, Alexander S, et al. Rapid increase in lymphogranuloma venereum in men who have sex with men, United Kingdom, 2003 to September 2015. Euro Surveill 2015;20(48):30076.

12. De Baetselier I, Tsoumanis A, Verbrugge R, et al. Lymphogranuloma venereum is on the rise in Belgium among HIV negative men who have sex with men: surveillance data from 2011 until the end of June 2017. BMC Infect Dis 2018;18(1):689.

13. de Barbeyrac B, Laurier-Nadalié C, Touati A, et al. Observational study of anorectal Chlamydia trachomatis infections in France through the lymphogranuloma venereum surveillance network, 2010-2015. Int J STD AIDS 2018;29(12):1215–24.

14. Neves JM, Ramos Pinheiro R, Côrte-Real R, et al. Lymphogranuloma venereum: a retrospective analysis of an emerging sexually transmitted disease in a Lisbon Tertiary Center. J Eur Acad Dermatol Venereol 2021;35(8):1712–6.

15. Pathela P, Jamison K, Kornblum J, et al. Lymphogranuloma Venereum: An Increasingly Common Anorectal Infection Among Men Who Have Sex With Men Attending New York City Sexual Health Clinics. Sex Transm Dis 2019;46(2):e14–7.

16. Peuchant O, Touati A, Laurier-Nadalié C, et al. Prevalence of lymphogranuloma venereum among anorectal Chlamydia trachomatis-positive MSM using pre-exposure prophylaxis for HIV. Sex Transm Infect 2020;96(8):615–7.

17. Prochazka M, Charles H, Allen H, et al. Rapid Increase in Lymphogranuloma Venereum among HIV-Negative Men Who Have Sex with Men, England, 2019. Emerg Infect Dis 2021;27(10):2695–9.

18. Parra-Sánchez M, García-Rey S, Pueyo Rodríguez I, et al. Clinical and epidemiological characterisation of lymphogranuloma venereum in southwest Spain, 2013-2015. Sex Transm Infect 2016;92(8):629–31.

19. Cole MJ, Field N, Pitt R, et al. Substantial underdiagnosis of lymphogranuloma venereum in men who have sex with men in Europe: preliminary findings from a multicentre surveillance pilot. Sex Transm Infect 2020;96(2):137–42.

20. de Voux A, Kent JB, Macomber K, et al. Notes from the Field: Cluster of Lymphogranuloma Venereum Cases Among Men Who Have Sex with Men - Michigan. MMWR Morbidity and mortality weekly report 2016;65(34):920–1.

21. Repiso-Jiménez JB, Millán-Cayetano JF, Salas-Márquez C, et al. Lymphogranuloma Venereum in a Public Health Service Hospital in Southern Spain: A Clinical and Epidemiologic Study. Actas Dermosifiliogr (Engl Ed). 2020;111(9):743–51.

22. Rönn MM, Ward H. The association between lymphogranuloma venereum and HIV among men who have sex with men: systematic review and meta-analysis. BMC Infect Dis 2011;11:70.

23. Sentís A, Martin-Sanchez M, Arando M, et al. Sexually transmitted infections in young people and factors associated with HIV coinfection: an observational study in a large city. BMJ Open 2019;9(5):e027245.
24. van Aar F, Kroone MM, de Vries HJ, et al. Increasing trends of lymphogranuloma venereum among HIV-negative and asymptomatic men who have sex with men, the Netherlands, 2011 to 2017. Euro Surveill 2020;25(14).
25. Bosma JW, van Tienhoven AJ, Thiesbrummel HF, et al. Delayed diagnosis of lymphogranuloma venereum in a hospital setting - a retrospective observational study. Int J STD AIDS 2021;32(6):517–22.
26. Gallegos M, Bradly D, Jakate S, et al. Lymphogranuloma venereum proctosigmoiditis is a mimicker of inflammatory bowel disease. World J Gastroenterol 2012;18(25):3317–21.
27. de Vrieze NHN, Versteeg B, Bruisten SM, et al. Low Prevalence of Urethral Lymphogranuloma Venereum Infections Among Men Who Have Sex With Men: A Prospective Observational Study, Sexually Transmitted Infection Clinic in Amsterdam, the Netherlands. Sex Transm Dis 2017;44(9):547–50.
28. Hughes Y, Chen MY, Fairley CK, et al. Universal lymphogranuloma venereum (LGV) testing of rectal chlamydia in men who have sex with men and detection of asymptomatic LGV. Sex Transm Infect 2022;98(8):582–5.
29. Saxon C, Hughes G, Ison C. Asymptomatic Lymphogranuloma Venereum in Men who Have Sex with Men, United Kingdom. Emerg Infect Dis 2016;22(1):112–6.
30. Craxford L, Fox A. Lymphogranuloma venereum: a rare and forgotten cause of rectal stricture formation. Int J STD AIDS 2018;29(11):1133–5.
31. Touati A, Laurier-Nadalié C, Bébéar C, et al. Evaluation of four commercial real-time PCR assays for the detection of lymphogranuloma venereum in Chlamydia trachomatis-positive anorectal samples. Clin Microbiol Infect 2021;27(6):909, e1-e5.
32. Kersh EN, Pillay A, de Voux A, et al. Laboratory Processes for Confirmation of Lymphogranuloma Venereum Infection During a 2015 Investigation of a Cluster of Cases in the United States. Sex Transm Dis 2017;44(11):691–4.
33. Allen H, Pitt R, Bardsley M, et al. Investigating the decline in Lymphogranuloma venereum diagnoses in men who have sex with men in the United Kingdom since 2016: an analysis of surveillance data. Sex Health 2020;17(4):344–51.
34. Lewis DA, Mitjà O. Haemophilus ducreyi: from sexually transmitted infection to skin ulcer pathogen. Curr Opin Infect Dis 2016;29(1):52–7.
35. Ricotta EE, Wang N, Cutler R, et al. Rapid divergence of two classes of Haemophilus ducreyi. J Bacteriol 2011;193(12):2941–7.
36. Grant JC, González-Beiras C, Amick KM, et al. Multiple Class I and Class II Haemophilus ducreyi Strains Cause Cutaneous Ulcers in Children on an Endemic Island. Clin Infect Dis 2018;67(11):1768–74.
37. Gangaiah D, Spinola SM. Haemophilus ducreyi Cutaneous Ulcer Strains Diverged from Both Class I and Class II Genital Ulcer Strains: Implications for Epidemiological Studies. PLoS Negl Trop Dis 2016;10(12):e0005259.
38. Janowicz DM, Ofner S, Katz BP, et al. Experimental infection of human volunteers with Haemophilus ducreyi: fifteen years of clinical data and experience. J Infect Dis 2009;199(11):1671–9.
39. González-Beiras C, Marks M, Chen CY, et al. Epidemiology of Haemophilus ducreyi Infections. Emerg Infect Dis 2016;22(1):1–8.
40. Centers for Disease Control and Prevention, Sexually Transmitted Disease Surveillance 2020, Available at: https://www.cdc.gov/std/statistics/2020/overview.htm, 2022. Accessed November 15, 2022.

41. Kularatne RS, Muller EE, Maseko DV, et al. Trends in the relative prevalence of genital ulcer disease pathogens and association with HIV infection in Johannesburg, South Africa, 2007-2015. PLoS One 2018;13(4):e0194125.
42. Mungati M, Machiha A, Mugurungi O, et al. The Etiology of Genital Ulcer Disease and Coinfections With Chlamydia trachomatis and Neisseria gonorrhoeae in Zimbabwe: Results From the Zimbabwe STI Etiology Study. Sex Transm Dis 2018;45(1):61–8.
43. Lautenschlager S, Kemp M, Christensen JJ, et al. European guideline for the management of chancroid. Int J STD AIDS 2017;28(4):324–9.
44. Bennett JD, Raphael, Blaser Martin. Mandell, Douglas, and Bennett's Principles and practice of infectious diseases. 9th edition. Elsevier Health Sciences; 2020.
45. Romero L, Huerfano C, Grillo-Ardila CF. Macrolides for treatment of Haemophilus ducreyi infection in sexually active adults. Cochrane Database Syst Rev 2017; 12(12):Cd012492.
46. Ray K, Bala M, Gupta SM, et al. Changing trends in sexually transmitted infections at a Regional STD Centre in north India. Indian J Med Res 2006;124(5):559–68.
47. Bright A. National Notifiable Diseases Surveillance System surveillance report: Sexually transmissible infections in Aboriginal and Torres Strait Islander people. Commun Dis Intell Q Rep 2015;39(4):E584–9.
48. Boulle A, Davies M-A, Hussey H, et al. Risk factors for COVID-19 death in a population cohort study from the Western Cape Province, South Africa. Clin Infect Dis 2020;73(7):e2005–15.
49. Daniele D, Wilkerson T. Surveillance Snapshot: Donovanosis Among Active Component Service Members, U.S. Armed Forces, 2011-2020. Msmr 2021; 28(12):22.
50. O'Farrell N, Moi H. European guideline on donovanosis. Int J STD AIDS 2016; 27(8):605–7.
51. O'Farrell N, Hoosen A, Kingston M. UK national guideline for the management of donovanosis. Int J STD AIDS 2018;29(10):946–8.
52. Rajam RV, Rangiah PN, World Health O. Donovanosis (granuloma inguinale, granuloma venereum/R. V. Rajam, P. N. Rangiah. Geneva: World Health Organization; 1954.
53. Isidro J, Borges V, Pinto M, et al. Phylogenomic characterization and signs of microevolution in the 2022 multi-country outbreak of monkeypox virus. Nat Med 2022;28(8):1569–72.
54. Update: multistate outbreak of monkeypox–Illinois, Indiana, Kansas, Missouri, Ohio, and Wisconsin. MMWR Morbidity and mortality weekly report 2003; 52(27):642–6.
55. Durski KN, McCollum AM, Nakazawa Y, et al. Emergence of Monkeypox - West and Central Africa, 1970-2017. MMWR Morbidity and mortality weekly report 2018;67(10):306–10.
56. Eteng WE, Mandra A, Doty J, et al. Notes from the Field: Responding to an Outbreak of Monkeypox Using the One Health Approach - Nigeria, 2017-2018. MMWR Morbidity and mortality weekly report 2018;67(37):1040–1.
57. Ogoina D, Izibewule JH, Ogunleye A, et al. The 2017 human monkeypox outbreak in Nigeria-Report of outbreak experience and response in the Niger Delta University Teaching Hospital, Bayelsa State, Nigeria. PLoS One 2019; 14(4):e0214229.
58. Yinka-Ogunleye A, Aruna O, Dalhat M, et al. Outbreak of human monkeypox in Nigeria in 2017–18: a clinical and epidemiological report. Lancet Infect Dis 2019;19(8):872–9.

59. Mauldin MR, McCollum AM, Nakazawa YJ, et al. Exportation of Monkeypox Virus From the African Continent. J Infect Dis 2022;225(8):1367–76.

60. Rao AK, Schulte J, Chen TH, et al. Monkeypox in a Traveler Returning from Nigeria - Dallas, Texas, 2021. MMWR Morbidity and mortality weekly report 2022;71(14):509–16.

61. Philpott D, Hughes CM, Alroy KA, et al. Epidemiologic and Clinical Characteristics of Monkeypox Cases - United States, May 17-July 22, 2022. MMWR Morbidity and mortality weekly report 2022;71(32):1018–22.

62. Thornhill JP, Barkati S, Walmsley S, et al. Monkeypox Virus Infection in Humans across 16 Countries - April-June 2022. N Engl J Med 2022;387(8):679–91.

63. Spicknall IH, Pollock ED, Clay PA, et al. Modeling the Impact of Sexual Networks in the Transmission of Monkeypox virus Among Gay, Bisexual, and Other Men Who Have Sex with Men - United States, 2022. MMWR Morbidity and mortality weekly report 2022;71(35):1131–5.

64. Lapa D, Carletti F, Mazzotta V, et al. Monkeypox virus isolation from a semen sample collected in the early phase of infection in a patient with prolonged seminal viral shedding. Lancet Infect Dis 2022;22(9):1267–9.

65. Palich R, Burrel S, Monsel G, et al. Viral loads in clinical samples of men with monkeypox virus infection: a French case series. Lancet Infect Dis 2023;23(1):80.

66. Curran KG, Eberly K, Russell OO, et al. HIV and Sexually Transmitted Infections Among Persons with Monkeypox - Eight U.S. Jurisdictions. MMWR Morbidity and mortality weekly report 2022;71(36):1141–7.

67. Hoffmann C, Jessen H, Wyen C, et al. Clinical characteristics of monkeypox virus infections among men with and without HIV: A large outbreak cohort in Germany. HIV Med 2022. https://doi.org/10.1111/hiv.13378.

68. Angelo KM, Smith T, Camprubí-Ferrer D, et al. Epidemiological and clinical characteristics of patients with monkeypox in the GeoSentinel Network: a cross-sectional study. Lancet Infect Dis 2022;23(2):196–206.

69. Adler H, Gould S, Hine P, et al. Clinical features and management of human monkeypox: a retrospective observational study in the UK. Lancet Infect Dis 2022; 22(8):1153–62.

70. Cash-Goldwasser S, Labuda SM, McCormick DW, et al. Ocular Monkeypox - United States, July-September 2022. MMWR Morbidity and mortality weekly report 2022;71(42):1343–7.

71. Miller MJ, Cash-Goldwasser S, Marx GE, et al. Severe Monkeypox in Hospitalized Patients — United States, August 10–October 10, 2022. MMWR Morb Mortal Wkly Rep 2022;71(44):1412–7.

72. Aden TA, Blevins P, York SW, et al. Rapid Diagnostic Testing for Response to the Monkeypox Outbreak - Laboratory Response Network, United States, May 17-June 30, 2022. MMWR Morbidity and mortality weekly report 2022;71(28):904–7.

73. Delaney KP, Sanchez T, Hannah M, et al. Strategies Adopted by Gay, Bisexual, and Other Men Who Have Sex with Men to Prevent Monkeypox virus Transmission - United States, 2022. MMWR Morbidity and mortality weekly report 2022;71(35): 1126–30.

74. Pittman PR, Hahn M, Lee HS, et al. Phase 3 Efficacy Trial of Modified Vaccinia Ankara as a Vaccine against Smallpox. N Engl J Med 2019;381(20):1897–908.

75. Overton ET, Stapleton J, Frank I, et al. Safety and Immunogenicity of Modified Vaccinia Ankara-Bavarian Nordic Smallpox Vaccine in Vaccinia-Naive and Experienced Human Immunodeficiency Virus-Infected Individuals: An Open-Label, Controlled Clinical Phase II Trial. Open Forum Infect Dis 2015;2(2):ofv040.

76. Hazra A, Rusie L, Hedberg T, et al. Human Monkeypox Virus Infection in the Immediate Period After Receiving Modified Vaccinia Ankara Vaccine. JAMA 2022; 328(20):2064–7.

77. Payne AB, Ray LC, Kugeler KJ, et al. Incidence of Monkeypox Among Unvaccinated Persons Compared with Persons Receiving ≥1 JYNNEOS Vaccine Dose - 32 U.S. Jurisdictions, July 31-September 3, 2022. MMWR Morbidity and mortality weekly report 2022;71(40):1278–82.

78. Frey SE, Wald A, Edupuganti S, et al. Comparison of lyophilized versus liquid modified vaccinia Ankara (MVA) formulations and subcutaneous versus intradermal routes of administration in healthy vaccinia-naïve subjects. Vaccine 2015; 33(39):5225–34.

79. Brooks JT, Marks P, Goldstein RH, et al. Intradermal Vaccination for Monkeypox — Benefits for Individual and Public Health. N Engl J Med 2022;387(13):1151–3.

80. Millman AJ, Denson DJ, Allen ML, et al. A Health Equity Approach for Implementation of JYNNEOS Vaccination at Large, Community-Based LGBTQIA+ Events - Georgia, August 27-September 5, 2022. MMWR Morbidity and mortality weekly report 2022;71(43):1382–883.

81. Soelaeman RH, Mendoza L, McDonald R, et al. Characteristics of JYNNEOS Vaccine Recipients Before and During a Large Multiday LGBTQIA+ Festival - Louisiana, August 9-September 5, 2022. MMWR Morbidity and mortality weekly report 2022;71(43):1379–81.

82. Mussini C, Guaraldi G, Orkin C. Monkeypox vaccination-an opportunity for HIV prevention. Lancet HIV 2022;9(11):e741–2.

83. Grosenbach DW, Honeychurch K, Rose EA, et al. Oral Tecovirimat for the Treatment of Smallpox. N Engl J Med 2018;379(1):44–53.

84. O'Laughlin K, Tobolowsky FA, Elmor R, et al. Clinical Use of Tecovirimat (Tpoxx) for Treatment of Monkeypox Under an Investigational New Drug Protocol - United States, May-August 2022. MMWR Morbidity and mortality weekly report 2022; 71(37):1190–5.

85. O'Shea J, Filardo TD, Morris SB, et al. Interim Guidance for Prevention and Treatment of Monkeypox in Persons with HIV Infection - United States, 2022. MMWR Morbidity and mortality weekly report 2022;71(32):1023–8.

86. Sherwat A, Brooks JT, Birnkrant D, et al. Tecovirimat and the Treatment of Monkeypox - Past, Present, and Future Considerations. N Engl J Med 2022;387(7): 579–81.

87. Baker RO, Bray M, Huggins JW. Potential antiviral therapeutics for smallpox, monkeypox and other orthopoxvirus infections. Antivir Res 2003;57(1–2):13–23.

88. Hutson CL, Kondas AV, Mauldin MR, et al. Pharmacokinetics and Efficacy of a Potential Smallpox Therapeutic, Brincidofovir, in a Lethal Monkeypox Virus Animal Model. mSphere 2021;6(1).

89. Muller EE, Kularatne R. The changing epidemiology of genital ulcer disease in South Africa: has donovanosis been eliminated? Sex Transm Infect 2020;96(8): 596–600.

90. González-Beiras C, Kapa A, Vall-Mayans M, et al. Single-Dose Azithromycin for the Treatment of Haemophilus ducreyi Skin Ulcers in Papua New Guinea. Clin Infect Dis 2017;65(12):2085–90.

91. Kularatne R, Venter JME, Maseko V, et al. Etiological Surveillance of Genital Ulcer Syndrome in South Africa: 2019 to 2020. Sex Transm Dis 2022;49(8):571–5.

92. Sousa JD, Müller V, Vandamme AM. The Impact of Genital Ulcers on HIV Transmission Has Been Underestimated-A Critical Review. Viruses 2022;14(3).

Advances in Diagnostics of Sexually Transmitted Infections

Mauricio Kahn, MD[a], Barbara Van Der Pol, PhD, MPH[a,b,*]

KEYWORDS

- Laboratory diagnostics • Molecular diagnostics • Point-of-care diagnostics
- Sexually transmitted infections • Sexually transmitted diseases

KEY POINTS

- Syndromic management is inadequate for the management of sexually transmitted infections (STIs).
- Knowledge of the performance characteristics of the available diagnostic tests must guide clinicians' interpretation of test results.
- Point-of-care diagnostic tests allow for a rapid treatment response and may be a helpful tool to optimize patient management and reduce STI transmission.

INTRODUCTION

Sexually transmitted infections (STIs) are caused by a variety of pathogens, many of which have shared symptoms and all of which have shared transmission routes as implied by the terminology. This review focuses on detection of etiologic agents of clinical syndromes that manifest as urethral or vaginal discharge, dysuria, pelvic pain, and genital ulcer disease (GUD). Infectious causes of discharge syndromes include *Chlamydia trachomatis*, *Neisseria gonorrhoeae*, *Trichomonas vaginalis*, and *Mycoplasma genitalium*. Bacterial vaginosis (BV) is a discharge-related syndrome typified by a shift in composition of the vaginal microbiome. This syndrome may or may not be the result of infection with specific organisms, but it is clearly related to sexual activity and therefore warrants discussion in this review. Vulvovaginal candidiasis (VVC) is caused by an overgrowth of *Candida* spp and, although not an STI, must be considered when attempting to determine the cause of discharge and is therefore also included. Genital lesions resulting from GUD are most frequently caused by

[a] Department of Medicine, Heersink School of Medicine, University of Alabama at Birmingham, Birmingham, AL, USA; [b] UAB School of Public Health, University of Alabama at Birmingham, Birmingham, AL, USA
* Corresponding author. 703 19th Streeet South, ZRB 242, Birmingham, AL 35294.
E-mail address: bvanderp@uab.edu
Twitter: @KahnMauricio (M.K.)

Infect Dis Clin N Am 37 (2023) 381–403
https://doi.org/10.1016/j.idc.2023.02.002
0891-5520/23/© 2023 Elsevier Inc. All rights reserved.

herpes simplex virus (HSV) types 1 and 2, followed by infection with *Treponema pallidum pallidum* (the causative agent of syphilis). Diagnostic options for each of these pathogens are described in this review.

C trachomatis is the most frequently reported bacterial infection in the United States.[1,2] It is estimated to be the most costly nonviral STI owing to its associated long-term complications in women if untreated (specifically, tubal infertility, ectopic pregnancy, chronic pelvic pain).[3] *N gonorrhoeae* is the second most commonly reported bacterial disease in the United States.[4] Higher rates of these diseases are reported in adolescents and young adults, racial or ethnic minorities, and men who have sex with men.[1] Both diseases have high global distribution prevalence, but precise estimates of prevalence are not possible owing to suboptimal reporting in many parts of the world. Furthermore, even in the United States, reported cases represent an underestimate of the true burden of disease because of lack of testing in many underserved populations.

T vaginalis is the most common nonviral STI in the world.[5] It affects women more frequently than men and is most frequently detected in perimenopausal women.[6] Its prevalence is difficult to estimate owing to a lack of general screening and no reporting mandate,[4] but it has been shown to be linked to adverse birth outcomes[7] and increased risk of HIV acquisition.[8] *M genitalium* is a bacterium that causes urethritis in men and cervicitis or pelvic inflammatory disease (PID) in women. Its prevalence in the US young adult population is estimated at 1%, lower than chlamydia and trichomoniasis, but higher than gonococcal infection.[9] It has been associated with PID, infertility, and adverse pregnancy outcomes.[10]

BV is the most common cause of vaginal discharge worldwide[11] and affects up to 50% of women in the United States, depending on their race or ethnicity.[12] VVC is a common cause of vaginal discharge. An estimated 75% of women will have 1 episode throughout their lifetime, and 40% to 45% will have 2 or more episodes.[4]

Syphilis is a systemic, multistage disease with protean manifestation that is prevalent worldwide and can be difficult to accurately diagnose. In 2016, 6.3 million new cases occurred worldwide.[13] Genital herpes is a chronic, lifelong viral STI caused by HSV characterized by a latent state and recurrent episodes of viral reactivation, especially in the year after initial infection.[14] About 11.9% of persons between the ages of 14 and 49 years in the United States have been exposed to HSV-2.[15] Both syphilis and genital herpes can be transmitted through the perinatal route and increase the risk of HIV transmission and acquisition.[16,17]

CLINICAL FINDINGS
Discharge/Dysuria

The majority of cases of urethritis are caused by *C trachomatis*, *N gonorrhoeae*, *T vaginalis*, or *M genitalium*. Viral infections such as HSV or adenovirus are less frequent causes of urethritis, but if all other tests are normal, these should be considered. Men with urethritis may report dysuria, pruritus, or penile discharge. Physical examination with mucoid or mucopurulent discharge confirms the diagnosis of urethritis. A swollen or erythematous urethral meatus supports the diagnosis. If discharge is not evident, clinicians can gently "milk" the penis to remove and collect any discharge for further testing. Clinicians place a gloved thumb along the ventral surface of the base of the penis and the forefinger in the dorsum, apply gentle pressure, and move the hand slowly toward the meatus.[18] Frankly purulent discharge is suggestive of gonorrhea, and no or minimal watery discharge suggests chlamydia. However, coinfections are common, so laboratory testing to confirm the etiologic agent or agents is warranted.[19]

Women with acute cervicitis may report yellow vaginal discharge or intermenstrual or postcoital bleeding. Some patients will also report urethritis, which usually has symptoms indistinguishable from cystitis. Examination of the vulva, along with a speculum examination of the vagina and cervix, should be performed. A bimanual pelvic examination to assess cervical motion tenderness, pelvic pain, or adnexal masses may provide helpful diagnostic clues for upper-genitourinary pathologic condition. Purulent or mucopurulent exudate in the endocervical canal, the presence of edematous ectopy, and easily induced endocervical bleeding (friability) are signs of cervicitis. Although a diagnosis of cervicitis is made clinically, additional testing is necessary to differentiate between infectious and noninfectious causes, and between etiologic organisms. Along with assessing for *C trachomatis* and *N gonorrhoeae*, clinicians should assess for concomitant *T vaginalis* and BV in patients with cervicitis, as the cause may be from a vaginitis-related dysbiosis; *M genitalium* should also be considered.

Patients with vaginal discharge may present with concomitant vaginal itching or erythema, dysuria, dyspareunia, bleeding, or pelvic pain. Clinicians should attempt to quantify and characterize the discharge and assess if symptoms are associated with sexual activity, menstruation, or recent procedures. No symptom is predictive of a particular cause, and noninfectious conditions may cause discharge. Differentiating between cervicitis and vaginitis is further complicated in clinical settings where a full pelvic examination is not routinely performed (eg, Emergency Departments). For this reason, syndromic management is not recommended.

Classically, patients with VVC report thick, cottage cheese–like discharge and intense pruritus, and may have signs of local inflammation on physical examination. Women with BV report malodorous discharge that is uniformly adherent to the vaginal wall, thin, and gray. Those with symptomatic *T vaginalis* report greenish, purulent, malodorous discharge and may have punctate cervical hemorrhage ("strawberry cervix") on speculum examination. However, clinical diagnosis in patients with vaginal discharge is unreliable,[20] and additional testing to determine a specific cause is necessary for adequate management. As a result of the shared symptoms and clinical signs as well as the high rates of coinfection,[21] women reporting any discharge-related complaints should be tested for chlamydia, gonorrhea, trichomonas, mycoplasma, BV, and VVC, if possible, in order to provide comprehensive sexual health care.

Vaginitis clinical examination

If pH paper is available, clinicians can measure the pH of vaginal secretions collected using a dry swab (moistened swabs can affect pH) against the vaginal sidewall or on residual material on the speculum. The specimen's pH remains stable at room temperature for 2 to 5 minutes. A pH test stick can be applied directly on the vaginal sidewall as an alternative. An elevated pH (>4.5) is almost always seen in BV, and frequently so in trichomoniasis. VVC is associated with a normal vaginal pH. However, noninfectious factors can alter vaginal pH, and the test is not diagnostic; moreover, a subset of women present with BV-VVC coinfection. Clinicians can also perform a potassium hydroxide (KOH) or amine test in the office. Vaginal samples are diluted in 10% KOH solution and may emit a fishlike odor immediately upon application of KOH. The Amsel criteria (discussed in later discussion) use vaginal pH, the KOH test, microscopy, and physical examination findings as diagnostic criteria for BV.

Genital Ulcer Disease

History and physical examination are generally inaccurate for the diagnosis of GUD, with the exception of classical herpetic vesicles that often define initial symptomatic episodes. The most common causes of genital ulcers are syphilis, HSV-1, and HSV-2. Classically, syphilitic ulcers are painless, indurated, and clean based, whereas herpetic ulcers are typically multiple, shallow, painful, and initially vesicular. However, diagnosing these conditions can be difficult because typical lesions are frequently absent when infected persons present to the clinic. In a study of 2393 HSV-negative participants followed by clinical experts in the field, 19% of patients were incorrectly diagnosed with genital herpes, and 60% of patients who acquired genital herpes during the study were not diagnosed.[22]

Less-common causes of genital ulcers include *C trachomatis* serovars L1-3 (lymphogranuloma venereum or LGV); *Haemophilus ducreyi* (chancroid); and *Klebsiella granulomatis* (granuloma inguinale or donovanosis). Chancroid ulcers are typically deep and purulent and associated with painful inguinal lymph nodes. Ulcers from granuloma inguinale are usually painless and described as beefy red.

DIAGNOSTIC TESTING IN PATIENTS' SYMPTOMS

Clinical observation is neither sensitive nor specific for diagnosing urethral or vaginal discharge, particularly in women. Symptoms are nonspecific, and syndromic management does not target the underlying infection as often as 75% of the time.[23–26] As a result, clinical diagnosis alone frequently results in overtreatment and undertreatment of infections. Clinicians should establish diagnostic strategies for STIs considering the clinical setting, available resources, and patient characteristics. Various laboratory-based and point-of-care (POC) diagnostic tests are available and may facilitate rapid, accurate treatment.

Determining which diagnostic test to use should consider the types of samples, test targets (single vs multiple organisms), time to results, clinical laboratory improvement amendment (CLIA) -waived status, instrument requirements, throughput, and cost. Clinicians need multiple diagnostic solutions to accommodate different patient care settings and needs. Thoughtful application of diagnostic tools can increase access to services, manage antimicrobial resistance, decrease stigma, and decrease the population prevalence of STIs.

At the Point of Care

POC testing is ideal when processing a single sample from 1 person at a time. Although the name implies a clinical care setting (eg, a primary care clinic), testing may also be done in the field (eg, HIV rapid testing). These tests are designed to be performed near-patient (on-site) and preferably require no laboratory training, and results should be available during the same visit. A CLIA certificate of waiver, given by the Food and Drug Administration (FDA) for simple laboratory examinations and tests that have an insignificant risk of an erroneous result, is critical to implement these tests in the field.

The major advantage of POC tests is the ability to test and treat during the same visit.[27,28] This is particularly beneficial in vulnerable and underserved populations who may not be able to return for test results at a later time. Rapidly available results lead to more accurately targeted treatment compared with a symptom-based approach.[29] Studies have shown that patients are willing to wait up to 20 minutes beyond the conclusion of their routine clinic visit for their POC test results.[30] These tests are often designed to use patient self-collected samples, which can increase patient engagement, enhance patient comfort, and improve clinical workflow.[4] Despite these benefits, POC testing is not appropriate in all settings. It requires clinical workflow optimization and periodic assessments of clinical utility and cost impacts. Before implementing POC tests, clinicians should develop strategies for follow-up care, treatment plans, and reporting protocols.

Microscopy

Microscopy is an inexpensive POC tool but requires trained personnel and microscopes in good repair. Although abnormal results may be immediately used to inform treatment, owing to low sensitivity, microscopy-negative samples should be referred to the laboratory for molecular testing. One exception is detection of gram-negative intracellular diplococci in the setting of urethral discharge, which is specific for the diagnosis of gonorrhea. In men, visible urethral discharge can be collected with a swab for microscopy. If no secretions are seen, clinicians can insert a swab 2 cm into the urethral meatus and rotate it, contacting the urethral wall before removing it. Swabs are then rolled across a microscope slide for evaluation. Collection of these samples causes discomfort and may be a disincentive for future testing, and thus, use of molecular testing with urine specimens is preferable when possible. Gram stain of urethral discharge with white blood cells (WBCs) containing intracellular gram-negative diplococci is 97.3% sensitive and 99.6% specific for gonococcal urethritis compared with molecular diagnostics. Gram stain is not recommended on pharyngeal, endocervical, and rectal specimens. Methylene blue or gentian violet stains showing intracellular purple diplococci have similar performance characteristics and provide more rapid results.[31] Observation of ≥2 polymorphonuclear leukocytes (PMNs) per oil immersion field is evidence of urethritis in men.[32] If a presumed diagnosis of gonococcal urethritis is made by microscopy, it is still necessary to test (or presumptively treat) for *C trachomatis*, as these 2 infections frequently coexist.

Quantification of PMNs on endocervical Gram stain is less helpful in diagnosing cervicitis. It has not been standardized and is neither sensitive nor specific.[33] Given the availability of better diagnostic tools, this is not a recommended diagnostic option. Examining vaginal fluid for leukorrhea (>10 leukocytes per high-power field [HPF]) is a more sensitive marker of cervical inflammation and has a high negative-predictive value for cervicitis.[34] However, because many STI may not result in cervicitis, the utility of this test is limited. For BV, VVC, and trichomonas, vaginal specimens are collected with a cotton-tipped swab and examined by diluting them in 1 to 2 drops of normal saline on a glass slide. A coverslip is placed on the slide and then visualized under the microscope at low and high power. This technique may reveal clue cells (epithelial cells with their borders obscured by small anaerobic coccobacilli) characteristic of BV, buds or hyphae suggestive of candidiasis, motile trichomonads, or PMNs that might indicate cervicitis.[4] Saline microscopy has a low sensitivity (26%–68%) for *T vaginalis* compared with nucleic acid amplification test (NAAT) and culture; if used, clinicians should evaluate slides immediately after specimen collection to avoid a rapid decrease in sensitivity.[4,35,36]

A KOH-diluted specimen should also be examined under the microscope. KOH can help visualize budding yeasts, hyphae, or pseudohyphae in VVC because it disrupts cellular material that may obscure fungal elements. Negative findings in KOH samples do not rule out infection because of poor sensitivity compared with culture (approximately 50% for Candida).[37]

The Amsel criteria for diagnosis of BV require 3 of the following 4 findings to make a diagnosis of BV[38]: Homogeneous, thin (milklike) vaginal discharge that smoothly coats the vaginal walls; clue cells on microscopy; pH of vaginal fluid greater than 4.5; and/or positive amine test after KOH. The sensitivity and specificity of the Amsel criteria are 37% to 70% and 94% to 99%, respectively, compared with the Nugent score, a research use diagnostic option.[39] The presence of concomitant *T vaginalis* or *Candida* sp lowers the diagnostic accuracy of the Amsel criteria, including the sensitivity of its components.[40]

Darkfield microscopy to detect *T pallidum* from lesion exudates or tissue is one of the definitive methods to diagnose early syphilis.[41] However, the lack of available equipment and trained personnel to perform and interpret this test limit its practical use.

Rapid antigen/antibody/metabolic activity detection

Antigen and metabolic activity tests are abnormal only during active infection. They usually require a high organism load and have limited sensitivity. Serology testing relies on detecting antibodies to an acute or previous infection. Serology is generally helpful for detection of viral infections (eg, HSV and HIV) and for epidemiologic studies of bacterial infections. Multiple samples over time are usually necessary for accurate identification of acute infections. Antibodies usually last lifelong, but this may not be true in patients who receive rapid treatment after infection.

If POC microscopy is unavailable, first-void urine can be tested for leukocyte esterase or spun and evaluated for pyuria. A positive leukocyte esterase or the presence of ≥10 WBCs/HPF is indirect evidence of urethritis.[4] A meta-analysis of 9 studies showed that the leukocyte esterase test has a median sensitivity of 71% and median specificity of 70% compared with molecular tests or culture.[42] The ideal urine sample for this test is the initial portion of the first urinary stream after awakening, collected without cleaning the urethral meatus (first-void urine). However, this is not practical, and sampling the initial portion (first catch) of the urinary stream at any time of the day is mainly used instead.[43]

Many antigen or antibody tests are based on lateral flow technology. The test is based on the movement of a liquid sample by capillary action through a polymeric (usually nitrocellulose) strip with attached capture moieties that interact with the target and provide a signal that can be detected visually within 10 to 30 minutes. This class of assay is generally low cost and easy to use with a long shelf life and no refrigeration requirement for storage, making them optimal for small or remote settings.[44] The most commonly used example is an at-home pregnancy test. Newer immunochromatographic tests for *chlamydia and for gonorrhea* are being developed to overcome the limited sensitivity of antigen assays developed in the 1990s. Studies of a new gonorrhea detection assay have estimated sensitivity of 60% to 94% and specificity of 89% to 97%.[42]

The Osom BV Blue test (Sekisui Diagnostics) is a POC chromogenic test that detects vaginal sialidase activity.[45] Its sensitivity is 91.7% to 94%, and specificity is 96% to -97.8% compared with the Nugent score for BV.[46,47] Osom also makes a trichomoniasis rapid antigen-detection test that uses immunochromatographic capillary flow dipstick technology and can be done with clinician-obtained vaginal specimens. Results take 10 to 15 minutes. The sensitivity is 82% to 95%, and specificity is 97% to 100% compared with wet mount, culture, and transcription-mediated amplification. This test should not be used in men.

The FemExam Test Card (Cooper Surgical) measures the presence of trimethylamine (a metabolite of *Gardnerella vaginalis*), proline aminopeptidase, and vaginal pH. Its sensitivity is 91% and specificity 61%, compared with the Nugent score.[48] It can be helpful in resource-limited settings, but it is not a preferred diagnostic method for BV.[4]

Multiple POC screening tests for syphilis are available. Most use immunochromatographic strips with attached treponemal antigens that react with the patient's serum antibodies.[49] These tests do not distinguish between active and treated infection because they detect lifelong antibodies and may not be adequate in at-risk populations. However, they can help initial treatment decisions in patients who might otherwise be lost to follow-up. Sensitivity for POC syphilis tests ranges from 74% to 90% in serum and 74% to 86% in whole blood, and specificity ranges from 94% to 99% in serum and 96% to 100% in whole blood.[50] Nontreponemal POC tests other than the reagin plasma reaction (RPR) test, which is labor intensive, are not available in the United States, and studies of dual nontreponemal/treponemal POC tests have shown mixed results.[51] Newer syphilis antibody tests paired with HIV antibody detection have high utility for outreach testing among people at risk for HIV.

Point-of-care molecular tests

POC tests for gonorrhea, chlamydia, and trichomonas allow optimal treatment at a single clinic visit and help improve antimicrobial stewardship. Molecular POC tests perform as well as laboratory-based molecular tests.[52] Currently, they are cost-prohibitive in most settings, but will likely be cost-effective when treatment accuracy is included in the calculation.[53] As more tests become available, market competition should result in decreasing prices, which may make these tests more widely available.

Cepheid GeneXpert CT/NG (Chepeid, Sunnyvale, CA) is an available POC test, although it is not rapid, with a modular cartridge-based platform that uses polymerase chain reaction (PCR) to detect nucleic acids of *C trachomatis* and *N gonorrhea*.[27] The test can use endocervical, vaginal, urine, and rectal samples. It can process multiple specimens simultaneously, and results are available within 90 minutes. For *C trachomatis*, sensitivity is 97.4% to 98.7% in women and 97.5% in male urine. Specificity estimates are ≥99.4%. For *N gonorrhea*, sensitivity is 95.6% to 100% in women and 98% in male urine. Specificity estimates are ≥99.8%. In rectal samples, sensitivity and specificity for *C trachomatis* are 86% and 99.2%, respectively, and sensitivity and specificity for *N gonorrhea* are 91.1% and 100%, respectively.[54] By using a second cartridge, samples can also be tested for the presence of trichomonas. Sensitivity and specificity estimates are 99.5% to 100% and 99.4% to 99.9%, respectively, compared with wet mount and culture.[55]

The binx io CT/NG (binx health, Boston, MA) detects *C trachomatis* and *N gonorrhea* within 30 minutes and can be done by non-laboratory-trained personnel.[28] This assay relies on a cartridge loaded with patient sample and placed into a small instrument, where a PCR reaction occurs with detection of product using electrochemical sensing. Assay performance characteristics are equivalent to commercially available laboratory-based molecular tests. For gonorrhea, sensitivity is 100% in women (vaginal swabs) and 97.3% in men (first-catch urine), and specificity is 99.9% in women and 100% in men. For chlamydia, sensitivity is 96.1% in women and 92.5% in men, and specificity is 99.1% in women and 99.3% in men.

The Visby Sexual Health (Visby, Santa Clara, CA) test also has good performance characteristics for detection of *C trachomatis*, *N gonorrhea*, and *T vaginalis* from self-obtained vaginal swabs in 30 minutes. For *C trachomatis*, sensitivity is 97.6%, and specificity is 98.3% compared with standard molecular tests. For *N gonorrhea*, sensitivity is 97.4% and specificity is 99.4%. For *T vaginalis*, sensitivity is 99.2%, and specificity is 96.9%[56] Interestingly, the Visby test has all of the mechanisms necessary for performing the PCR reaction in the test cartridge, so no instrumentation is required. Detection of the amplified product is done by use of a lateral flow readout, and the entire test is disposable.

The Solana trichomonas assay (Quidel, San Diego, CA) detects *T vaginalis* DNA qualitatively in female vaginal and urine specimens. Results take less than 40 minutes. Its sensitivity is greater than 98% compared with NAAT for vaginal and greater than

92% for urine specimens.[57] A similar test, the AmpliVue trichomonas assay (Quidel), qualitatively detects T vaginalis in vaginal samples, with a sensitivity of 90.7% and specificity of 98.9% compared with NAAT.[58] These tests have not been widely adopted because microscopy, although substantially less sensitive, is very inexpensive, and because a test that does not include chlamydia and gonorrhea has limited application.

Laboratory-Based Diagnostic Tests

Laboratory-based diagnostics guided by clinical symptoms offer improvements over clinical evaluation only. They are geared for high throughput and may take place on-site with relatively rapid results or in a reference laboratory. They can be a part of telehealth medicine or direct-to-consumer (DTC) services. In general, the delay in time to results is offset by the substantially lower cost of testing. Different strategies for testing patients with symptoms for whom treatment should be provided as soon as possible compared with screening asymptomatic patients according to recommendations will result in mixed use of both POC and laboratory-based testing. Furthermore, the laboratory generally has more resources and may be able to provide testing for additional pathogens or evaluate positive samples for markers of antimicrobial resistance. Therefore, even in cases whereby a POC test is used while the patient waits, further testing in the laboratory may be required.

Serology

Serologic tests to detect antibodies to HSV-1 and HSV-2 can help diagnose genital HSV if lesions are absent at the time of evaluation. Antibodies develop during the first few (2–6) weeks after infection and persist indefinitely. Clinicians should use type-specific assays that distinguish between HSV-1 and HSV-2.[59,60] Available assays usually test for the HSV-specific glycoproteins G2 (HSV-2) and G1 (HSV-1). For HSV-2, antibodies can be checked in capillary blood or serum. Sensitivity varies from 80% to 98%, and false negatives may occur at the early stages of infection.[60–62] Providers should consider repeat testing after 12 weeks of presumed exposure if clinical suspicion is high.

The HerpeSelect HSV-2 (Focus, Cypress, CA) enzyme immunoassay (EIA) test is commonly used for serologic testing but has poor specificity (57.4%), particularly at low index values (the ratio of the patient result compared with a negative control).[63] A confirmatory test using a different method should be performed to finalize results. Tests like the Biokit or Western blot assays improve the accuracy of HSV-2 serologic testing.[64] The HerpeSelect HSV-2 immunoblot should not be used for confirmation of the HerpeSelect EIA because it uses the same antigen targets.[4] Serologic testing should be avoided if confirmatory tests are unavailable. Immunoglobulin M (IgM) testing for HSV-1 or HSV-2 is not recommended because it is not type-specific and does not differentiate between primary and recurrent episodes.

The presence of antibodies against HSV-2 indicates prior anogenital infection. However, detecting HSV-1 antibodies does not distinguish between previous oral and genital infections. Ideally, clinicians should confirm the diagnosis of genital HSV with virologic tests (culture or PCR) from active genital lesions.[4] Nonetheless, a positive serologic test can be helpful in patients with a history of genital ulcers without a previous workup or with a negative workup for GUD. It can also help in patients with atypical or late presentations without visible ulcers to sample.

A presumptive diagnosis of syphilis can be made using nontreponemal and treponemal antibodies. Using a single type of test is inadequate and can result in false-negative or false-positive results. In addition, diagnosis and staging of syphilis rely on a detailed medical and sexual history, and laboratory tests alone are insufficient.

Nontreponemal antibody tests use a cardiolipin-cholesterol-lecithin antigen that reacts with the patient's serum. They include the RPR, venereal disease research laboratory, and toluidine red unheated serum test. Serum is diluted to obtain the highest reactive titer, and results are reported quantitatively. The number of antibodies (IgM and IgG) detected may correlate with disease activity. Nontreponemal tests help monitor treatment response. Although titers can decrease over time without treatment, appropriate therapy increases the rate of decline. Providers should use the same serologic test from the same manufacturer to assess treatment response.[4] Nontreponemal tests can be used as the initial syphilis screening test in patients with genital ulcers. They are low cost and easy to perform. However, false positives can occur with other infections, autoimmune conditions, vaccinations, injection drug use, pregnancy, and older age.[65] False-negative results may be seen in immunocompromised hosts or early in the disease.

Treponemal tests detect antibodies against specific treponemal antigens and are generally more specific than nontreponemal assays. They include the fluorescent treponemal antibody absorption, microhemagglutination test for antibodies to *T pallidum*, *T pallidum* particle agglutination assay, *T pallidum* EIA, and chemiluminescence immunoassay (CIA). These are qualitative tests only. Automated EIAs or CIAs can be used for screening purposes.[66,67] Clinicians can use treponemal tests to confirm syphilis in patients with a reactive nontreponemal test, or the reverse algorithm can be performed that uses treponemal-specific tests first and only uses nontreponemal tests for confirmation. This algorithm works best in populations with low risk of previous infection (eg, pregnant women). If used for screening purposes, providers should confirm a positive treponemal test with a nontreponemal assay. If the nontreponemal test is normal, a second, different treponemal test should be performed. If the second treponemal test is abnormal, a diagnosis of syphilis (latent syphilis of unknown duration) is made.

Culture

Although culture is possible for many STIs, the disadvantages compared with molecular testing are numerous, and this option should be used only when antimicrobial resistance (ie, for gonorrhea) or speciation (ie, for yeast) is clinically relevant.

Gonorrhea culture is no longer recommended other than as a tool for antimicrobial resistance testing of isolates. Clinicians should pursue culture and antimicrobial susceptibilities for *N gonorrhea* when they suspect treatment failure and antibiotic resistance in patients with urethritis. Samples are obtained from urethral swabs by inserting the swab tip 2 to 3 cm into the urethral meatus. Specimens from the rectum, oropharynx, endocervix, or conjunctiva can also be used for culture.[4] Swabs should have plastic or wire shafts and rayon or Dacron tips because other materials may be toxic to *N gonorrhea*.[68] For optimal yield, direct inoculation into modified Thayer-Martin agar and prompt incubation in an increased CO_2 environment at 35°C to 37°C is recommended.[68] Transport systems that may maintain *N gonorrhea* viability for less than 48 hours in ambient temperatures are available. *N gonorrhea* culture sensitivity ranges from 85% to 95% with optimal conditions,[69] but declines to 65% to 85% in asymptomatic women[70] or when culture optimization is impossible. Results are only available in 48 hours, and sensitivities take longer.

Yeast culture remains the standard for diagnosis of VVC, although molecular methods provide rapid and sensitive information.[4] Culture should be considered when the patient presentation is suggestive of VVC (normal pH), and no pathogens are seen on microscopy. Vaginal samples can be inoculated into Sabouraud agar, Nickerson medium, or Microstix-Candida mediums for culture, as these perform equally well.[71] Positive results should only be considered relevant in symptomatic patients. Cultures become particularly important in women with complicated VVC to assess for antimicrobial resistance. They are also important to confirm the diagnosis of non-*albicans Candida* because some species, like *Candida glabrata*, do not form hyphae or pseudohyphae and are difficult to visualize on microscopy.[4]

Culture for HSV can be obtained in vesicular fluid from active genital lesions. Samples are placed in viral culture media and then transported to the laboratory. Culture sensitivity is low compared with PCR, particularly in recurrent lesions or those starting to heal.[72] Use of the ELVIS system (Quidel, San Diego, CA, USA), which uses a genetically modified cell line that produces a colorimetric change in cells infected with HSV, allows for results to be available in less than 24 hours. HSV-2 will generate a fluorescent light, whereas staining is required to detect HSV-1. A normal test does not rule out infection because viral shedding is intermittent.

Molecular tests

NAATs amplify and detect DNA or RNA target sequences specific to an organism of interest. These tests do not require viable organisms and usually have high sensitivity because they can theoretically detect as few as a single copy of a target nucleic acid,[68] which supports the use of less-invasively collected specimens. However, molecular testing may detect dead organisms that do not represent an active infection or produce a false-positive result by amplifying sequences from closely related species.

NAATs are the recommended diagnostic method and are considered the gold standard for genital and extragenital *N gonorrhea* and *C trachomatis* infections. They can be performed in endocervical, vaginal, and urine samples in women and urine and urethral samples in men. Rectal and pharyngeal swabs can be tested in men and women. Swabs should have a plastic or wire shaft and rayon or Dacron tip to prevent organism inhibition, which happens with other materials.[68] Patient self-collection is ideal with urine, vaginal, rectal, or oropharyngeal swabs.[73] Turnaround time to results is usually 1 to 2 days. Chlamydia, gonorrhea, trichomonas, and mycoplasma testing can all be performed from a single sample (urine or vaginal swabs). This substantially improves clinical efficiency, but providers must place specific orders so that inappropriate testing is not performed (eg, mycoplasma among asymptomatic women or trichomonas from nongenital samples). Many newer assays are under development or evaluation and may be available in the near future.

NAATs for *C trachomatis* and *N gonorrhea* should be performed in all men with urethritis. Testing can be done with a urethral swab, but it is unnecessary. First-catch urine, the first 10 to 30 mL, is the ideal sample type for detection of genital infection in men.[43] It is important to remember that urine will not detect infections in other anatomic sites (eg, the rectum and pharynx). Sensitivity for *chlamydia/gonorrhea* detection is better with NAATs than with other classes of tests but varies between NAAT types (all >92% sensitivity).[68] Clinicians should consult product inserts for each test manufacturer before collecting any samples, as sampling methods and performance characteristics may vary. NAAT for *T vaginalis* in urine samples from men with recurrent or persistent urethritis may be helpful if the local prevalence is high. Testing should also be considered if the patient's partner has a known infection with *T vaginalis*.

NAATs for *C trachomatis* and *N gonorrhea* are the preferred diagnostic test in women with cervical infection, whether cervical inflammation is present or not.[68] Testing can be done in vaginal swabs, cervical swabs, or first-void urine. Cervical samples are obtained by rotating a swab within the endocervical canal while applying lateral pressure. Self-collected vaginal swabs have equivalent sensitivity and specificity as those collected by a clinician.[73] They are optimal for NAAT testing and are highly accepted by women with urogenital symptoms and for screening.[68,74] Clinicians should use vaginal swabs for testing whenever possible because urine specimens may miss up to 10% of infections.[68] Liquid-based cytology specimens from PAP smears may be used for NAAT testing for *C trachomatis*, although they may have lower sensitivity than vaginal swabs.[75]

Testing of all anatomic exposure sites is essential. Compared with culture, NAATs have improved sensitivity and specificity for detecting *N gonorrhea* and *C trachomatis* at rectal and oropharyngeal sites.[68,76] Because clinically significant oropharyngeal *Chlamydial* infection is uncommon, testing for *C trachomatis* is not recommended at this site. Self-collected rectal and pharyngeal swabs have comparable performance to clinician-collected specimens, and this strategy is acceptable in men who have sex with men.[73,77] Laboratories that test extragenital sites using NAATs should have previously evaluated their test on nongenital samples, as performance characteristics may vary. For example, NAATs that detect commensal *Neisseria* species may have low specificity for *N gonorrhea* in oropharyngeal specimens.[68]

Available *C trachomatis* NAATs do not differentiate between serovars when abnormal. If clinicians suspect LGV proctitis, they must request an LGV-specific NAAT, which is only available in referral centers. In patients with severe rectal symptoms like rectal discharge, bleeding, tenesmus, or ulcers, empiric treatment of LGV should be considered instead of waiting for LGV-specific results. Non-LGV *C trachomatis* rectal infections are usually asymptomatic.[78] As well as *N gonorrhea* and *C trachomatis*, patients presenting with proctitis should be evaluated for HSV (NAAT in rectal lesions) and *T pallidum* (serology).

Testing for *M genitalium* should be considered in selected patients. NAAT testing is FDA-cleared for use in urine, urethral, endocervical, and vaginal swab samples. Preferred specimens are first-void urine in men and vaginal swabs in women. Extragenital testing is not recommended.[4] Men with recurrent or persistent nongonococcal urethritis and women with recurrent cervicitis or PID should be tested for *M genitalium* using an FDA-approved NAAT. Sensitivity ranges from 78% to 100%, and providers should consult with their laboratory to obtain information about the test in use.

NAATs can also be used diagnose BV and VVC with vaginal samples from symptomatic women. Samples can be clinician- or patient-collected. Some tests assess for the presence of a single pathogen, and others evaluate for various pathogens simultaneously. Providers should consult with the laboratory to determine what assay is being used and to understand the assay performance characteristics. There are currently 3 assays that have claims for detection of agents of BV and VVC (BD Vaginal Panel, Aptima BV and CVTV, and Cepheid MVP). Each has performance superior to clinical evaluation and can be performed with the vaginal swab collected for STI testing. Several other vaginitis NAATs are under evaluation and will be available in the near future.

When lesions are present, NAATs are the preferred diagnostic test for genital HSV using swabs from genital ulcers or other mucocutaneous lesions. FDA-cleared assays can distinguish between HSV-1 and HSV-2 infections with sensitivity ranges from 91% to 100% and high specificity.[4]

LGV-specific molecular testing (serovars L1, L2, and L3) is the only definitive method to diagnose LGV, which may present in genital ulcers. However, results are not readily available, and a positive *C trachomatis* NAAT, along with clinical suspicion and exclusion of other causes of genital ulcers, can be more practical for diagnosis.

NAATs for *T pallidum* are not commercially available, but certain laboratories have validated PCR tests that can help diagnose syphilis. Compared with darkfield microscopy and serology, sensitivity ranges from 70% to 95% and specificity from 92% to 98%.[79,80] Performance characteristics are potentially higher than darkfield microscopy alone.[81] The difficulty with NAATs for detection of syphilis is a lack of data about where the organism is located during different stages of infection. As a result, although positive results are meaningful, normal results may not be clinically useful in ruling syphilis. Sensitivity in blood or cerebrospinal fluid is much lower (24%–32%).[82]

RESISTANCE-GUIDED THERAPY

Resistance-guided therapy (RGT) using molecular diagnostics is becoming more readily available and can facilitate staged treatment strategies. RGT optimizes antibiotic selection and predicts the efficacy of specific treatments against agents like *N gonorrhea* and *M genitalium*.[83,84] These tests are usually only available in reference laboratories and have a longer turnaround time. For gonorrhea, studies have shown that the presence of a wild-type gyrA serine *N gonorrhea* genotype predicts the efficacy of treatment with ciprofloxacin.[83] Additional studies are ongoing to assess options that permit use of oral therapies for treatment of gonococcal infections.

Testing for *M genitalium* macrolide or quinolone resistance markers is currently limited to research settings.[4] If RGT is available, macrolide resistance should be tested because it leads to better treatment outcomes in patients with urethritis, cervicitis, or proctitis.[84,85] For patients with wild-type organisms, a week of doxycycline followed by extended azithromycin has a high clinical cure rate (>90%). Similarly, patients with a macrolide resistance marker have excellent outcomes when 1 week of doxycycline is followed by moxifloxacin. This type of staged and targeted treatment is only possible with the support of laboratory testing.

SCREENING OF ASYMPTOMATIC POPULATIONS

All sexually active women younger than 25 years should have annual screening for *N gonorrhea* and *C trachomatis*.[86] These are the 2 most common bacterial infections diagnosed in the United States[2] and are more prevalent in persons under the age of 25. Asymptomatic *C trachomatis* is common in men and women but can lead to long-term complications like infertility in women. Screening young women for *T vaginalis* should be considered in high-prevalence settings or patients with risk factors.[4] Women older than 25 should be screened for STIs if they are at increased risk. According to national guidelines, cervical cancer screening should be pursued beginning at age 21.[87] Any men or women with elevated potential for exposure (eg, injection drug users, incarcerated persons, and men on PreExposure Prophylaxis [PrEP]) should also be screened. Screening in the general population is not recommended for genital herpes,[88] *M genitalium*,[89] BV, trichomoniasis, or VVC.[4]

Patients who ask for STI screening should be offered tests for chlamydia, gonorrhea, trichomonas (for vaginal samples), syphilis, and HIV because they may recognize potential behavioral risks. Urine samples from persons with a penis and vaginal swabs from those with a vagina should be used for chlamydia, gonorrhea, and trichomonas NAATs. Serum should be sampled and tested for treponemal or nontreponemal syphilis antibodies and with an HIV antigen/antibody immunoassay.

All pregnant women should be screened for HIV, hepatitis B (surface antigen, surface antibody, and core antibody),[87] and syphilis at their first prenatal visit.[90] Pregnant women living with HIV should also be tested for genital *C trachomatis*, *N gonorrhea*,

Table 1
Available diagnostic tests for sexually transmitted infections

Potential Infection	Signs/Symptoms	Clinical Presentation	Microscopy	Molecular Testing	Antigen/ Metabolic Product	Antibody	Culture	Comments
Chlamydia	Cervicitis Urethritis Epididymitis PID Proctitis LGV Asymptomatic in 70% of women and 50% of men[a]	Poor	Poor	POC or laboratory Excellent	POC Poor, but in development	Poor	Poor	
Gonorrhea	Cervicitis Urethritis Epididymitis PID Proctitis Pharyngitis Disseminated Infection Up to 68% of women[93] and 42%–88% of men[94,95] are asymptomatic	Poor	High if symptomatic	POC or laboratory Excellent	POC Poor, but in development	n/a	Moderate but useful for antimicrobial susceptibility testing	
Trichomonas	Vaginal discharge, irritation, or odor Urethritis (in men) Asymptomatic in at least 50% of women and 70%–80% of men[a]	Moderate if symptomatic	Moderate if symptomatic	POC or laboratory Excellent	Good	n/a	Good	

(continued on next page)

Table 1
(continued)

Potential Infection	Signs/Symptoms	Clinical Presentation	Microscopy	Molecular Testing	Antigen/ Metabolic Product	Antibody	Culture	Comments
Mycoplasma genitalium	Urethritis Cervicitis PID Asymptomatic in 27% of men[96] and up to 77% of women[97]	Poor	Poor	Laboratory only Excellent	n/a	n/a	Very poor	
Bacterial vaginosis	Vaginal discharge, irritation, or odor 50%–70% of women are asymptomatic[98]	Moderate	Moderate	Laboratory only Excellent	Moderate	n/a	Poor	Requires good microscopy skills and is best when no coinfections
Vulvovaginal candidiasis	Vaginal discharge, irritation, or odor Present in 6%–12% of asymptomatic women[99]	Moderate	Moderate	Laboratory only Excellent	n/a	n/a	Good	
Syphilis	Genital ulcers Protean manifestations in its secondary stage (rash, condyloma lata, hepatitis,) Early neurologic disease (meningitis, stroke, cranial	Moderate	Not generally available	Good, research use only	n/a	POC, Good Laboratory, excellent	New opportunities coming	Requires sexual exposure history in addition to test results

neuritis, ocular involvement)
Late neurologic disease (general paresis, tabes dorsalis)
Gumma
Cardiovascular disease
Difficult to estimate the proportion of asymptomatic patients due to the multistage nature of the disease. As many as 50.8% of patients are diagnosed without active symptoms[100]

| Herpes simplex virus | Genital vesicles that progress to ulcers Urethritis Proctitis 12%–23% have asymptomatic viral shedding[101] | Moderate | n/a | Laboratory only Excellent | n/a | Moderate |

[a] Data obtained from the Pan American Health Organization.

and *T vaginalis* at their initial prenatal visit. Repeat syphilis testing in the third trimester and at delivery can prevent congenital syphilis cases[91] and should be pursued.

Clinicians should screen all patients aged 15 to 65 years for HIV and those aged 18 to 79 years for hepatitis C at least once in their lifetime. Testing for hepatitis C is done using serum hepatitis C antibodies. Additional screening recommendations vary according to assigned sex at birth. Transgender and gender-diverse persons should have recommendations adopted based on anatomy.[4]

Men who have sex with men should undergo periodic testing for syphilis, *C trachomatis*, and *N gonorrhea*. Extragenital testing at all exposure sites is important, and clinicians may miss about 70% of gonococcal and chlamydial infections if they perform urogenital-only testing.[4] Rectal testing by NAAT for *C trachomatis* and *N gonorrhea* and pharyngeal testing by NAAT for *N gonorrhea* are recommended. Testing for evidence of prior infection with hepatitis A (IgG antibody) and hepatitis B should also be performed, and vaccination should be provided in nonimmune individuals. Men who have sex with women should be screened for STIs if they are at increased risk.

THE FUTURE OF SEXUALLY TRANSMITTED INFECTION DETECTION TESTS

DTC testing has gained popularity among patients in the setting of the SARS-CoV-2 global pandemic. Self-testing and home-testing are alternative names. In DTC testing, patients request a test, self-collect their samples at home, and ship them to a centralized laboratory without involving their health care providers.[92] Physicians should confer with local health departments, outreach programs, or research centers to see if they offer DTC testing. They must have access to DTC test performance characteristics to interpret their results and may need additional testing before making a diagnosis. High-risk patients, such as pregnant women, should not use DTC testing.

Over-the-counter (OTC) home testing may be the future of STI diagnostics. When available, guidance should be provided to patients regarding the timing of testing after a high-risk exposure. Requirements for biohazard management and refrigeration or storage should be specified. Tests should be easy to use and interpret. Patients with positive test results should be linked to care, and their results should be reported to the local health department. Clinicians should plan a management strategy according to the OTC test results and develop a system for reporting them. Some concerns with this approach include cost and equity, specimen integrity, assay performance, inappropriate test requests, and inadequate treatment and notification to public health agencies.

SUMMARY

STIs remain a public health problem worldwide. Syndromic management of STIs may lead to complications, such as antimicrobial resistance, and is no longer recommended. Accurate diagnostic tests and rapid implementation of targeted treatments for patients and their partners are essential to stop or slow down the spread of STIs. It is hoped this will lead to a reduction in associated long-term complications, including infertility, adverse pregnancy outcomes, and congenital infections. Clinicians should be familiar with the performance characteristics of the tests available to them **(Table 1)** and determine individual patient risk factors to select the optimal diagnostic strategy. They should be aware of adequate sampling techniques and test characteristics for different types of samples. Providers should review the performance data of novel diagnostic assays before implementing them in their practice. These measures should allow for quality interpretation of test results and subsequent implementation of adequate treatments to reduce STI transmission.

POC tests are tools to provide rapid, targeted treatments for populations at risk for loss to follow-up or living in remote or rural areas. However, their cost may be a barrier to access in some settings. Patient self-collected samples and platforms that test for multiple pathogens simultaneously have made STI testing more convenient and accepted by patients. DTC and OTC home tests are likely to become more available and gain popularity in the next few years. Patients and clinicians should be appropriately guided on the interpretation and follow-up protocols for abnormal results before the widespread adoption of these diagnostics.

CLINICS CARE POINTS

- Syndromic management based on clinical observations is no longer recommended.
- Individual patient characteristics and risk factors should guide the selection of diagnostic tests.
- Sexually transmitted infection diagnostic test performance characteristics vary depending on the type of assay, manufacturer, and sample type. Clinicians should consult with their laboratory for optimal diagnostic yield.
- Point-of-care sexually transmitted infection diagnostic tests are helpful tools to reduce sexually transmitted infection transmission if they are accessible to clinicians.
- Dissemination of public health strategies will be key to supporting patients who opt for direct-to-consumer and over-the-counter sexually transmitted infection diagnostics.

DISCLOSURES

M. Kahn has nothing to disclose. B. Van Der Pol reports receiving grant funding to her institution or personal consulting or honorarium fees from Abbott, BD Diagnostics, binx health, bioMérieux, Cepheid, Hologic, Preventx, Rheonix, Roche Molecular, and Visby.

REFERENCES

1. Centers for Disease Control and Prevention. Sexually Transmitted Disease Surveillance. 2019. Available at: https://www.cdc.gov/std/statistics/2019/announcement. htm. Accessed October 26, 2022.
2. Kreisel KM, Weston EJ, St. Cyr SB, et al. Estimates of the prevalence and incidence of chlamydia and gonorrhea among US men and women, 2018. Sexual Trans Dis 2021;48(4):222–31.
3. Kumar S, Chesson HW, Spicknall IH, et al. The estimated lifetime medical cost of chlamydia, gonorrhea, and trichomoniasis in the United States, 2018. Sex Transm Dis 2021;48(4):238–46.
4. Workowski KA, Bachmann LH, Chan PA, et al. Sexually transmitted infections treatment guidelines, 2021. MMWR Recomm Rep (Morb Mortal Wkly Rep) 2021;70(4):1–187.
5. Van Der Pol B. *Editorial Commentary: Trichomonas vaginalis* Infection: the most prevalent nonviral sexually transmitted infection receives the least public health attention. Clin Infect Dis 2007;44(1):23–5.
6. Stemmer SM, Mordechai E, Adelson ME, et al. Trichomonas vaginalis is most frequently detected in women at the age of peri-/premenopause: an unusual

pattern for a sexually transmitted pathogen. Am J Obstet Gynecol 2018;218(3): 328.e1–13.

7. Van Gerwen OT, Craig-Kuhn MC, Jones AT, et al. Trichomoniasis and adverse birth outcomes: a systematic review and meta-analysis. BJOG 2021;128(12): 1907–15.

8. Masha SC, Cools P, Sanders EJ, et al. Trichomonas vaginalis and HIV infection acquisition: a systematic review and meta-analysis. Sex Transm Infect 2019; 95(1):36–42.

9. Manhart LE, Holmes KK, Hughes JP, et al. Mycoplasma genitalium among young adults in the United States: an emerging sexually transmitted infection. Am J Public Health 2007;97(6):1118–25.

10. Lis R, Rowhani-Rahbar A, Manhart LE. Mycoplasma genitalium infection and female reproductive tract disease: a meta-analysis. Clin Infect Dis 2015;61(3): 418–26.

11. Peebles K, Velloza J, Balkus JE, et al. High global burden and costs of bacterial vaginosis: a systematic review and meta-analysis. Sex Transm Dis 2019;46(5): 304–11.

12. Allsworth JE, Peipert JF. Prevalence of bacterial vaginosis: 2001-2004 National Health and Nutrition Examination Survey data. Obstet Gynecol 2007;109(1): 114–20.

13. Rowley J, Vander Hoorn S, Korenromp E, et al. Chlamydia, gonorrhoea, trichomoniasis and syphilis: global prevalence and incidence estimates, 2016. Bull World Health Organ 2019;97(8):548–562P.

14. Johnston C, Magaret A, Son H, et al. Viral shedding 1 year following first-episode genital HSV-1 infection. JAMA 2022;328(17):1730.

15. McQuillan G, Kruszon-Moran D, Flagg EW, et al. Prevalence of herpes simplex virus type 1 and type 2 in persons aged 14-49: United States, 2015-2016. NCHS Data Brief 2018;(304):1–8.

16. Solomon MM, Mayer KH, Glidden DV, et al. Syphilis predicts HIV incidence among men and transgender women who have sex with men in a preexposure prophylaxis trial. Clin Infect Dis 2014;59(7):1020–6.

17. Freeman EE, Weiss HA, Glynn JR, et al. Herpes simplex virus 2 infection increases HIV acquisition in men and women: systematic review and meta-analysis of longitudinal studies. AIDS 2006;20(1):73–83.

18. Babu TM, Urban MA, Augenbraun MH. Urethritis. In: Bennett JE, Dolin R, Blaser MJ, Mandell, Douglas, editors. Bennett's Principles and Practice of Infectious Diseases. Ninth Edition. Philadelphia, PA: Elsevier; 2019. p. 1452–61.

19. Getman D, Jiang A, O'Donnell M, et al. Mycoplasma genitalium prevalence, co-infection, and macrolide antibiotic resistance frequency in a multicenter clinical study cohort in the United States. J Clin Microbiol 2016;54(9):2278–83.

20. Broache M, Cammarata CL, Stonebraker E, et al. Performance of a vaginal panel assay compared with the clinical diagnosis of vaginitis. Obstet Gynecol 2021;138(6):853–9.

21. Van Der Pol B, Daniel G, Kodsi S, et al. Molecular-based testing for sexually transmitted infections using samples previously collected for vaginitis diagnosis. Clin Infect Dis 2019;68(3):375–81.

22. Langenberg AG, Corey L, Ashley RL, et al. A prospective study of new infections with herpes simplex virus type 1 and type 2. Chiron HSV Vaccine Study Group. N Engl J Med 1999;341(19):1432–8.

23. Cheng Y, Paintsil E, Ghebremichael M. Syndromic versus laboratory diagnosis of sexually transmitted infections in men in Moshi district of Tanzania. AIDS Res Treat 2020;2020:7607834.

24. Maina AN, Mureithi MW, Ndemi JK, et al. Diagnostic accuracy of the syndromic management of four STIs among individuals seeking treatment at a health centre in Nairobi, Kenya: a cross-sectional study. Pan Afr Med J 2021;40:138.

25. Barry MS, Ba Diallo A, Diadhiou M, et al. Accuracy of syndromic management in targeting vaginal and cervical infections among symptomatic women of reproductive age attending primary care clinics in Dakar, Senegal. Trop Med Int Health 2018;23(5):541–8.

26. Loh AJW, Ting EL, Wi TE, et al. The diagnostic accuracy of syndromic management for genital ulcer disease: a systematic review and meta-analysis. Front Med 2021;8:806605.

27. Gaydos CA, Van Der Pol B, Jett-Goheen M, et al. Performance of the Cepheid CT/NG Xpert Rapid PCR Test for Detection of Chlamydia trachomatis and Neisseria gonorrhoeae. J Clin Microbiol 2013;51(6):1666–72.

28. Van Der Pol B, Taylor SN, Mena L, et al. Evaluation of the performance of a point-of-care test for chlamydia and gonorrhea. JAMA Netw Open 2020;3(5):e204819.

29. Harding-Esch EM, Nori AV, Hegazi A, et al. Impact of deploying multiple point-of-care tests with a "sample first" approach on a sexual health clinical care pathway. A service evaluation. Sex Transm Infect 2017;93(6):424–9.

30. Gettinger J, Van Wagoner N, Daniels B, et al. Patients are willing to wait for rapid sexually transmitted infection results in a university student health clinic. Sex Transm Dis 2020;47(1):67–9.

31. Taylor SN, DiCarlo RP, Martin DH. Comparison of methylene blue/gentian violet stain to gram's stain for the rapid diagnosis of gonococcal urethritis in men. Sex Transm Dis 2011;38(11):995–6.

32. Rietmeijer CA, Mettenbrink CJ. Recalibrating the gram stain diagnosis of male urethritis in the era of nucleic acid amplification testing. Sex Transm Dis 2012; 39(1):18–20.

33. Marrazzo JM, Handsfield HH, Whittington WLH. Predicting chlamydial and gonococcal cervical infection: implications for management of cervicitis. Obstet Gynecol 2002;100(3):579–84.

34. Marrazzo JM, Martin DH. Management of women with cervicitis. Clin Infect Dis 2007;44(Suppl 3):S102–10.

35. Hobbs MM, Seña AC. Modern diagnosis of *Trichomonas vaginalis* infection: Table 1. Sex Transm Infect 2013;89(6):434–8.

36. Kingston MA, Bansal D, Carlin EM. "Shelf life" of *Trichomonas vaginalis*. Int J STD AIDS 2003;14(1):28–9.

37. Trubiano JA, Thursky KA, Stewardson AJ, et al. Impact of an integrated antibiotic allergy testing program on antimicrobial stewardship: a multicenter evaluation. Clin Infect Dis 2017;65(1):166–74.

38. Amsel R, Totten PA, Spiegel CA, et al. Nonspecific vaginitis. Diagnostic criteria and microbial and epidemiologic associations. Am J Med 1983;74(1):14–22.

39. Coleman JS, Gaydos CA. Molecular diagnosis of bacterial vaginosis: an update. In: Kraft CS, editor. J Clin Microbiol 2018;56(9). 003422-e418.

40. Belley-Montfort L, Lebed J, Smith B, et al. P248 Sensitivity of the Amsel's criteria compared to the Nugent score in absence and in presence of trichomonas vaginalis (TV) and/or candida SPP among women with symptomatic vaginitis/vaginosis. Sex Transm Infect 2015;91(Suppl 1):A97.

41. Theel ES, Katz SS, Pillay A. Molecular and direct detection tests for treponema pallidum subspecies pallidum: a review of the literature, 1964-2017. Clin Infect Dis 2020;71(Suppl 1):S4–12.
42. Watchirs Smith LA, Hillman R, Ward J, et al. Point-of-care tests for the diagnosis of Neisseria gonorrhoeae infection: a systematic review of operational and performance characteristics. Sex Transm Infect 2013;89(4):320–6.
43. Wisniewski CA, White JA, Michel CEC, et al. Optimal method of collection of first-void urine for diagnosis of Chlamydia trachomatis infection in men. J Clin Microbiol 2008;46(4):1466–9.
44. Koczula KM, Gallotta A. Lateral flow assays. Essays Biochem 2016;60(1): 111–20.
45. Bradshaw CS, Morton AN, Garland SM, et al. Evaluation of a Point-of-Care Test, BVBlue, and Clinical and Laboratory Criteria for Diagnosis of Bacterial Vaginosis. J Clin Microbiol 2005;43(3):1304–8.
46. Myziuk L, Romanowski B, Johnson SC. BVBlue test for diagnosis of bacterial vaginosis. J Clin Microbiol 2003;41(5):1925–8.
47. Sumeksri P, Koprasert C, Panichkul S. BVBLUE test for diagnosis of bacterial vaginosis in pregnant women attending antenatal care at Phramongkutklao Hospital. J Med Assoc Thai 2005;88(Suppl 3):S7–13.
48. West B, Morison L, Van Der Loeff MS, et al. Evaluation of a New Rapid Diagnostic Kit (FemExam) for Bacterial Vaginosis in Patients With Vaginal Discharge Syndrome in The Gambia. Sex Transm Dis 2003;30(6):483–9.
49. Seña AC, White BL, Sparling PF. Novel Treponema pallidum serologic tests: a paradigm shift in syphilis screening for the 21st century. Clin Infect Dis 2010; 51(6):700–8.
50. Jafari Y, Peeling RW, Shivkumar S, et al. Are Treponema pallidum specific rapid and point-of-care tests for syphilis accurate enough for screening in resource limited settings? Evidence from a meta-analysis. PLoS One 2013;8(2):e54695.
51. Causer LM, Kaldor JM, Conway DP, et al. An evaluation of a novel dual treponemal/nontreponemal point-of-care test for syphilis as a tool to distinguish active from past treated infection. Clin Infect Dis 2015;61(2):184–91.
52. Herbst de Cortina S, Bristow CC, Joseph Davey D, et al. A systematic review of point of care testing for chlamydia trachomatis, neisseria gonorrhoeae, and trichomonas vaginalis. Infect Dis Obstet Gynecol 2016;2016:4386127.
53. Rönn MM, Menzies NA, Gift TL, et al. Potential for point-of-care tests to reduce chlamydia-associated burden in the United States: a mathematical modeling analysis. Clin Infect Dis 2020;70(9):1816–23.
54. Goldenberg SD, Finn J, Sedudzi E, et al. Performance of the GeneXpert CT/NG assay compared to that of the Aptima AC2 assay for detection of rectal Chlamydia trachomatis and Neisseria gonorrhoeae by use of residual Aptima Samples. J Clin Microbiol 2012;50(12):3867–9.
55. Gaydos CA, Beqaj S, Schwebke JR, et al. Clinical validation of a test for the diagnosis of vaginitis. Obstet Gynecol 2017;130(1):181–9.
56. Morris SR, Bristow CC, Wierzbicki MR, et al. Performance of a single-use, rapid, point-of-care PCR device for the detection of Neisseria gonorrhoeae, Chlamydia trachomatis, and Trichomonas vaginalis: a cross-sectional study. Lancet Infect Dis 2021;21(5):668–76.
57. Gaydos C, Schwebke J, Dombrowski J, et al. Clinical performance of the Solana® Point-of-Care Trichomonas Assay from clinician-collected vaginal swabs and urine specimens from symptomatic and asymptomatic women. Expert Rev Mol Diagn 2017;17(3):303–6.

58. Gaydos CA, Hobbs M, Marrazzo J, et al. Rapid diagnosis of trichomonas vaginalis by testing vaginal swabs in an isothermal helicase-dependent AmpliVue assay. Sex Transm Dis 2016;43(6):369–73.

59. Song B. HSV type specific serology in sexual health clinics: use, benefits, and who gets tested. Sex Transm Infect 2004;80(2):113–7.

60. Whittington WLH, Celum CL, Cent A, et al. Use of a glycoprotein g-based type-specific assay to detect antibodies to herpes simplex virus type 2 among persons attending sexually transmitted disease clinics. Sex Transm Dis 2001; 28(2):99–104.

61. Turner KR, Wong EH, Kent CK, et al. Serologic herpes testing in the real world: validation of new type-specific serologic herpes simplex virus tests in a public health laboratory. Sex Transm Dis 2002;29(7):422–5.

62. Eing BR, Lippelt L, Lorentzen EU, et al. Evaluation of confirmatory strategies for detection of type-specific antibodies against herpes simplex virus type 2. J Clin Microbiol 2002;40(2):407–13.

63. Agyemang E, Le QA, Warren T, et al. Performance of commercial enzyme-linked immunoassays for diagnosis of herpes simplex virus-1 and herpes simplex virus-2 infection in a clinical setting. Sex Transm Dis 2017;44(12):763–7.

64. Morrow R, Friedrich D. Performance of a novel test for IgM and IgG antibodies in subjects with culture-documented genital herpes simplex virus-1 or -2 infection. Clin Microbiol Infect 2006;12(5):463–9.

65. Tuddenham S, Katz SS, Ghanem KG. Syphilis laboratory guidelines: performance characteristics of nontreponemal antibody tests. Clin Infect Dis 2020; 71(Supplement_1):S21–42.

66. Centers for Disease Control and Prevention (CDC). Syphilis testing algorithms using treponemal tests for initial screening–four laboratories, New York City, 2005-2006. MMWR Morb Mortal Wkly Rep 2008;57(32):872–5.

67. Centers for Disease Control and Prevention (CDC). Discordant results from reverse sequence syphilis screening–five laboratories, United States, 2006-2010. MMWR Morb Mortal Wkly Rep 2011;60(5):133–7.

68. Centers for Disease Control and Prevention. Recommendations for the laboratory-based detection of Chlamydia trachomatis and Neisseria gonorrhoeae–2014. MMWR Recomm Rep (Morb Mortal Wkly Rep) 2014; 63(RR-02):1–19.

69. Bignell C, Ison CA, Jungmann E. Gonorrhoea. Sex Transm Infect 2006;82(Suppl 4):iv6–9.

70. Schink JC, Keith LG. Problems in the culture diagnosis of gonorrhea. J Reprod Med 1985;30(3 Suppl):244–9.

71. Sobel JD. Vulvovaginal candidosis. Lancet 2007;369(9577):1961–71.

72. Wald A, Huang ML, Carrell D, et al. Polymerase chain reaction for detection of herpes simplex virus (HSV) DNA on mucosal surfaces: comparison with HSV isolation in cell culture. J Infect Dis 2003;188(9):1345–51.

73. Lunny C, Taylor D, Hoang L, et al. Self-collected versus clinician-collected sampling for chlamydia and gonorrhea screening: a systemic review and meta-analysis. PLoS One 2015;10(7):e0132776.

74. Hobbs MM, van der Pol B, Totten P, et al. From the NIH: proceedings of a workshop on the importance of self-obtained vaginal specimens for detection of sexually transmitted infections. Sex Transm Dis 2008;35(1):8–13.

75. Chernesky M, Freund GG, Hook E, et al. Detection of Chlamydia trachomatis and Neisseria gonorrhoeae infections in North American women by testing

SurePath liquid-based Pap specimens in APTIMA assays. J Clin Microbiol 2007; 45(8):2434–8.

76. Cosentino LA, Danby CS, Rabe LK, et al. Use of nucleic acid amplification testing for diagnosis of extragenital sexually transmitted infections. J Clin Microbiol 2017;55(9):2801–7.

77. van der Helm JJ, Hoebe CJPA, van Rooijen MS, et al. High performance and acceptability of self-collected rectal swabs for diagnosis of chlamydia trachomatis and neisseria gonorrhoeae in men who have sex with men and women. Sex Transm Dis 2009;36(8):493–7.

78. Ward H, Alexander S, Carder C, et al. The prevalence of lymphogranuloma venereum infection in men who have sex with men: results of a multicentre case finding study. Sex Transm Infect 2009;85(3):173–5.

79. Leslie DE, Azzato F, Karapanagiotidis T, et al. Development of a real-time PCR assay to detect Treponema pallidum in clinical specimens and assessment of the assay's performance by comparison with serological testing. J Clin Microbiol 2007;45(1):93–6.

80. Heymans R, van der Helm JJ, de Vries HJC, et al. Clinical value of Treponema pallidum real-time PCR for diagnosis of syphilis. J Clin Microbiol 2010;48(2): 497–502.

81. Gayet-Ageron A, Sednaoui P, Lautenschlager S, et al. Use of Treponema pallidum PCR in testing of ulcers for diagnosis of primary syphilis. Emerg Infect Dis 2015;21(1):127–9.

82. Grange PA, Gressier L, Dion PL, et al. Evaluation of a PCR test for detection of treponema pallidum in swabs and blood. J Clin Microbiol 2012;50(3):546–52.

83. Klausner JD, Bristow CC, Soge OO, et al. Resistance-Guided Treatment of Gonorrhea: A Prospective Clinical Study. Clin Infect Dis 2021;73(2):298–303.

84. Read TRH, Fairley CK, Murray GL, et al. Outcomes of resistance-guided sequential treatment of *Mycoplasma genitalium* infections: a prospective evaluation. Clin Infect Dis 2019;68(4):554–60.

85. Durukan D, Read TRH, Murray G, et al. Resistance-guided antimicrobial therapy using doxycycline–moxifloxacin and doxycycline–2.5 g azithromycin for the treatment of mycoplasma genitalium infection: efficacy and tolerability. Clin Infect Dis 2020;71(6):1461–8.

86. LeFevre ML. U.S. Preventive Services Task Force. Screening for Chlamydia and gonorrhea: U.S. Preventive Services Task Force recommendation statement. Ann Intern Med 2014;161(12):902–10.

87. US Preventive Services Task Force, Curry SJ, Krist AH, et al. Screening for cervical cancer: US preventive services task force recommendation statement. JAMA 2018;320(7):674.

88. US Preventive Services Task Force, Bibbins-Domingo K, Grossman DC, et al. Serologic screening for genital herpes infection: US preventive services task force recommendation statement. JAMA 2016;316(23):2525–30.

89. Golden MR, Workowski KA, Bolan G. Developing a public health response to mycoplasma genitalium. J Infect Dis 2017;216(suppl_2):S420–6.

90. Lin JS, Eder M, Bean S. Screening for syphilis infection in pregnant women: a reaffirmation evidence update for the U.S. Preventive services task force. Agency for Healthcare Research and Quality (US); 2018. Available at: http://www.ncbi.nlm.nih.gov/books/NBK525910/. Accessed August 23, 2022.

91. Matthias JM, Rahman MM, Newman DR, et al. Effectiveness of prenatal screening and treatment to prevent congenital syphilis, Louisiana and Florida, 2013-2014. Sex Transm Dis 2017;44(8):498–502.

92. Exten C, Pinto CN, Gaynor AM, et al. Direct-to-consumer sexually transmitted infection testing services: a position statement from the American Sexually Transmitted Diseases Association. Sex Transm Dis 2021;48(11):e155–9.

93. Farley TA, Cohen DA, Elkins W. Asymptomatic sexually transmitted diseases: the case for screening. Prev Med 2003;36(4):502–9.

94. Handsfield HH, Lipman TO, Harnisch JP, et al. Asymptomatic gonorrhea in men. Diagnosis, natural course, prevalence and significance. N Engl J Med 1974; 290(3):117–23.

95. Klouman E, Masenga EJ, Sam NE, et al. Asymptomatic gonorrhoea and chlamydial infection in a population-based and work-site based sample of men in Kilimanjaro, Tanzania. Int J STD AIDS 2000;11(10):666–74.

96. Falk L, Fredlund H, Jensen JS. Symptomatic urethritis is more prevalent in men infected with Mycoplasma genitalium than with Chlamydia trachomatis. Sex Transm Infect 2004;80(4):289–93.

97. Falk L, Fredlund H, Jensen JS. Signs and symptoms of urethritis and cervicitis among women with or without Mycoplasma genitalium or Chlamydia trachomatis infection. Sex Transm Infect 2005;81(1):73–8.

98. Klebanoff MA, Schwebke JR, Zhang J, et al. Vulvovaginal symptoms in women with bacterial vaginosis. Obstet Gynecol 2004;104(2):267–72.

99. Tibaldi C, Cappello N, Latino MA, et al. Vaginal and endocervical microorganisms in symptomatic and asymptomatic non-pregnant females: risk factors and rates of occurrence. Clin Microbiol Infect 2009;15(7):670–9.

100. Lang R, Read R, Krentz HB, et al. A retrospective study of the clinical features of new syphilis infections in an HIV-positive cohort in Alberta, Canada. BMJ Open 2018;8(7):e021544.

101. Koelle DM, Benedetti J, Langenberg A, et al. Asymptomatic reactivation of herpes simplex virus in women after the first episode of genital herpes. Ann Intern Med 1992;116(6):433–7.

Approach to Managing Sex Partners of People with Sexually Transmitted Infections

Emily Hansman, BA[a],*, Jeffrey D. Klausner, MD, MPH[b]

KEYWORDS

- Partner management • Sexually transmitted infections • Expedited partner therapy

KEY POINTS

- The treatment of sex partners is essential in the management of STIs and is the responsibility of the health care provider.
- Expedited partner therapy is superior to standard partner referral and should be practiced for index patients diagnosed with chlamydia and/or gonorrhea.
- Other strategies to improve partner management include patient- and partner-centered counseling, provision of supplementary written information, and use of technology to facilitate notification.

INTRODUCTION

The tracing and treatment of sex partners of patients is an essential component of sexually transmitted infection (STI) management. The regular implementation of this concept dates back nearly a century, to US Surgeon General Thomas Parran's 1937 introduction of a systematic nationwide plan to combat syphilis, which included the concept of partner treatment.[1] The decades since have witnessed the growth and subsequent decline of public health departments' involvement in the treatment of other STIs, including chlamydia, gonorrhea, and HIV infection. In more recent years, the responsibility of partner treatment has shifted from the public health department to the individual health care provider. In 1995, 92% of public health programs offered partner services for syphilis, 67% for gonorrhea, and 52% for chlamydia.[2] However, by 2003, whereas 89% of public health departments still offered partner services for syphilis, only 17% and 12% did for gonorrhea and chlamydia, respectively.[3] In the setting of decreased public health department involvement, current methods of

a David Geffen School of Medicine University of California Los Angeles, Los Angeles, CA, USA;
b University of Southern California Keck School of Medicine, 1845 North Soto Street, Health Sciences Campus, Los Angeles, CA 90032, USA
* Corresponding Author. 1845 North Soto Street, Health Sciences Campus, Los Angeles, CA 90032
E-mail address: ehansman@mednet.ucla.edu

Infect Dis Clin N Am 37 (2023) 405–426
https://doi.org/10.1016/j.idc.2023.02.003
0891-5520/23/© 2023 Elsevier Inc. All rights reserved.

id.theclinics.com

partner referral have had limited success, with only 37% to 60% of partners being reached.[4–6] Despite these shifts, the evaluation, treatment, and counseling of sex partners of persons who are infected with an STI is still considered one of the Centers for Disease Control and Prevention's (CDC) five major strategies in the prevention and control of STIs.[7] This strategy necessitates that providers have a strong command of STI partner management, including expedited partner therapy (EPT), to ensure successful STI treatment and reduce reinfection.

Per the CDC definition, partner services refers to the continuum of clinical evaluation, counseling, diagnostic testing, and treatment designed to increase the number of infected persons brought to treatment and to reduce transmission among sexual networks.[7] Comprehensive partner management involves a cascade of events including[8]

1. Elicitation of sex partners
2. Establishing contactable sex partners
3. Notifying sex partners
4. Sex partners' testing
5. Sex partners' treatment

The range of services offered and the role of the individual provider varies by geographic location, infection type, resources, and patient risk factors. This article provides an overview of clinical recommendations regarding partner management, with particular emphasis on EPT, and an update on new and emerging evidence in the field.

GOALS OF PARTNER MANAGEMENT

The benefits of successful partner management are numerous, and extend to the patient, the partner, the community, and the health care system.[9] For the patient, partner treatment serves to reduce reinfection rates. For the partner, timely notification and treatment can prevent infection and/or serious illness, and treat curable infections. For the community, partner services can diminish transmission of infections among sexual networks. Finally, for the health care system, partner treatment may be a more cost effective and targeted approach to STI management than general screening and prevention programs. In one model, improving the number of partners treated from 0.4 to 0.8 per index case was more cost-effective than increasing screening.[10]

Notably, the benefit of partner management varies by disease. Characteristics of infections for which partner management has the greatest benefit include those that (1) are curable, (2) have the potential for high morbidity if untreated, and (3) have a long latency period before such adverse effects occur.[11] Syphilis is therefore an example of an STI for which partner services should be a high priority. Similarly, chlamydia and gonorrhea are infections with an important role for partner management.

METHODS OF PARTNER MANAGEMENT

Traditionally, there are four different approaches to partner management, each with strengths and weaknesses in certain clinical contexts.

Provider referral refers to the process where the health care provider elicits the sex partners' contact information from the index patient, and then attempts to contact the partner, independent of the index patient. Variations on this model include approaches in which public health departments or other staff, notably, STI disease intervention specialists, have responsibility for notifying sex partners of exposure.

Patient referral involves the index patient directly notifying their sex partners. This is typically done following counseling provided by the provider at the time of diagnosis. Material aids, such as a contact tracing card or pamphlet, may be used to facilitate communication of key information, and to aid the partner in seeking care. Formerly, patient referral required the index patient to notify the sex partner directly, either in person, or by telephone, text, and so forth. However, in recent years, the development of various online platforms (see the section on information technology) has allowed for anonymous communication between the patient and the partner without involvement of the provider. At the time of diagnosis, patients should be counseled on all notification options available to them.

Contractual referral is a hybrid of patient and provider referral. In this method, the index patient agrees to notify their sex partner within a specified time frame. After the expiration of that time frame, if the partner has not presented for examination and treatment, the provider attempts to contact the partner.

EPT is a practice where the index patient is given a prescription or a medication to give to their sex partners without the provider having the opportunity to examine the sex partner first. EPT is discussed in detail later.

A summary of these four methods, including their advantages and disadvantages, is presented in **Fig. 1**. A Cochrane Review did not identify a single optimal strategy for any particular STI[12] and many factors are involved in determining the strategy of choice for a given clinical scenario.

STRATEGIES IN PARTNER MANAGEMENT

The success of achieving partner treatment varies not only between the four methods described previously, but by details in the approach to notification and treatment. Because there is generally insufficient evidence to determine the most effective individual components of an enhanced partner referral intervention, providers should be aware of the variety of enhanced partner referral strategies that have been demonstrated to increase the success of partner management, and adopt these strategies when possible.[12]

Partner Type

The approach a provider adopts for partner management can and should vary by partner type. As part of the sexual history, the provider should elicit not only the number of sex partners but the nature of the index patient's relationship with each partner. Classically, partner type has been dichotomized as "regular" partners versus "casual" partners, or "main" partner versus "other" partners in those with multiple partners.[13,14] When greater detail is captured, in clinical and research settings, partner type was frequently categorized by marital status or living arrangement, details that may not be clinically relevant. Estcourt and colleagues[15] have proposed an updated classification of partner types that provides greater nuance and more accurately captures clinically relevant information (**Fig. 2**). The five main partner types include.

1. Established partner
2. New partner
3. Occasional partner
4. One-off partner
5. Sex worker

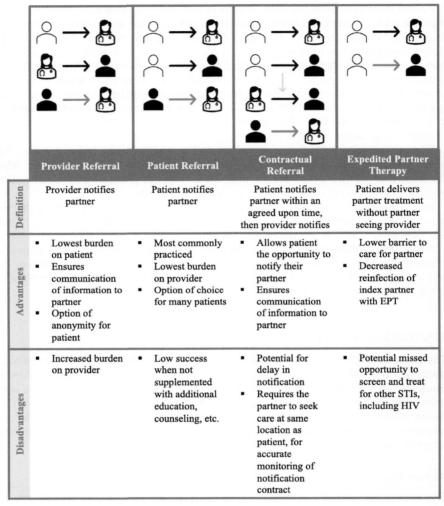

	Provider Referral	**Patient Referral**	**Contractual Referral**	**Expedited Partner Therapy**
Definition	Provider notifies partner	Patient notifies partner	Patient notifies partner within an agreed upon time, then provider notifies	Patient delivers partner treatment without partner seeing provider
Advantages	▪ Lowest burden on patient ▪ Ensures communication of information to partner ▪ Option of anonymity for patient	▪ Most commonly practiced ▪ Lowest burden on provider ▪ Option of choice for many patients	▪ Allows patient the opportunity to notify their partner ▪ Ensures communication of information to partner	▪ Lower barrier to care for partner ▪ Decreased reinfection of index partner with EPT
Disadvantages	▪ Increased burden on provider	▪ Low success when not supplemented with additional education, counseling, etc.	▪ Potential for delay in notification ▪ Requires the partner to seek care at same location as patient, for accurate monitoring of notification contract	▪ Potential missed opportunity to screen and treat for other STIs, including HIV

⌒ Patient   ▲ Partner   ⚕ Provider

→ Interaction for diagnosis or notification   ⇢ Interaction for treatment

Fig. 1. Approaches to partner management.

These types vary in characteristics, such as sexual exclusivity and likelihood of sex reoccurring, and their association with risk of reinfection, onward transmission, and engagement with partner notification.

Based on the partner type elicited, the provider should adapt their approach to partner counseling and management, because the ease of notification for the index patient, and their motivation to notify, varies by partner type. For example, counseling focused on the index patient's emotions will likely be more important with established partners and new partners, whereas counseling on the health consequences and risk of reinfection may be more relevant with occasional partners. EPT may be more

PARTNER TYPES
FOR CLINICAL PRACTICE

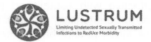

When to use: This grid may be used in any setting to support discussions about sexual partners and relationships. It may be particularly useful for STI partner notification and contact tracing and to discuss people's sexual networks. However, in cases of sexual assault, alternatives may be more appropriate.

How to use: This grid may be used in any setting to support discussions about sexual partners and relationships. It may be particularly useful for STI partner notification and contact tracing and to discuss people's sexual networks. However, in cases of sexual assault, alternatives may be more appropriate.

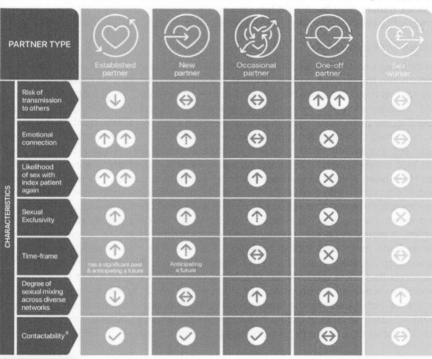

Fig. 2. Sex partner types for clinical practice. (*From* Estcourt CS, Flowers P, Cassell JA, et al. Going beyond 'regular and casual': development of a classification of sexual partner types to enhance partner notification for STIsSexually Transmitted Infections 2022;98:108-114.)

effective with established partners and occasional partners, whereas the more resource-intensive provider referral may be necessary for one-off partners where the index patient has lower motivation for notification. In the interest of providing more complete sexual health care, a provider might encourage the index patient to bring their established partner to clinic with them, whereas relying on EPT may be more appropriate with other partner types.[15–17]

By gathering a complete sexual history with details on the varying relationship types an index patient may have, and tailoring partner services accordingly, providers may increase the likelihood of successful partner treatment.

Supplementary Materials

The provision of additional educational materials to index patients and partners has been shown to increase partner treatment success compared with standard partner referral, and may be as effective as EPT in certain settings.[6,12] One common practice is to include written information regarding the infection, mode of transmission (including the prevalence of asymptomatic infection to assist in minimizing the potential for blame), potential symptoms and complications, and instructions on accessing treatment. For infections or practice settings in which EPT is not possible, contact slips that contain basic information and are presented in clinic to obtain appropriate care have been shown to increase partner treatment success.[18] Where EPT is practiced, the quality of information provided with the medication can impact the likelihood of successful delivery and receipt of patient-delivered partner therapy.[19]

Although the provision of written information is the most commonly used supplementary material in partner management, the scientific literature suggests that other interventions may merit further attention. For example, the provision of chlamydia home-sampling diagnostic kits to partners has been studied in several trials with mixed results.[12] One study found that home-sampling kits that could be mailed to a laboratory increased the proportion of index patients with at least one partner tested, compared with sampling kits that needed to be brought to a health care provider.[20] However, other studies found no reduction in reinfection or increase in partners notified or treated when compared with standard partner referral.[12,21,22]

Information Technology

The use of information technology, including short-message-service, email, mobile apps, and automated Web sites, has been studied as a means of enhancing or replacing more traditional forms of partner management. Use of those services may provide patients with anonymity and streamline the process of partner notification without placing enhanced burden of notification on the provider. Although the promise of such technology applications is clear, the evidence of effectiveness has been mixed. In a 2016 review, e-notification was found to have high level of interest and acceptability among patients; however, evidence on the actual use of such technology was limited, and the impact varied.[23] Partner notification success ranged from 10% to 97% with the use of information technology in one review.[24] The qualities of those methods that make them appealing tools for notification in some scenarios (fast, anonymous, impersonal), may be the same qualities that make them undesirable in other settings[25] and use of such services should be tailored appropriately.

Examples of Web sites or applications providing partner notification services that have been studied include inSPOT.org in the United States, letthemknow.org.au and whytest.org in Australia, and suggestatest.nl in the Netherlands. Currently in the United States, tellyourpartner.org is the primary Web site for electronic sex partner notification. Several studies found that advertising, including banner ads on popular

Web sites, newspaper ads, and radio public service announcements, increased the number of notification messages sent to sex partners on those platforms.[26,27]

For the right clinical scenario, particularly with partner types who may be less likely to be otherwise notified,[23] use of these technologies may increase the likelihood of successful partner treatment. Additionally, the use of technology saved between $22,795 and $45,362 in direct and indirect medical costs to programs.[24] Given that reduced cost, those technologies should be considered as part of partner management even if they do not demonstrate superior performance to other notification methods. Providers should consider those options and use shared decision making to determine the most suitable approach for a given patient.

Counseling

It is perhaps not surprising that increased time spent counseling patients on the importance of notifying sex partners has been correlated with improved notification outcomes.[28] Designated time for education and questions and answers between providers and patients have resulted in greater number of sex partners notified per patient.[6,29,30] However, although counseling is an essential component in the provision of responsible clinical care, there may be a limit to the impact of counseling on partner management success, because several studies have demonstrated no difference in partner outcomes with increased education and counseling.[6,31,32]

The differing impact of counseling on partner management may be related to the quality of counseling provided. Enhanced counseling should be tailored by partner type, in addition to individual patient experience and other factors. Patients should be given opportunity to ask questions and shared clinical decision making should be used when determining the most appropriate method of partner notification.

Given that most STI care in most areas is taking place in the outpatient primary care setting, the demand on the provider's time is a significant limitation in the ability to provide robust partner counseling. Providers should be aware that Internal Classification of Diseases-10 codes Z70.1 ("Counseling related to patient's sexual behavior and risk factors") and Z70.8 ("Other sex counseling") is used to bill for time spent on STI counseling, including counseling on partner notification and treatment.

CLINICAL GUIDANCE

CDC guidance for the clinical management of the sex partners of patients diagnosed with various STIs are described in **Table 1**.[7] In general, partners should be treated with the same treatment regimen that is recommended for index patients, except in cases where the sex partner may be pregnant and doxycycline is contraindicated. Index patients and partners should be counseled to abstain from condomless sex until both have completed treatment. In cases where the index patient has had no sexual exposure in the stated time, the most recent sex partner should be considered. In areas where EPT is permissible by law (**Fig. 3**), an effort should be made for partners to be evaluated by a clinician; however, if treatment is likely to be delayed, EPT should be offered with appropriate counseling.

EXPEDITED PARTNER THERAPY

EPT (also referred to as accelerated partner therapy) refers to the process where the sex partner is treated without being seen by a provider. The two primary methods of EPT involve the index patient delivering the partner a prescription that the partner will then fill at a pharmacy, or, more commonly, delivering the medication to the partner directly, which may be referred to as patient-delivered partner therapy.

Table 1
Clinical guidelines for partner management of STD syndromes, diseases, and pathogens

Disease	Partner Identification Period	Treatment	Recommendation	Notes
Syndromes				
Nongonococcal urethritis	60 d	Treat with drug regimen effective against chlamydia	Evaluate and treat presumptively according to pathogen	EPT is used if linkage to care is delayed or unlikely
Cervicitis	60 d	Treat according to pathogen	Evaluate, test and provide presumptive treatment if chlamydia, gonorrhea, or trichomoniasis identified in index patient	EPT is considered for chlamydia or gonorrhea
Pelvic inflammatory disease	60 d	See chlamydia and gonorrhea	Treat partners presumptively for chlamydia and gonorrhea regardless of pathogens isolated	EPT is used if linkage to care delayed or unlikely
Epididymitis	60 d	See chlamydia and gonorrhea	If confirmed or suspected to be caused by *Neisseria gonorrhoeae* or *Chlamydia trachomatis* treat partners presumptively	EPT is used if linkage to care delayed or unlikely
Pathogen				
Chancroid	10 d	Azithromycin 1g PO single dose Or Ceftriaxone 250 mg IM single dose Or Ciprofloxacin 500 mg PO BID, 3 d Or Erythromycin base 500 mg PO TID, 7d	Examine and treat presumptively	

...rpes	Current partners of symptomatic index patients	Acyclovir 400 mg PO TID, 7–10 d Or Famciclovir 250 mg PO TID, 7–10 d Or Valacyclovir 1g PO BID, 7–10 d	Evaluate and counsel all partners Symptomatic partners: treat; regimen listed is for first clinical episode, alternative regimens used for suppression or recurrent episodes Asymptomatic partners: gather history on genital symptoms, offer type-specific serologic testing	No available evidence on postexposure prophylaxis or pre-exposure prophylaxis, therefore should not be offered as prevention strategy
Granuloma inguinale	60 d	Azithromycin 1g PO weekly or 500 mg daily, minimum 3 wk, until all lesions healed	Examine and treat if evidence of disease	Empiric treatment not recommended
Lymphogranuloma venereum	60 d	Doxycycline 100 mg PO BID for 21 d (symptomatic) or 7 d (asymptomatic)	Evaluate, examine, and test for chlamydial infection; treat presumptively	
Syphilis	Primary syphilis: 3 mo Secondary syphilis: 6 mo Early latent syphilis: 1 y	Penicillin G IM, dose varies Doxycycline 100 mg PO BID for 14 d if penicillin allergy	Evaluate clinically and serologically <90 d: treat presumptively >90 d: treat if positive, if test results not immediately available, or if follow-up is uncertain Long-term partners of patients with late latent syphilis: evaluate with serologic testing and treat if positive	Among populations with high syphilis infection rates: consider presumptive treatment of partners of patients with high titers and unknown symptom duration
Chlamydia	60 d	Doxycycline 100 mg PO BID for 7 d	Presumptive treatment	EPT should be offered as permitted by law For MSM, shared clinical decision-making regarding EPT is

(continued on next page)

Table 1
(continued)

Disease	Partner Identification Period	Treatment	Recommendation	Notes
				recommended given risk of coexisting infections
Gonococcal infection	60 d	If chlamydia excluded: cefixime 800 mg single dose / If chlamydia not excluded: cefixime PLUS doxycycline 100 mg PO BID for 7 d	Presumptive treatment	EPT should be offered as permitted by law / For MSM, shared clinical decision-making regarding EPT is recommended, given risk of coexisting infections
Mycoplasma genitalium	Current partners	Resistance-guided therapy based on index patient / Generally, doxycycline followed by azithromycin in macrolide-sensitive strains or moxifloxacin in macrolide-resistant strains	Test partners, treat if positive	No studies have determined whether reinfection is reduced with partner treatment[a] / If testing partner not possible, can provide EPT
Bacterial vaginosis			Routine treatment of sex partners is not recommended[b]	
Trichomoniasis	Current partners	Metronidazole 500 mg PO BID for 7 d for women, 2 g PO single dose for men	Presumptive treatment	EPT is offered as permitted by law[c]
Vulvovaginal candidiasis			Not typically acquired through sexual intercourse, partner treatment not recommended	A minority of male partners have balanitis, and may benefit from a topical antifungal for symptomatic relief

Condition	Interval	Treatment	Management	Decontamination
Human papilloma virus			Sex partners do not need to be tested for human papilloma virus	Duration of viral persistence after warts have resolved is unknown, no recommendation is made regarding future partners. Female partners should continue cervical cancer screening at same interval as average-risk women
Pediculosis pubis	1 mo	Permethrin 1% cream Or Pyrethrin with piperonyl butoxide Both applied to affected areas, washed off after 10 min	Presumptive treatment	Decontaminate bedding and clothing
Scabies	1 mo	Permethrin 5% cream applied to entire body from neck down, washed off after 8–14 h Or Ivermectin 200 μg/kg PO, repeat in 14 d Or Ivermectin 1% lotion applied to entire body from neck down, washed off after 8–14 h, repeat in 1 wk if symptoms persist	Examine, treat those identified as being infested	

a No studies have determined whether reinfection is reduced with partner treatment.[77,78]
b Pilot found that male partner treatment of women with recurrent bacterial vaginosis decreased bacterial diversity.[79]
c No partner management intervention has been demonstrated to be superior in reducing reinfection.[34,35] Larger study found that this did not reduce bacterial vaginosis recurrence in female partners, but were less likely to experience treatment failure.[80]

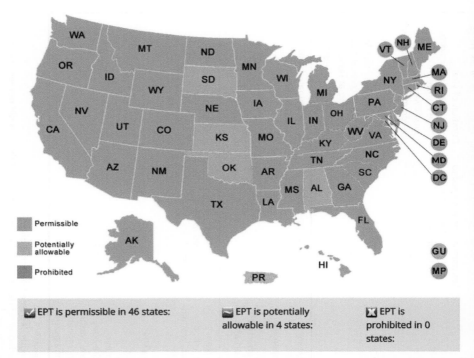

Fig. 3. Legal status of expedited partner therapy by state. (*From* Centers for Disease Control and Prevention (CDC). Legal Status of Expedited Partner Therapy. Sexually Transmitted Diseases (STSs). Available at https://www.cdc.gov/std/ept/legal/default.htm.)

Although EPT has garnered increasing attention in recent years, this is not a new practice. For decades, providers have been providing treatment for the male sex partners of women diagnosed with trichomoniasis.[33] As partner management was increasingly recognized as a critical component of STI care, public health department programs for partner management of syphilis, chlamydia, and gonorrhea grew more robust.[3] However, other STIs were less commonly addressed by formal programs, placing the onus for partner management on the provider. Additionally, trichomoniasis was one of the few common STIs at the time that was managed with an oral pill rather than an injection. That constellation of factors rendered trichomoniasis well-suited for management via EPT.[33] Although more recent studies have not demonstrated a superiority of any method of partner management in trichomoniasis,[34,35] EPT is still frequently regarded as standard practice for partner management in trichomoniasis.

EPT is now most commonly used for chlamydia and gonorrhea, and has been officially supported by various authorities, including the CDC,[7] World Health Organization,[36] American Medical Association,[37] American College of Obstetricians and Gynecologists,[38] and the Society for Adolescent Medicine,[39] for use in partner management of chlamydia and gonorrhea. In the United States, use of EPT is regulated at the state level. Currently EPT is permissible in 46 states and potentially allowable in 6 states and territories (Alabama, Kansas, South Dakota, Oklahoma, Puerto Rico, and Guam). No jurisdiction prohibited EPT (see **Fig. 3**). Detailed state-by-state guidance is provided by the CDC (https://www.cdc.gov/std/ept/legal/default.htm).

The initial evidence for the use of EPT in chlamydia and gonorrhea was derived from three randomized controlled trials conducted in the United States on the impact of EPT in reducing chlamydial and gonococcal reinfection.[40–42] All of these studies found more sex partners were treated when EPT was offered, and two reported statistically significant reductions in recurrent or persistent infection.[41,42] Subsequent reviews have maintained support for EPT. A 2007 meta-analysis demonstrated a 27% reduced risk of persistent or recurrent infection in patients with chlamydia or gonorrhea[6] and a 2013 Cochrane Review found that EPT reduced reinfection by 29% compared with standard partner referral. Both reviews included several studies conducted in low- and middle-income countries, where EPT is potentially of the greatest benefit.[29,43] In trials where EPT was not found to reduce reinfection, the authors still acknowledge the existence of other advantages of EPT, including simplicity and cost.[44,45] In sum, multiple studies demonstrate the utility of EPT in increasing partner treatment and decreasing recurrent infection in index patients.

EPT has additionally been compared with other forms of enhanced partner notification (provision of education materials, videos, home-sampling kits, disease-specific Web sites, reminders by telephone, theory-based counseling) with equivocal to favorable performance. EPT increased the mean number of sex partners treated per original patient by 54% when compared with inSPOT, a World Wide Web–based partner notification service,[46] and resulted in greater proportion of patients reporting successful partner treatment when compared with booklet-enhanced partner referral (55.8% vs 45.6%).[42] However, reviews have found that EPT was not superior to enhanced partner referral.[6,12]

There is evidence that EPT improves outcomes not only for individual patients but also on a population scale. In a model of chlamydia cases by state as a function of year, legal status of EPT, and the interaction between year and legality, the incidence of chlamydia in states with prohibitive EPT legislation grew significantly faster compared with states where EPT was permissible.[47] This suggests that EPT, and EPT legislation, have an important role to play in facilitating detection of infection, promoting their treatment, and thus slowing the spread of STIs. Additionally, EPT is less costly from a health care system perspective when compared with standard referral, and is less costly for an individual depending on how many partners are treated.[48]

Guidance on the use of EPT in partner management for different sexually transmitted disease syndromes and pathogens is outlined in **Table 1**. In brief, EPT is recommended for chlamydia and gonorrhea, including syndromes (urethritis, cervicitis, pelvic inflammatory disease) in which a pathogen has not been identified but there is high suspicion for *Chlamydia trachomatis* or *Neisseria gonorrhoeae*. EPT may be used for trichomoniasis, although it has not been shown to be superior to traditional forms of partner management.[34,35] In general, directly providing oral medication is preferable to providing a prescription, and should be pursued when possible, given the challenges that some patients may face in filling prescriptions for EPT.[49] Most guidelines recommend that EPT should be pursued when the provider reasonably believes that a partner would be unwilling or unable to seek treatment, thus delaying care; the preferred alternative is a standard evaluation by a clinician.[7,37] However, it is up to the discretion of the provider to determine what scenarios would meet this criteria, giving the provider the opportunity for routine use of EPT in the appropriate clinical context.

When using EPT, providers should counsel patients on their STI diagnosis and partner notification. At minimum patients should be instructed on the medication being provided, including possible adverse drug reactions, medication interactions, and/or allergies. Written education materials should be provided along with the medication that summarizes this information. Patients should additionally be instructed to encourage sex partners receiving EPT to consult a clinician, because EPT is intended to supplement and expedite, not replace, standard clinical care. Specifically, partners should be encouraged to seek STI testing, because coinfections with multiple STIs are common and screening for such conditions as HIV infection or syphilis may be necessary.

There are several limitations and risks that should be considered in the use of EPT. Providers' reservations with EPT may stem from concerns around the risk of unmonitored adverse events, including allergic reactions, given the sex partner's unknown medical history.[50] These events are rare but possible, and providers can minimize the risk of such adverse events by providing thorough counseling to the index patient and clear written instructions for the partner, including allergy warnings, drug-drug interactions, and potential side effects of the medication.

A second set of concerns regarding EPT involves the potential for overtreatment and potential effects on fostering antimicrobial resistance, particularly with *N gonorrhoeae*. However, the data have not born this out. In several studies of *N gonorrhoeae* genotypes between index cases and sex partners, the proportion of pairs with concordant genotypes ranged from 88% to 98%.[51–53] That suggests that a treatment that is effective in the index patient would be similarly effective in the sex partner in most cases, and that resistance-guided therapy could be used to guide EPT.[54]

A final concern around EPT relates to the lost opportunity for STI and HIV screening by eliminating the need for the partner to visit a clinic for treatment, particularly given the prevalence of coinfections of multiple STIs or HIV.[55] The prevalence of coinfection varies, ranging from 0.8% among heterosexual males to 13.8% among men who have sex with men (MSM) in one study.[56] Those different frequencies of undetected coinfection have resulted in differing recommendations for EPT for certain high-risk populations.[7] However, as further discussed later, any decision to use or not use EPT must balance these concerns against the equally legitimate and perhaps more probable risk of partner nontreatment and index patient reinfection or recurrent infection, and continued community transmission.

SPECIAL POPULATIONS AND CONSIDERATIONS

The discussion in this article thus far has focused primarily on the management of partners of index patients who are heterosexual, nonpregnant adults with minimal additional risk factors. However, there are several populations that merit additional attention with regards to partner management. These include MSM, adolescents, pregnant women, and victims of intimate partner violence (IPV).

Men Who Have Sex with Men

Male partners of MSM who have been diagnosed with an STI are at increased risk of also having other STIs, including syphilis or undiagnosed HIV infection.[56–58] Therefore, the importance of a complete clinical examination and opportunity for STI screening is critical in this population. Additionally, the three trials that formed the basis for the recommendation of EPT in the management of chlamydia and gonorrhea did not include MSM.[40–42] For those reasons, the CDC does not routinely recommend EPT for the male partners of MSM. Instead, there is a recommendation for shared clinical decision making between the provider and the patient to determine the most appropriate approach to partner management. EPT may still be used, but it is essential that the increased risk of undetected infection in sex partners is discussed with the patient and clear information about the benefits of screening is communicated to the sex partner.

With increased use of HIV pre-exposure prophylaxis among MSM, the dynamics of STI care for this community may be changing, and pre-exposure prophylaxis users have increased contact with health care and opportunities for infection screening. Therefore, use of EPT among MSM merits further research, because qualitative work and case studies have demonstrated that community members are largely unaware of EPT but potentially interested, and providers are motivated to provide EPT to MSM.[59,60]

Adolescents

Broadly speaking, partner management is conducted similarly in adolescents as in adults. Partner types and ease of notifying may vary from adult populations, and the provider's approach to counseling should reflect this difference in context and motivation. The success of partner notification among adolescents may be more influenced by such factors as self-efficacy, fear of a negative interaction, and relationship quality.[61,62] With respect to partner referral method, adolescents were less interested in EPT and more comfortable with advising sex partners to seek traditional clinical encounters.[63] Additionally, adolescents frequently have a hard time filling prescriptions, thus patient-delivered partner therapy is more likely to succeed than EPT with a prescription only.[64]

Cases of suspected child abuse or sexual assault should be reported immediately to the appropriate authorities. Partner management should not be pursued in this context.

Pregnant Patients

Successful management of STIs during pregnancy is particularly critical, given the consequences of untreated STIs, including preterm birth, low birth weight, and vertical transmission, among others.[65,66] As with adolescents, counseling should reflect the differing motivations a pregnant person may have, including a desire to protect the health of their pregnancy, because this may be a more effective way to encourage partner notification. For scenarios in which EPT is permissible, the heightened consequence of a delay in care, particularly in sex partners with whom the patient is still sexually active, should be taken into consideration and reflected in decisions regarding the use of EPT.

The success of partner notification among pregnant women diagnosed with an STI may vary by context, with some studies indicating no difference in notification between pregnant and nonpregnant women, and other studies reporting a higher notification among pregnant women.[67,68] Data are limited on how the increased risk of IPV during pregnancy may impact a patient's motivation to notify their partner of an STI.[67,69]

Intimate Partner Violence

In the United States, the lifetime prevalence of IPV among women is 43.6%.[70] Given this high prevalence, providers should consider screening for IPV as part of routine STI care, with emphasis on behaviors related to STI risk and sexual coercion.[7,71] Although data regarding the rate of IPV that is directly attributable to partner notification are limited,[72,73] there is a potential risk, particularly among partners with a previous history of IPV.[74] Providers need to assess the risk for IPV and adjust partner counseling accordingly, given the potential risk to the index patient in notifying an abusive partner of an STI diagnosis. Again, counseling and management approaches should be tailored to the circumstances and providers should be cognizant of the sensitivity of the discussion.

ROLE OF THE HEALTH DEPARTMENT

Historically, the approach to partner management by clinicians had been to rely on public health departments for STI contact tracing and partner management.[3,75] However, given increasing lack of resources, other priorities, and staff shortages, many public health departments no longer provide routine partner services.[55] Clinicians providing STI care should therefore be aware of the services their local public health department does and does not offer, and generally, should assume that the responsibility for partner management lies with them and the patient.

Areas where the public health department still plays a role in most areas of the United States include early syphilis and new HIV diagnoses.[3] However, health department notification should be viewed as supplementary to the role of the health care provider and should not negate the need for thorough patient counseling on partner notification and treatment. Health departments should play a role in partner services for cephalosporin-resistant gonorrhea, given the increasing public health concerns presented by rising antimicrobial resistance.[3] For other STIs, including chlamydia, trichomoniasis, and cephalosporin-sensitive gonorrhea, the public health department is typically not involved in partner services.[3]

Providers should be aware of the reporting process and requirements for various STIs in their geographic area of practice. Providers should inform patients that their name, contact information, and disease including treatment status may be shared with the local health department. Syphilis, gonorrhea, chlamydia, chancroid, and HIV are reportable diseases in every state. Other reporting requirements for STIs differ by state. Additionally, providers should understand the reporting process, because this may be provider based, laboratory based, or both.

LEGAL CONSIDERATIONS

With respect to partner services, providers face the conflicting ethical obligations of patient confidentiality and duty to warn. At a minimum, the provider has the obligation to inform patients of their ability to infect others, and to recommend that they disclose their infection to sex partners and take steps to reduce the risk of transmission, including completing treatment when indicated and using condoms. Although physicians face an ethical duty to warn, there is no legal duty to warn for STIs except in rare circumstances of HIV infection among married couples in certain states; partner notification is therefore a voluntary process.[76] When health departments perform contact tracing, this is done in a manner that maintains patient confidentiality.

However, three states (California, Nebraska, and Indiana) have formal regulatory guidance for partner management of certain STIs.[76] The specific STIs vary by state but generally include syphilis, gonococcal infection, chlamydia, granuloma inguinale, lymphogranuloma venereum, and chancroid. The regulations broadly consist of the provider making a reasonable effort, with cooperation from the patient, for the sex partner to be informed and treated, and reporting the case to the local health department. Providers in those states should familiarize themselves with these requirements.

EPT may play an important role in the legal responsibilities of providers in partner management. It is currently cited as a reason why a "duty to warn" for STIs is not necessary, because partners can access treatment in this fashion. Historically, concerns about the legal implications of EPT have reflected the risk of providing medication to a patient that the clinician has not evaluated; given the increasing acceptance and use of EPT, an argument could be made that failure to offer EPT to a patient when clinically appropriate could render the provider liable for inadequately managing the care of partners. Currently, few such cases have been successfully prosecuted.

SUMMARY

Partner management of STIs is essential to identify and treat new cases, to prevent reinfection in the index case, to interrupt chains of transmission, to reduce STI-related morbidity, and to target STI screening and treatment interventions. However, partner treatment success remains low, in the United States and globally. The responsibility for partner notification and treatment falls on the patient and the health care provider, and the provider has an obligation to practice evidence-based care to improve partner treatment outcomes. Optimal care of the patient with an STI requires management of the patient and their sex partner. In this sense, STIs are unique from other diseases that providers encounter in that care for the patient in front of them requires care of two individuals: the index patient and their sex partner. Without taking responsibility for the management of the sex partner, the provider is not adequately managing the STI.

Research has focused on interventions to improve partner treatment success. EPT, specifically patient-delivered partner therapy, and enhanced partner referral are both superior to standard partner referral, and their use should be encouraged. Future research should attempt to elucidate the components of enhanced partner notification that are of highest impact, and focus on the use of EPT in high-risk populations and/or low resource settings where it may have the greatest impact.

CLINICS CARE POINTS

- The treatment of sex partners is essential in the management of STIs and is the responsibility of the health care provider. Approaches to partner management include patient referral, provider referral, contractual referral, and expedited partner therapy.

- The necessary care for partners varies by disease. Chlamydia, gonorrhea, trichomoniasis, chancroid, and syphilis should be treated presumptively.

- Expedited partner therapy is superior to standard partner referral and should be practiced for index patients diagnosed with chlamydia and/or gonorrhea.

- Other strategies to improve partner management include patient- and partner-centered counseling, provision of supplementary written information, and use of technology to facilitate notification.

- Partner type may influence partner treatment outcomes. Providers should seek to understand the nature of the index patient's relationship with their partner and services should be tailored appropriately.

DISCLOSURE

The authors have nothing to disclose.

FUNDING

This project was supported by the National Institutes of Health (NIH) under Award Number R21HD100821 and Fogarty International Center of the NIH under Award Number D43TW009343 and the University of California Global Health Institute

(UCGHI). The content is solely the responsibility of the authors and does not necessarily represent the official views of the NIH or UCGHI.

REFERENCES

1. Parran T. Shadow on the land: syphilis. New York: Reynal & Hitchcock; 1937.
2. Landry DJ, Forrest JD. Public health departments providing sexually transmitted disease services. Fam Plann Perspect 1996;28(6):261–6.
3. Golden MR, Hogben M, Handsfield HH, et al. Partner notification for HIV and STD in the United States: low coverage for gonorrhea, chlamydial infection, and HIV. Sex Transm Dis 2003;30(6):490–6.
4. Armstrong H, Fernando I. An audit of partner notification for syphilis and HIV. Int J STD AIDS 2012;23(11):825–6.
5. Low N, Welch J, Radcliffe K. Developing national outcome standards for the management of gonorrhoea and genital chlamydia in genitourinary medicine clinics. Sex Transm Infect 2004;80(3):223–9.
6. Trelle S, Shang A, Nartey L, et al. Improved effectiveness of partner notification for patients with sexually transmitted infections: systematic review. BMJ 2007; 334(7589):354.
7. Workowski KA, Bachmann LH, Chan PA, et al. Sexually transmitted infections treatment guidelines, 2021. MMWR Recomm Rep (Morb Mortal Wkly Rep) 2021;70(4):1–187.
8. Wayal S, Estcourt CS, Mercer CH, et al. Optimising partner notification outcomes for bacterial sexually transmitted infections: a deliberative process and consensus, United Kingdom, 2019, Euro Surveill, 2022;27(3):1-6.
9. Low N, Broutet N, Adu-Sarkodie Y, et al. Global control of sexually transmitted infections. Lancet 2006;368(9551):2001–16.
10. Althaus CL, Turner KM, Mercer CH, et al. Effectiveness and cost-effectiveness of traditional and new partner notification technologies for curable sexually transmitted infections: observational study, systematic reviews and mathematical modelling. Health Technol Assess 2014;18(2):1–100, vii-viii.
11. Klausner JD, Hook EW. Current diagnosis & treatment of sexually transmitted diseases. New York, NY: McGraw Hill Professional; 2007.
12. Ferreira A, Young T, Mathews C, et al. Strategies for partner notification for sexually transmitted infections, including HIV. Cochrane Database Syst Rev 2013; 2013(10):Cd002843.
13. Nelson LE, Morrison-Beedy D, Kearney MH, et al. Sexual partner type taxonomy use among black adolescent mothers in the United States. Can J Hum Sex 2011; 20(1):1–10.
14. Macaluso M, Demand MJ, Artz LM, et al. Partner type and condom use. Aids 2000;14(5):537–46.
15. Estcourt CS, Flowers P, Cassell JA, et al. Going beyond 'regular and casual': development of a classification of sexual partner types to enhance partner notification for STIs. Sex Transm Infect 2022;98(2):108–14.
16. Yu Y-Y, Frasure-Williams JA, Dunne EF, et al. Chlamydia partner services for females in California family planning clinics. Sex Transm Dis 2011;38(10):913–8.
17. Mickiewicz T, Al-Tayyib A, Thrun M, et al. Implementation and effectiveness of an expedited partner therapy program in an urban clinic. Sex Transm Dis 2012; 39(12):923–9.

18. Hansman E, Wynn A, Moshashane N, et al. Experiences and preferences with sexually transmitted infection care and partner notification in Gaborone, Botswana. Int J STD AIDS 2021;32(13):1250–6.
19. McBride K, Goldsworthy RC, Fortenberry JD. Formative design and evaluation of patient-delivered partner therapy informational materials and packaging. Sex Transm Infect 2009;85(2):150–5.
20. Ostergaard L, Anderson B, Moller JK, et al. Managing partners of people diagnosed with *Chlamydia trachomatis*: a comparison of two partner testing methods. Sex Transm Infect 2003;79(5):358–61.
21. Mathews C, Coetzee N. Partner notification. BMJ Clin Evid 2009;2009:1–39.
22. Andersen B, Ostergaard L, Moller JK, et al. Home sampling versus conventional contact tracing for detecting *Chlamydia trachomatis* infection in male partners of infected women: randomised study. BMJ 1998;316(7128):350–1.
23. Pellowski J, Mathews C, Kalichman MO, et al. Advancing partner notification through electronic communication technology: a review of acceptability and utilization research. J Health Commun 2016;21(6):629–37.
24. Kachur R, Hall W, Coor A, et al. The use of technology for sexually transmitted disease partner services in the United States: a structured review. Sex Transm Dis 2018;45(11):707–12.
25. Hopkins CA, Temple-Smith MJ, Fairley CK, et al. Telling partners about chlamydia: how acceptable are the new technologies? BMC Infect Dis 2010;10(1):58.
26. Bourne C, Zablotska I, Williamson A, et al. Promotion and uptake of a new online partner notification and retesting reminder service for gay men. Sex Health 2012; 9(4):360–7.
27. Rietmeijer CA, Westergaard B, Mickiewicz TA, et al. Evaluation of an online partner notification program. Sex Transm Dis 2011;38(5):359–64.
28. Wilson TE, Hogben M, Malka ES, et al. A randomized controlled trial for reducing risks for sexually transmitted infections through enhanced patient-based partner notification. Am J Public Health 2009;99(S1):S104–10.
29. Moyo W, Chirenje ZM, Mandel JS, et al. Impact of a single session of counseling on partner referral for sexually transmitted disease treatment, Harare, Zimbabwe. AIDS Behav 2004;6:237–43.
30. Faxelid E, Tembo G, Ndulo J, et al. Individual counseling of patients with sexually transmitted diseases. A way to improve partner notification in a Zambian setting? Sex Transm Dis 1996;23(4):289–92.
31. Katz BP, Danos CS, Quinn TS, et al. Efficiency and cost-effectiveness of field follow-up for patients with *Chlamydia trachomatis* infection in a sexually transmitted diseases clinic. Sex Transm Dis 1988;15(1):11–6.
32. Ellison G, Moniez V, Stein J. A randomized controlled trial of a standardised health message vs patient-centred counseling to improve STD partner notification. Ann Hum Biol 2001;30.
33. Handsfield HH, Hogben M, Schillinger JA, et al. Expedited partner therapy in the management of sexually transmitted diseases. Atlanta, GA: US Department of Health and Human Services/Centers for Disease Control and Prevention; 2006.
34. Kissinger P, Schmidt N, Mohammed H, et al. Patient-delivered partner treatment for *Trichomonas vaginalis* infection: a randomized controlled trial. Sex Transm Dis 2006;33(7):445–50.
35. Schwebke JR, Desmond RA. A randomized controlled trial of partner notification methods for prevention of trichomoniasis in women. Sex Transm Dis 2010;37(6): 392–6.

36. Global HIV WHO. HaSTIP and Guidelines Review Committee, Guidelines for the management of symptomatic sexually transmitted infections. Geneva: WHO Guidelines; 2021.

37. Association AM. Code of Medical Ethics Opinion 8.9 Expedited Partner Therapy. Available at: https://www.ama-assn.org/delivering-care/ethics/expedited-partner-therapy. Accessed 2022.

38. Gynecologists ACoOa. Expedited partner therapy. ACOG committee opinion No. 737. Obstet Gynecol; 2018.

39. Burstein GR, Eliscu A, Ford K, et al. Expedited partner therapy for adolescents diagnosed with chlamydia or gonorrhea: a position paper of the Society for Adolescent Medicine. J Adolesc Health 2009;45(3):303–9.

40. Schillinger JA, Kissinger P, Calvet H, et al. Patient-delivered partner treatment with azithromycin to prevent repeated *Chlamydia trachomatis* infection among women: a randomized, controlled trial. Sex Transm Dis 2003;30(1):49–56.

41. Golden MR, Whittington WL, Handsfield HH, et al. Effect of expedited treatment of sex partners on recurrent or persistent gonorrhea or chlamydial infection. N Engl J Med 2005;352(7):676–85.

42. Kissinger P, Mohammed H, Richardson-Alston G, et al. Patient-delivered partner treatment for male urethritis: a randomized, controlled trial. Clin Infect Dis 2005; 41(5):623–9.

43. Nuwaha F, Kambugu F, Nsubuga PSJ, et al. Efficacy of patient-delivered partner medication in the treatment of sexual partners in Uganda. Sex Transm Dis 2001; 28(2):105–10.

44. Cameron ST, Glasier A, Scott G, et al. Novel interventions to reduce re-infection in women with chlamydia: a randomized controlled trial. Hum Reprod 2009;24(4): 888–95.

45. Estcourt CS, Stirrup O, Copas A, et al. Accelerated partner therapy contact tracing for people with chlamydia (LUSTRUM): a crossover cluster-randomised controlled trial. Lancet Public Health 2022;7(10):e853–65.

46. Kerani RP, Fleming M, DeYoung B, et al. A randomized, controlled trial of inSPOT and patient-delivered partner therapy for gonorrhea and chlamydial infection among men who have sex with men. Sex Transm Dis 2011;38(10):941–6.

47. Mmeje O, Wallett S, Kolenic G, et al. Impact of expedited partner therapy (EPT) implementation on chlamydia incidence in the USA. Sex Transm Infect 2018; 94(7):545–7.

48. Gift TL, Kissinger P, Mohammed H, et al. The cost and cost-effectiveness of expedited partner therapy compared with standard partner referral for the treatment of chlamydia or gonorrhea. Sex Transm Dis 2011;38(11):1067–73.

49. Borchardt LN, Pickett ML, Tan KT, et al. Expedited partner therapy: pharmacist refusal of legal prescriptions. Sex Transm Dis 2018;45(5):350–3.

50. McCool-Myers M, Goedken P, Henn MC, et al. Who is practicing expedited partner therapy and why? Insights from providers working in specialties with high volumes of sexually transmitted infections. Sex Transm Dis 2021;48(7):474–80.

51. Viscidi RP, Demma JC, Gu J, et al. Comparison of sequencing of the *por* gene and typing of the *opa* gene for discrimination of *Neisseria gonorrhoeae* strains from sexual contacts. J Clin Microbiol 2000;38(12):4430–8.

52. Bilek N, Martin IM, Bell G, et al. Concordance between *Neisseria gonorrhoeae* genotypes recovered from known sexual contacts. J Clin Microbiol 2007; 45(11):3564–7.

53. Chen H, Wu Z, Chen R, et al. Typing of *Neisseria gonorrhoeae* Opa and NG-MAST gene of 12 pairs of sexual contact gonorrhea patients in China. J Huazhong Univ Sci Technolog Med Sci 2008;28(4):472–5.
54. Allan-Blitz L-T, Adamson PC, Klausner JD. Resistance-guided therapy for *Neisseria gonorrhoeae*. Clin Infect Dis 2022;75(9):1655–60.
55. Erbelding EJ, Zenilman JM. Toward better control of sexually transmitted diseases. N Engl J Med 2005;352(7):720–1.
56. McNulty A, Teh MF, Freedman E. Patient delivered partner therapy for chlamydial infection: what would be missed? Sex Transm Dis 2008;35(9):834–6.
57. Stekler J, Bachmann L, Brotman RM, et al. Concurrent sexually transmitted infections (STIs) in sex partners of patients with selected STIs: implications for patient-delivered partner therapy. Clin Infect Dis 2005;40(6):787–93.
58. Schillinger J, Jamison K, Slutsker J, et al. P075 STI and HIV infections among MSM reporting exposure to gonorrhea or chlamydia: implications for expedited partner therapy. Conference Abstract 2019;2019.
59. Gamarel KE, Mouzoon R, Rivas A, et al. Healthcare providers and community perspectives on expedited partner therapy (EPT) for use with gay, bisexual and other men who have sex with men. Sex Transm Infect 2020;96(2):101–5.
60. Braun HM, Taylor JL. It's time to expand chlamydia treatment for gay and bisexual men. Ann Fam Med 2021;19(2):168–70.
61. Fortenberry JD, Brizendine EJ, Katz BP, et al. The role of self-efficacy and relationship quality in partner notification by adolescents with sexually transmitted infections. Arch Pediatr Adolesc Med 2002;156(11):1133.
62. Rosenthal SL, Baker JG, Biro FM, et al. Secondary prevention of STD transmission during adolescence: partner notification. Adolesc Pediatr Gynecol 1995; 8(4):183–7.
63. Shamash Z, Catallozzi M, Dayan PS, et al. Preferences for expedited partner therapy among adolescents in an urban pediatric emergency department: a mixed-methods study. Pediatr Emerg Care 2021;37(3):e91–6.
64. Slutsker JS, Tsang LB, Schillinger JA. Do prescriptions for expedited partner therapy for chlamydia get filled? Findings from a multi-jurisdictional evaluation, United States, 2017-2019. Sex Transm Dis 2020;47(6):376–82.
65. Blas MM, Canchihuaman FA, Alva IE, et al. Pregnancy outcomes in women infected with *Chlamydia trachomatis*: a population-based cohort study in Washington State. Sex Transm Infect 2007;83(4):314–8.
66. Mullick S, Watson-Jones D, Beksinska M, et al. Sexually transmitted infections in pregnancy: prevalence, impact on pregnancy outcomes, and approach to treatment in developing countries. Sex Transm Infect 2005;81(4):294–302.
67. Thurman AR, Holden AEC, Shain R, et al. Partner notification of sexually transmitted infections among pregnant women. Int J STD AIDS 2008;19(5):309–15.
68. Offorjebe OA, Wynn A, Moshashane N, et al. Partner notification and treatment for sexually transmitted infections among pregnant women in Gaborone, Botswana. Int J STD AIDS 2017;28(12):1184–9.
69. Silverman JG, Decker MR, Reed E, et al. Intimate partner violence victimization prior to and during pregnancy among women residing in 26 U.S. states: associations with maternal and neonatal health. Am J Obstet Gynecol 2006;195(1):140–8.
70. Smith SG, Zhang X, Basile KC, et al. The national intimate partner and sexual violence survey: 2015 data brief - updated release. National Center for Injury Prevention and Control, Centers for Disease Control and Prevention; 2018.

71. Rosenfeld EA, Marx J, Terry MA, et al. Intimate partner violence, partner notification, and expedited partner therapy: a qualitative study. Int J STD AIDS 2016; 27(8):656–61.
72. KISSINGER PJ, NICCOLAI LM, MAGNUS M, et al. Partner notification for HIV and syphilis: effects on sexual behaviors and relationship stability. Sex Transm Dis 2003;30(1):75–82.
73. Thurman AR, Shain RN, Holden AEC, et al. Partner notification of sexually transmitted infections: a large cohort of Mexican American and African American women. Sex Transm Dis 2008;35(2):136–40.
74. Klabbers RE, Muwonge TR, Ayikobua E, et al. Understanding the role of interpersonal violence in assisted partner notification for HIV: a mixed-methods study in refugee settlements in West Nile Uganda. J Glob Health 2020;10(2):020440.
75. Henderson RH. Control of sexually transmitted diseases in the United States: a federal perspective. Br J Vener Dis 1977;53(4):211.
76. Duty to Warn. Centers for Disease Control and Prevention. Available at: https://www.cdc.gov/std/treatment/duty-to-warn.htm. Accessed 2022.
77. Cina M, Baumann L, Egli-Gany D, et al. *Mycoplasma genitalium* incidence, persistence, concordance between partners and progression: systematic review and meta-analysis. Sex Transm Infect 2019;95(5):328–35.
78. Slifirski JB, Vodstrcil LA, Fairley CK, et al. *Mycoplasma genitalium* infection in adults reporting sexual contact with infected partners, Australia, 2008-2016. Emerg Infect Dis 2017;23(11):1826–33.
79. Plummer EL, Vodstrcil LA, Danielewski JA, et al. Combined oral and topical antimicrobial therapy for male partners of women with bacterial vaginosis: acceptability, tolerability and impact on the genital microbiota of couples - A pilot study. PLoS One 2018;13(1):e0190199.
80. Schwebke JR, Lensing SY, Lee J, et al. Treatment of male sexual partners of women with bacterial vaginosis: a randomized, double-blind, placebo-controlled trial. Clin Infect Dis 2021;73(3):e672–9.

Moving?

Make sure your subscription moves with you!

To notify us of your new address, find your **Clinics Account Number** (located on your mailing label above your name), and contact customer service at:

Email: journalscustomerservice-usa@elsevier.com

800-654-2452 (subscribers in the U.S. & Canada)
314-447-8871 (subscribers outside of the U.S. & Canada)

Fax number: 314-447-8029

Elsevier Health Sciences Division
Subscription Customer Service
3251 Riverport Lane
Maryland Heights, MO 63043

*To ensure uninterrupted delivery of your subscription, please notify us at least 4 weeks in advance of move.

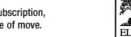

Printed and bound by CPI Group (UK) Ltd, Croydon, CR0 4YY

08/05/2025

01864749-0006